1001

great ways to
♡ get better

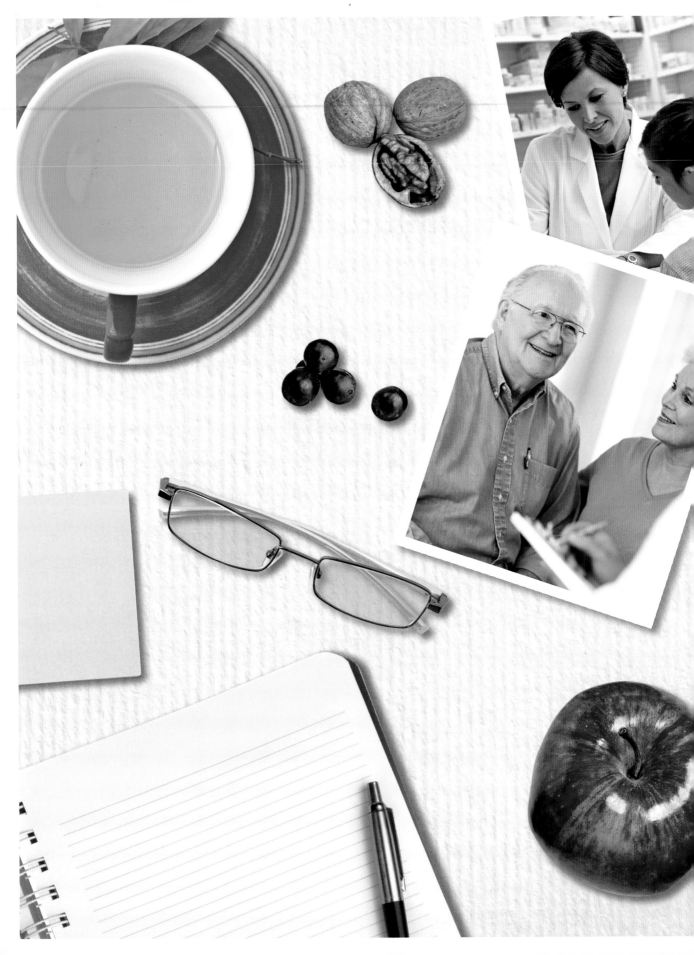

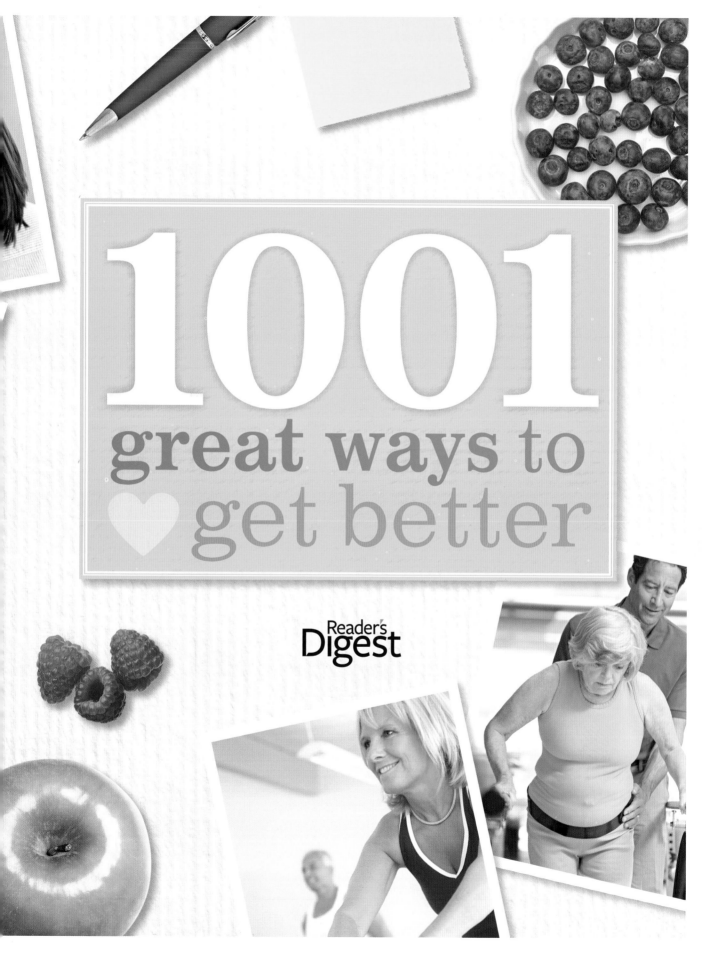

1001
great ways to get better

Reader's Digest

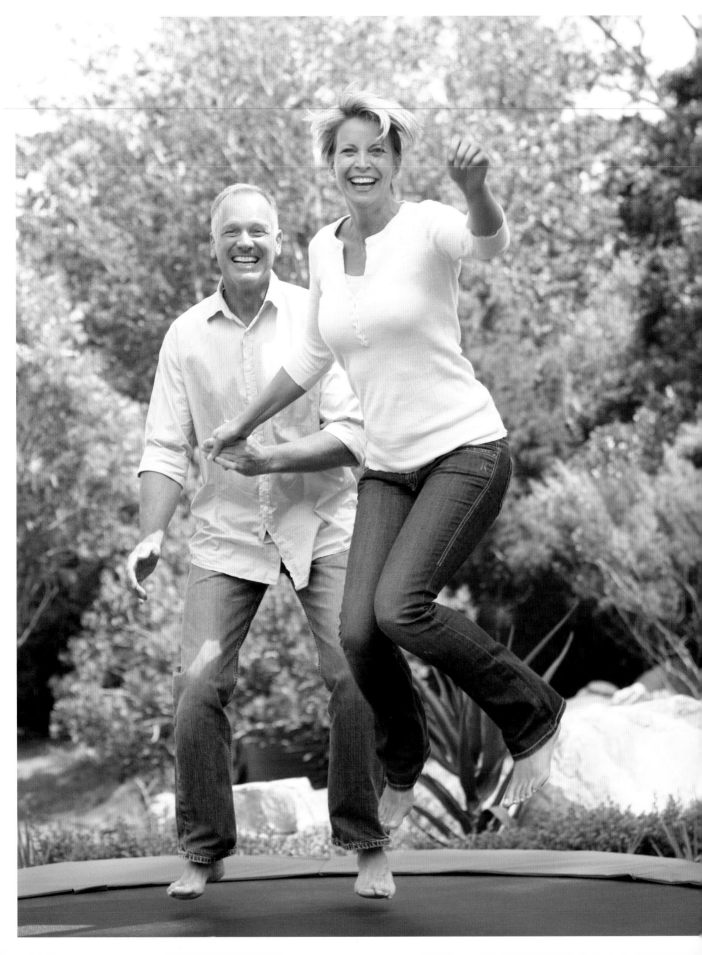

CONTENTS

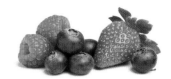

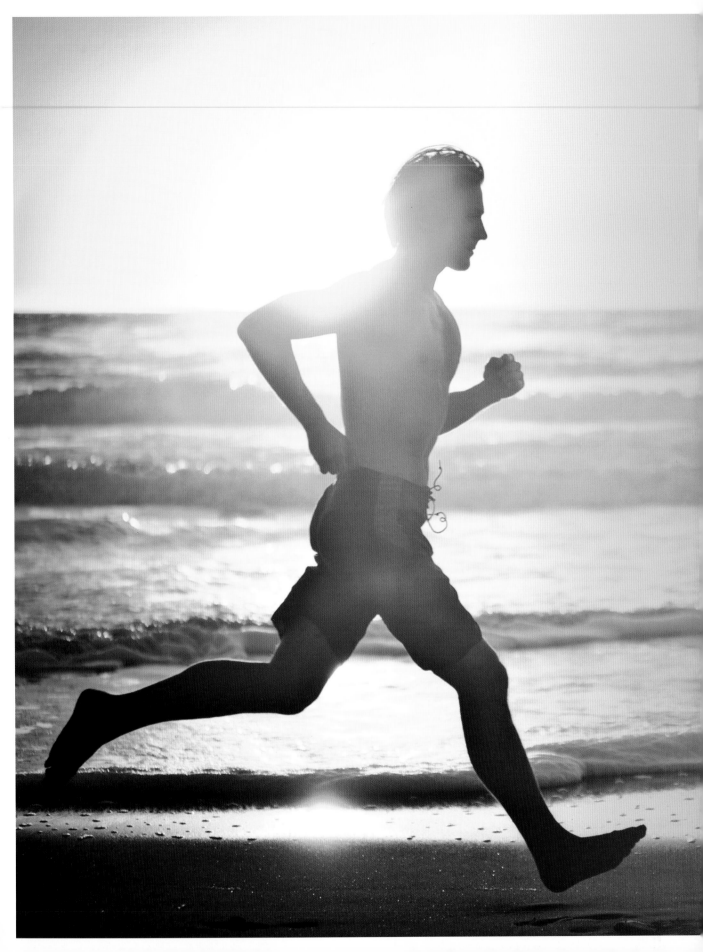

Foreword

On average, Australians see a GP about five times a year –
for the rest of the time, looking after ourselves is largely
our own responsibility.

That task may seem easy when you are in good health. But accidents
happen, you may need an operation, or you may join the ranks of the
one in three Australian adults who have at least one chronic health
condition, such as asthma, diabetes or arthritis. Although medical science
has developed many effective health strategies, ranging from changes in
diet to medications and surgical procedures, the reality is that we need to
look after ourselves, day in and day out, if we're going to get healthy and
stay healthy.

This is where 'self care' comes in – all the things you do for your own or
your family's wellbeing, in addition to the treatments prescribed by doctors
and other health professionals, such as pharmacists and physiotherapists.
Human beings have amazing self-healing powers, and this is where this
book can really help. It's packed with practical, effective tips and advice
that can complement medical treatments or help get the most out of those
treatments. The aim is not only to get you feeling better faster but also to
help you cope more positively along the way.

So *1001 Great Ways to Get Better* is a book for people who want to
be proactive; not just in looking after everyday illnesses such as coughs
and colds, but also in boosting the effectiveness of medical treatments
for more serious illness. There's plenty of effective, scientifically based
advice that includes mental strategies – to combat pain and stress, for
instance. Reader's Digest has done a marvellous job of collecting so many
of them together in this empowering book and I recommend it for every
home library.

Dr Kathy Kramer MBBS/BA, BScMed(Hons) (USyd)
General practitioner

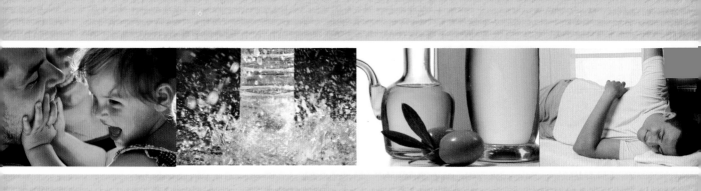

part 1

taking charge of getting better

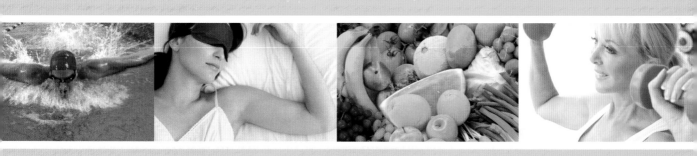

Fight back ... and win

Few people are lucky enough to go through life without at least a skirmish with sickness. Whether the problem is minor or major, understanding your condition and your own role in the healing process puts *you* in control and can ensure a faster, better recovery.

When you're ill, your doctors can only do so much. The rest is up to you. *1001 Great Ways To Get Better* is the first book to focus on how you can give yourself the best chance of a full and fast recuperation from any kind of problem, whether a headache, hernia or heart attack. It arms you with the tools you need to regain your health or – for chronic conditions – to manage the illness to limit its impact. You'll be amazed at how much you can achieve.

The book explains how to work with your medical team from the moment you fall ill. You'll discover how best to respond to a diagnosis, what to expect from different treatments and what questions will put you in the driving seat. You'll also learn from nurses and other health professionals the crucial actions you can take for yourself and those for whom you are caring to help ensure the best and speediest recovery.

Health in your hands

While GPs and consultants may provide the crucial initial diagnosis and treatment, most have neither the time nor the resources to play an active role in their patients' recovery. That is why this book is so important. *1001 Great Ways To Get Better*:

● **Gets you back on your feet** after minor and major illnesses and accidents with dozens of tried-and-tested tips and strategies.
● **Explains exercise techniques** recommended by physiotherapists and carers for recuperation from a wide range of common ailments, conditions and operations.
● **Offers dozens of complementary solutions** to lift your spirits, soothe pain and help you to relax and sleep.
● **Gives you the tools and strategies** to care effectively for your family – young and old – at home.
● **Provides inspirational case histories** from people who have recovered from a range of debilitating conditions.

Research increasingly shows that the lifestyle choices that people make can have a major effect on how they cope with and recover from illness. This book helps you to make the right choices at every stage of your journey to better health.

WHAT CAUSES ILLNESS?

Why, when a group of people are exposed to the same common cold virus, do some individuals suffer a raging sore throat and streaming nose, while others have mild symptoms or are totally unaffected? There are no simple answers to these questions: genes, environment and lifestyle all play a part – and each affects the others in ways we are only now beginning to understand. While we have little control over some factors, such as our genes and environment, there is much we can do to influence how our bodies respond, for example, to infection, trauma and potential allergens. We can also learn to deal with our emotions to protect our mental health.

LIFESTYLE MATTERS

According to the Cancer Council, a third of all cancers could be prevented by lifestyle changes. Emerging research shows that the same kinds of changes – avoiding cigarettes and alcohol, eating healthily and exercising – can also affect survival rates in people who have already developed the disease. And according to INTERHEART, a 2004 study, as many as 90 per cent of first heart attacks could be prevented by lifestyle changes. Even people with a genetic predisposition to a particular illness shouldn't assume that the outcome is inevitable.

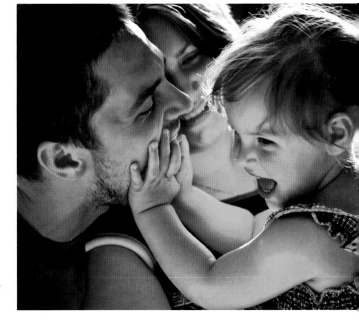

Families with a history of heart disease once believed that nothing could be done to prevent successive generations succumbing to this condition, often dying prematurely. But today those with raised cholesterol can slash the chances of a heart attack by taking appropriate medication, improving their diet and increasing the amount of exercise they take.

Disease prevention rightly commands massive attention. But until we can protect against every illness – an unlikely achievement – we need to continue to focus on boosting our chances of recovery. Doctors hold some of the keys to that process (see *Getting the best from your treatment*, page 12), but many others are in our own hands – known collectively as the 'four pillars of health' (see page 14).

Getting the best from your treatment

No matter what your health problem, your medical team is your best ally. And there's evidence that developing a good relationship with the doctors who are caring for you can itself bring health benefits.

PARTNERS IN CARE

None of us can predict exactly how we'll react in the first few moments after being given a diagnosis, especially if the condition is a serious one. For this reason, when you have a doctor's appointment, make sure you take somebody with you if there's a chance that you'll be given bad news. Have a list of questions ready (see *Questions to ask*, left) and leave a space on the page for your doctor's replies or ask your companion to write them down for you.

ACTIVE ENGAGEMENT

There is no need to be concerned that asking questions about your illness and the treatment options will annoy your doctor. The vast majority of health professionals welcome patients' involvement in their own care; treatment is more likely to be effective – and recovery swifter – in these cases. What's more, research suggests that if you feel you are playing an active role in your treatment, you are likely to be more satisfied with the care provided by your doctor.

HOW TO FIND OUT MORE

Being well informed about your condition helps you know what questions to ask and what treatment to expect. A range of possible sources of information are listed under *Helpful organisations* (page 340). But take care when surfing the web on health issues. There's a great deal of alarming, misleading and downright inaccurate material online, information that can do more harm than good.

Questions to ask

When you visit your doctor – whether your GP or a specialist – arrive prepared with a list of questions, such as:

- *What have I got?*
- *What's the cause?*
- *What are the symptoms, how will things develop and over what time scale?*
- *Will this resolve itself/get worse/ become chronic?*
- *What treatments are available?*
- *Is there a cure?*
- *Where can I get more information?*
- *What happens next?*

TREATMENT CHOICES ON THE ROAD TO RECOVERY

Having made a diagnosis, your GP (or specialist) will consider possible treatments. Some straightforward conditions – such as flu – simply require time and a few simple home remedies (see *Bouncing back from everyday ailments*, pages 36–65). For such illnesses, you're largely in charge of your recovery.

In other cases – for example, a heart condition – your doctor may prescribe medication (see *Mending your heart*, pages 120–141) and you will need to take it as advised. But there will be additional measures, such as diet changes and exercise, that will help you return to health. Surgery may be the primary treatment in other cases, and there is often much you can do before and after the operation to maximise the speed of your recovery (see *Before and after surgery*, pages 196–213).

A SECOND OPINION

Because a relationship of trust is key to the success of your treatment, it's important that you share any concerns that you may have about any aspect of your care with your GP or consultant. If you're still unhappy, you can ask for a second opinion. If your GP practice has several doctors, you can simply ask to see someone else in the practice. If you want to switch consultants, your GP will have to write another referral letter for you. Finding a doctor you like, respect and trust can make all the difference to how you feel about the health care you receive, so it is often worth the initial inconvenience of seeking alternative medical advice.

The four pillars of health

Expert diagnosis, timely treatment and effective medication play key roles in getting better from any ailment. But human beings are not machines and the recovery process is not necessarily automatic. Your physical state, the strength of your immune system and also your willpower are vital factors.

The following pages focus on four key aspects of your lifestyle, where the changes you make can provide a significant boost to your physical and mental defences as you recover from illness or injury, helping you to return to full health.

ATTITUDE COUNTS

While nobody should claim that you can think yourself well, there's little doubt that mental attitude plays an important part in many common ills. One US study analysed the records of more than 1,000 patients suffering from symptoms such as chest pain, headache, back pain, abdominal pain and weight loss, and discovered actual physical causes for only 16 per cent of them. The rest were thought to have 'psychosocial causes' (linked to the emotional condition and social background of the patient). And it is also clear that the way you deal with illness or trauma can affect its outcome.

The connection between attitude and life expectancy has been shown in several studies. One involving nearly 100,000 women, published in the journal *Circulation* in 2009, showed that the most optimistic people were 14 per cent less likely to die from any cause over the eight-year study than those who were the most pessimistic, even when other factors such as wealth and lifestyle were taken into account.

DIET REPAIRS

A healthy diet plays a key role in keeping illness at bay – for example, one third of all cancers are thought to be due, at least in part, to poor nutrition. What you eat also has a significant effect on the way your body copes when under attack. In particular, foods that contain the right nutrients can boost the functioning of the immune system, helping it to fight off infection.

A good diet can give you energy and provide the nutrients you need to help cell regeneration and speed up tissue repair, while a poor one can impair recovery and increase the risk that complications may develop. In this chapter you'll find out how a balanced diet that contains foods from each of the main food groups can set you on the road to optimum health.

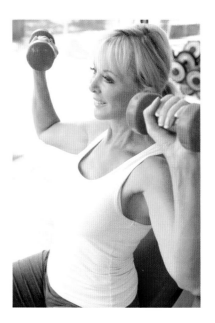

EXERCISE STRENGTHENS

Rest is important in the first stages of many illnesses, but once you're through the worst, a return to activity is an important part of the recovery process, boosting morale as well as muscles. But you don't have to join a gym or take up a sport; informal types of exercise are just as beneficial. Gardening, housework and walking the dog can all help in the management of a huge range of health problems including depression, back pain, diabetes, heart disease and osteoporosis. As a general rule, aim for 30 minutes of moderate activity – something that makes you slightly breathless – five days a week.

SLEEP HEALS

Have you noticed that you succumb to bugs more quickly when you're tired? Research at Carnegie Mellon University in the USA has shown that the less we sleep, the more likely we are to develop a cold. This may be because lack of sleep impairs the immune system and therefore compromises the body's ability to fight off viruses. And another US study highlighted the correlation between poor sleep and the subsequent occurrence of gastrointestinal symptoms in women suffering from irritable bowel syndrome (IBS).

Every body needs down time in which to repair itself, and a body damaged by illness or injury will need more rest than most. Good-quality sleep is essential for the health of the cerebral cortex in the brain. If you're sleep-deprived, you'll feel physically and mentally below par. There's also evidence that those who experience poor sleep feel more pain and are less able to muster the coping skills needed to put into action strategies for recovery.

1: Attitude

A positive attitude is a key predictor of recovery from many illnesses, especially those that require the determination to make major lifestyle changes. But more than that, your expectations can actually have a powerful effect on the course of your disease.

POSITIVE OR NEGATIVE?

Research shows that an optimistic outlook is good for health. For example, in a recent study from Columbia University, New York, people leading happy lives were found to be less prone to heart disease. The reasons for this are not clear. Perhaps people with a positive outlook are better at handling stressful situations, decreasing the harmful effects of stress on the body, or perhaps they lead healthier lives. Conversely, people who feel hopeless and helpless about life or who blame outside forces for what happens to them tend to cope less well with ill health.

ALTERING YOUR THINKING

A sense of no longer being in control is a key aspect of the increased vulnerability that many people feel when suffering from a serious disorder. You cannot change your personality type, but you can alter the way you deal with illness. Cardiac rehabilitation programs, for example, can make heart attack patients less anxious and therefore more willing to take exercise, which promotes recovery. Try these strategies to distract yourself from unhelpful negative thoughts:

Give yourself thinking time Allow yourself 15 minutes each day to focus on your illness instead of letting your thoughts return to the topic throughout the day.

Take one day at a time Concentrate on how you'll deal with today rather than dwelling on an uncertain future.

Surround yourself with positive people Spend time with people who are constructive, support you, make you laugh and give you good advice. Avoid doom-mongers, who may undermine you with their negativity.

Practise mindfulness Essentially this means consciously savouring every moment to the full with your senses, from smelling the soap in the shower to listening to the hiss of the steam iron and feeling the texture of food in your mouth.

HOW YOUR MIND AFFECTS YOUR BODY

You have raging toothache and sit down to watch your favourite TV sitcom. For half an hour you forget about your pain. When the show ends, the agony starts up again. Why? There are a number of factors that come into play, and how the mind influences the body continues to fascinate research scientists. It's a potent force: a study at the University of Rochester in the USA found that men who believed they had a lower than average risk of coronary artery disease were three times less likely to die of heart attack and stroke.

God, grant me the serenity
To accept the things I cannot change;
Courage to change the things I can;
And wisdom to know the difference.

'Serenity Prayer' Reinhold Niebuhr

PLACEBO AND NOCEBO

In every clinical trial for a new medication, some patients who are given a placebo or dummy pill show an improvement in symptoms – because they expect to. Even placebo operations can work: a procedure for angina that was believed to relieve pain by 60 per cent was discontinued many years ago when simply cutting the skin was found to have a similar success rate.

The placebo response is not just about the power of positive thinking. It is now known that dummy medicines cause chemical changes in the brain. Professor Fabrizio Benedetti of the University of Turin, Italy, has found that patients with Parkinson's disease, whose symptoms improved after being given a placebo during a drug trial, showed a rise in dopamine levels similar to that of those in the study who had taken the active drug.

Powerful medicine

America's prestigious Mayo Clinic lists the possible benefits of thinking positively as:

- better psychological and physical wellbeing
- lower rates of depression
- better coping skills during hardship and times of stress
- greater resistance to the common cold
- reduced risk of death from cardiovascular disease.

ATTITUDE

The placebo effect is a chemical response triggered by expectation. Who gives the 'drug', the language used and the setting in which this takes place can all influence the strength of the reaction. The effect probably plays a role in every medical interaction. When Professor Benedetti's patients received a proven painkiller without their knowledge, it didn't work. As the journal *New Scientist* reported, this is because the placebo effect and the active medication work together to stimulate production of natural pain-relieving chemicals called endorphins. The same may be true of other medications.

By contrast, the nocebo effect can be damaging. Anxiety can lead patients to experience symptoms and unpleasant side effects because they expect to do so. Again, the effect is real; as well as the sensations reported, measurable changes in brain chemistry have been found.

Nocebo is often seen in chemotherapy patients. Approximately a third of people having chemo treatment experience anticipatory nausea and around one in ten actually vomits before treatment. Psychological approaches, including the use of hypnosis and relaxation techniques, can switch off or reduce the nocebo response (see also *Coping with chemotherapy*, page 185).

Managing stress

The link between stress and illness is something most people understand all too well. Your boss is giving you hell, the baby is keeping you up every night, your brother is going through an acrimonious divorce – and to cap it all you go down with flu.

Scientific studies confirm this picture. Work at Ohio State University in the USA suggests that stressed people are more susceptible to infection and that their wounds take longer to heal. According to the British Heart Foundation (BHF), stressful experiences such as divorce or workplace problems can increase the risk of diabetes, especially for people with a family history of the disease. Stress may also affect how well a person's diabetes is controlled. And a 2010 study published in the *European Heart Journal* showed that full-time workers who do more than 3 hours of overtime a day are 60 per cent more likely to suffer from heart problems. The researchers suggest that the underlying causes may be high blood pressure, reduced sleep and mental stress.

It's thought that long-term stress on the nervous system interferes with the production of substances in the body that stimulate and coordinate white blood cell activity and help fight disease – what we call the immune system.

LAUGHTER IS THE BEST MEDICINE...

How providing something to laugh about has helped those recovering from cancer

John Cremer, a speaker and trainer who has run improvised comedy sessions for cancer patients, describes the benefits of laughter.

66 People made other people laugh and then they were off, laughing themselves. You could see the whole structure of their faces change. Their eyes were brighter and there was more eye contact. They became more upright and confident.

Quite a few people talked about getting real pain relief from the endorphin release they experienced. One woman said she had noticeably less pain for ten days after each session.

The brain creates habitual neural pathways in people who are gravely ill or severely depressed, and laughter disrupts these patterns, setting up something new. 99

BE CALM, BE HAPPY, GET WELL

If the bad news is that stress can impede the immune system and make us more susceptible to illness, the good news is that calming the mind may reverse its effects. The beneficial effects of laughter are described on page 141 and you'll find plenty more helpful suggestions on the following pages for reducing stress. What's more, taking time out to have a relaxing complementary therapy treatment can also help relieve stress. Many people find reflexology, massage and aromatherapy helpful. Acupuncture and hypnosis may also be worth trying. You'll find more relaxation tips in the section on sleep (see pages 30–31).

YOU NEED A FRIEND

When we're feeling ill, the support of friends can provide a wonderful boost. This help can be invaluable when you've come home from hospital after a major operation. Research has shown that being in the company of others can bring health benefits. In one American trial, group therapy designed to reduce psychological distress in patients with melanoma seemed to boost levels of T-cells and increase survival time. It is also true that those who do not have such support are likely to suffer from worse health than people whose life is filled with friends and family. According to *The Lonely Society*, a report published by the UK Mental Health Foundation in 2010, persistent loneliness affects stress hormones, the immune system and cardiovascular function and can have a 'cumulative effect equivalent in impact to being a smoker'. Research on animals suggests that isolation can make us more prone to infection. Infant monkeys separated from their mothers, especially if they are caged alone rather than in groups, generate fewer infection-fighting T-cells and fewer antibodies in response to viruses.

Support comes in many guises. Here are some ideas for getting in touch with people who may be able to help:

- Ask your GP or search on the internet for a health charity related to your condition, which may run self-help groups either online or locally. Arthritis Australia, for example, publicises events for local groups on its website (www.arthritisaustralia.com.au).
- Search online for internet chat forums that can link you to other people with similar health problems. Exchanging ideas and sharing experiences with others can make all the difference.
- Ask your local health authority for a list of local support groups.
- If you are religious, visiting places of worship can be comforting and you may also make new friends.
- Helping others is a great way to help yourself. Decades of research has shown that volunteering improves happiness, health and even longevity.

GET CREATIVE

By providing enjoyable and satisfying distraction from your illness, creative pursuits can help to reduce stress levels and bring a variety of health benefits.

Express yourself Try your hand at creative writing, but this needn't be more ambitious than keeping a diary of your experiences. According to a report in the Royal College of Psychiatrists' journal *Advances in Psychiatric Treatment*, 'Writing about traumatic, stressful or emotional events has been found to result in improvements in both physical and psychological health.'

Tune in to music Make time to listen to the type of music you most enjoy. Offering pre-operative patients the music of their choice has been shown to reduce anxiety and the need for analgesics. And a 2010 Finnish study showed that playing music to stroke patients induced brain changes that could lead to improved function.

Find your inner artist Why not have a go at painting or sculpture?

Art for Health, a report on 15 community arts projects written for the NHS, the British health service, states that, 'The arts clearly have the potential to make a major contribution to our health, wellbeing and life skills.' The projects, which ranged from painting to quilting, helped participants to have a more positive outlook, reduced isolation and anxiety and gave increased confidence, sociability and self-esteem.

ENVIRONMENT AND MOOD

Florence Nightingale was among the first to recognise the importance of a patient's surroundings on healing, writing in her *Notes on Hospitals* that 'variety of form and brilliancy of colour in the objects presented to patients is the actual means of recovery'. There's plenty you can do at home to create surroundings that are conducive to health for yourself or those you are caring for (see also *Changing rooms*, page 270):

- Keep curtains drawn right back, put mirrors opposite windows and cut away foliage that blocks light coming into your home. Natural light is good for body, mind and soul.
- If possible, spend time where you can see green space. Studies show that looking at plants and nature reduces stress and increases positive feelings. If you don't have a garden, buy some house plants.
- Surround yourself with colours you like – buy some new cushions, artwork or a throw in your favourite shades.
- Use an essential oil diffuser to provide scents that you find relaxing or stimulating, as you prefer.

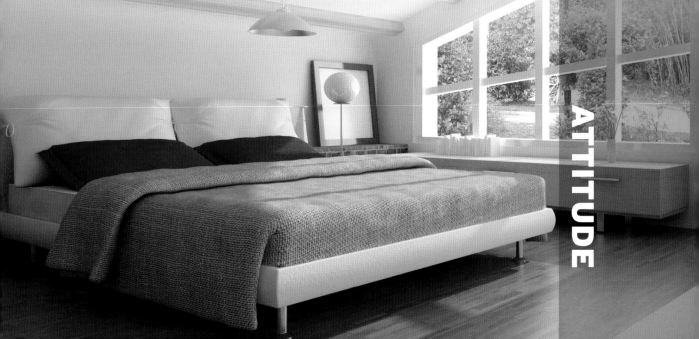

ATTITUDE

2: Diet

Nobody doubts that what we eat affects our health. Every week there's a new story showing a link between diet and disease. And when you are recovering from illness, it is simple good sense to give your body the best nutrition you can provide.

EATING FOR RECOVERY

'It is extremely important that you are well nourished and hydrated while recovering from illness,' says Rick Wilson, Director of Nutrition and Dietetics at King's College Hospital, London. 'Our bodies are in a constant state of turnover, making an average of 3 million new cells every second. The raw material for manufacturing these new cells comes from the food we eat. When you're recovering from illness, it's essential that the body's defences get the raw materials they need to do their job properly.'

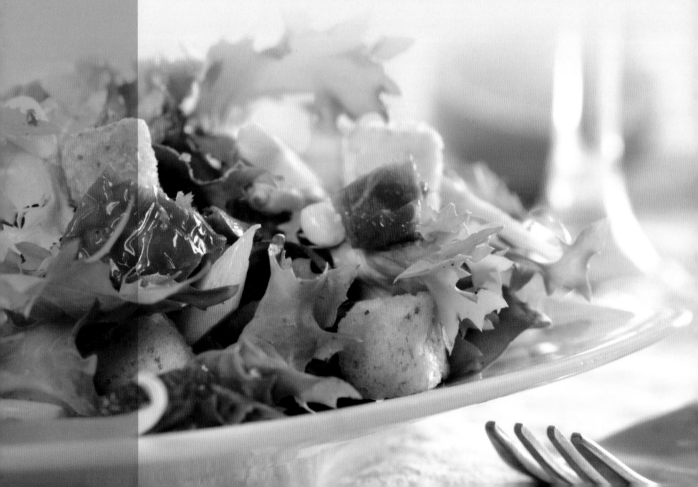

ExpertView

EATING FOR HEALTH

How a simple change in eating habits
restored a 65 year-old's zest for life

**Director of Nutrition Rick Wilson tells
the story of Bill, 65, who was feeling
exhausted and breathless. His wife
had died the previous year and he
gradually found it more difficult to
do the things he enjoyed:**

66 He had put off going to the doctor
because he thought his symptoms were
caused by his loss. But tests revealed he
was anaemic. Bill confessed that he hadn't
eaten very well since his wife died. He did
not know how to cook and could not see
any point in making a meal for one.

Bill's iron stores had become depleted,
causing his symptoms. His doctor
prescribed a course of iron and
multivitamin tablets, and he was told
about a basic cooking course run by the
local health authority.

Bill learned about iron-rich foods such as
red meat, fortified breakfast cereals and
dark green leafy vegetables. Within six
months, he had far more energy and felt
generally better. He made new friends at
the cooking class and has even been known
to hold small dinner parties for them. 99

GET NOURISHED; STAY WELL

A balanced diet gives us the best chance of staying well, of avoiding
obesity – a risk factor for many diseases – and of beating illness when
it strikes. The World Health Organization has estimated that 40 per cent
of ill health in the developed world is caused by poor diet. This includes
major problems such as heart disease, diabetes and cancer, but also,
perhaps surprisingly, varicose veins, appendicitis and haemorrhoids
(piles). Research shows that within 48 hours of dietary neglect, the
immune system starts to display signs of being under strain and
becomes less effective at combating disease.

The basics of good diet as outlined by expert bodies such as the UK
government's Department of Health and the Food Standards Agency
(FSA) apply to everybody, unless you are getting over a major illness,
accident or surgery. The plate illustrated on page 109 provides a guide
for healthy eating for most people at most stages of life. See also
A healing diet, page 271.

DIET

A HEALTHY DIET - THE BASICS

Give your body all the nutrients it needs by consuming a well-balanced diet – which is as much about what you don't eat as what you do eat. It's not an exact science and there is no need to be overly precise about what you eat at every meal; it's more useful to look at the general picture over a day. But here are some basic guidelines to help you get it right.

Food	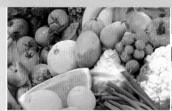 Fruit and vegetables	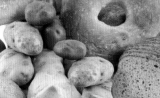 Starchy foods	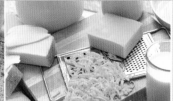 Milk and dairy
Why?	These plant foods are a good source of vitamins and minerals, as well as antioxidants, which fight disease-causing free radicals.	Starchy (high carbohydrate) foods give us energy and provide fibre (roughage), essential for digestion and the health of the bowel. Nutrients found in starchy foods include calcium, iron and B vitamins.	Dairy foods are a good source of protein, vitamins A and B_{12}, and calcium for strong bones.
What?	Have plenty of different varieties (leaves, legumes, roots and stems) and try them raw or cooked, dried, canned or frozen. When cooking, use as little water as possible, don't overcook.	Pasta, rice, potatoes, oats, bread, grains and legumes. Wholegrain pasta, rice and bread deliver more fibre. Sugar is pure carbohydrate but contains no additional nutrients or fibre.	This category includes milk and milk products, including cheese and yoghurt. Adults should go for reduced-fat products. Vegans should choose fortified soy or rice milk.
How much?	About a third of what you eat should be fruit and veg. Have at least seven portions a day. A portion is one apple or two plums or three heaped tablespoons of vegetables. Juice counts for only one portion a day, no matter how much you drink.	About a third of what you eat (by volume) should be starchy foods. Intake of sugar-rich foods should be kept to a minimum.	Dairy products should make up no more than about a seventh of an adult's daily food intake in terms of volume. See also *Fats and oils*, facing page.

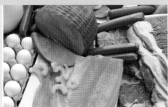 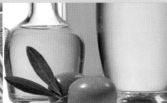 

Meat, fish, eggs, legumes	Fat and oils	Fluids
All these foods are high in protein. Fish and shellfish are rich in niacin (vitamin B2), selenium and iodine. Oily fish are rich in omega-3 fatty acids. Red meat contains iron, selenium, zinc and B vitamins. Eggs contain vitamins A, D and B2.	Fats help the body absorb some nutrients and provide essential fatty acids that we cannot make ourselves. But caution is needed because fats are high in kilojoules and therefore contribute to weight gain.	Most of the chemical reactions that occur in cells need water. Low fluid levels in the body can impair a wide range of functions, causing symptoms such as headaches, nausea and constipation.
Go for the lean cuts of red meat and choose poultry without the skin. White fish is low in fat, but does not have the same health benefits as oily fish. Non-animal sources of protein such as legumes (beans) contain virtually no fat.	Fats are either saturated (mostly animal fats) or unsaturated (most, but not all, vegetable oils). Too much saturated fat can raise blood cholesterol levels. Get most of your fat intake from unsaturated fats.	Water contains no kilojoules and cannot damage the teeth. Have tea, coffee, milk and juice in moderation. Keep fizzy drinks to a minimum - they are usually high in sugar.
Protein-rich foods should make up about a seventh of your daily food intake. Women of childbearing age and below are advised to have no more than two portions of oily fish a week as they can contain low levels of pollutants.	No more than 35 per cent of your total daily kilojoules should come from fat, and no more than 11 per cent from saturated fat.	You need a total of about 1.2 litres of fluid every day - some of which will come from food - to prevent dehydration.

DIET

Know your units

Regularly drinking more than the recommended alcohol limits over a long period puts you at increased risk of liver damage, some cancers, high blood pressure, heart disease, stroke and depression. The National Health and Medical Research Council (NHMRC) recommends that both men and women drink no more than two standard drinks on any day. A standard drink is definted as containing 10 g of alcohol (equivalent to 12.5 ml of pure alcohol).

What is a standard drink?

Beer 1 can or stubbie
(mid-strength or light beer, 3.5% alcohol)

Wine 100 ml glass
(9.5-13% alcohol)

Spirits 1 nip
(30 ml; 37-40% alcohol)

You can find an easy-to-use visual guide to standard drinks at www.nhmrc.gov.au/_files_nhmrc/file/your_health/healthy/alcohol/std-drinks-large.jpg

WHEN YOU'RE UNWELL

If you are clinically malnourished when you become ill – and overweight people are at as much risk as anyone else – you are more likely to develop complications. Because ill health may also diminish your appetite, causing you to skip meals, eating a healthy diet when you are well is doubly important.

You may regard losing weight when you're unwell as an unexpected bonus, but in fact it's bad news. Shedding 10 per cent of your body weight or more in three months or less is considered harmful. What is shed is not fat, but muscle, which you need in recovery to build up your strength. For example, you need strong respiratory muscles to breathe and cough to clear your lungs; you need muscles in your legs to enable you to regain mobility. Symptoms of malnourishment include depression and lack of motivation, both of which can prevent you from taking part in vital rehabilitation programs after illness.

If you're caring for someone who is recuperating from surgery or an illness, think carefully about how to provide easy-to-eat meals, such as homemade soups and smoothies. There's plenty of advice for boosting the nutritional value of meals for those recovering from illness on pages 271–4.

KEEP IT LOW

Whether you are recovering from a current illness or just trying to keep in the best possible health, as well as maximising your intake of 'good' foods, it's important to limit how much you consume of certain foods or ingredients that may have a damaging effect on your health. The most important of these are:

Sugar It's bad for teeth and contains 'empty' kilojoules that can lead to weight gain without providing any nutritional benefit. It's rapid absorption can also lead to special problems for those with diabetes (see *Eating your way better*, pages 108–112).

Salt Too much salt raises blood pressure, tripling your risk of heart disease or stroke. Eat no more than 6 g (1 teaspoon) of salt (the equivalent of 2.3 g of sodium) a day, taking into account salt in processed food. Those with high blood pressure or heart problems may need to reduce their salt intake further.

Alcohol Heavy drinking leads to an increased risk of cancer, liver disease, stroke, high blood pressure and mental health problems. The recommended limits for men and women are given in the panel, left. Don't be tempted to save up your alcohol units for a weekend of heavy drinking. Binge drinking brings added risks such as accidents, falls and reckless behaviour.

3: Exercise

Fitness is a vital tool in the recovery process. Thousands of scientific studies demonstrate that exercise not only plays a part in keeping a whole range of illnesses at bay, it can also help people to manage chronic conditions and prevent them worsening.

FITNESS BENEFITS

You can reap numerous physical and psychological benefits by being physically active. Medical experts agree that taking regular exercise can:

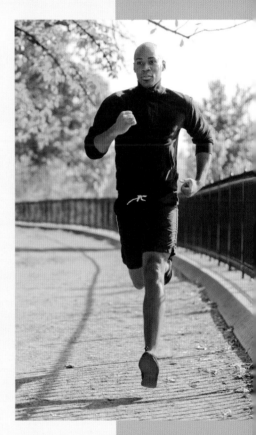

- Reduce your chances of developing heart disease and stroke and help you to stay well if you are already a sufferer. It can bring down blood pressure and raise levels of HDL – 'good' cholesterol. Inactive people are almost twice as likely to die from these conditions as people who keep fit (see *Exercise your heart*, page 134, and *An active recovery*, page 159).
- Maintain healthy blood glucose levels, cutting your risk of diabetes. This is especially important if you're at risk of developing type 2 diabetes because you're overweight, have high blood pressure or have a close family member with the condition. Exercise also helps people with diabetes keep glucose levels down and stay well (see *Get active*, page 112).
- Protect against some cancers, notably cancer of the colon, the uterus (womb) and – in post-menopausal women – the breast. See also *How exercise helps*, page 178.
- Improve your mental health and relieve stress. A 2010 study of university students carried out by the University of Gloucestershire showed that those who took more exercise had better mental health (see *Exercise to keep your spirits high*, page 260).
- Increase bone density, helping to prevent osteoporosis in the future (young people) and slowing bone loss (older people).

Exercise and obesity

Keeping active delivers a double health advantage; it has a direct effect on all kinds of diseases and also indirectly benefits wellbeing by helping to control weight. Being overweight or obese is a risk factor for many illnesses, including heart disease, diabetes and arthritis. For example,

EXERCISE

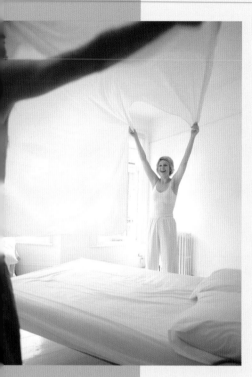

people who are likely to develop diabetes can reduce the chances of getting it by half if they lose just 5 per cent of their body weight. Excess weight also makes these conditions harder to manage. According to medical experts, obesity can shorten the life expectancy of adults over the age of 40 by about seven years.

HOW TO KEEP ACTIVE

The National Physical Activity Guidelines for Australians recommend at least 30 minutes of moderate-intensity physical activity on most days, preferably all days. To gain the full health benefit, the activity should make you feel warm and slightly out of breath. You don't have to take the 30 minutes of exercise all in one session; you could do it in shorter periods over the course of the day.

Many forms of exercise can provide health benefits so how you keep active is largely a matter of personal preference. Water-based exercise is recommended for many medical conditions including musculoskeletal problems and rehabilitation after surgery because, as well as providing aerobic exercise, it strengthens a wide range of muscles without the risk of jarring or falls.

There's no need to join a gym or a class to get the right amount of exercise. The important thing is to build activity into your daily routine. A system developed by the Mayo Clinic in the USA called NEAT (Non-Exercise Activity Thermogenesis) focuses on the exercise value of everyday activities. Here are some NEAT-inspired suggestions for ways to increase your activity levels:

At work Get off the bus before your destination and walk the rest of the way. Take the stairs instead of the lift as much as possible at work. Get active in your lunch break – power walk to a sandwich shop rather than eating in the company canteen.

At home Run up and down the stairs a few times. Put some elbow grease into housework. The most demanding activities include vacuuming, mopping, changing the bed linen, cleaning the windows and scrubbing the bath and oven.

Out and about with the kids Walk your children to school or to the shops. Put your toddler in a jogging stroller and go running.

In the garden Pruning, trimming, digging, weeding, raking, shovelling and planting incorporate many of the exercises and elements of a workout at the gym. You can use as much energy performing some gardening tasks as you do when walking, cycling or swimming.

In your spare time Choose an activity you enjoy – swimming, dancing, yoga, cycling, walking – and build it into your daily or weekly routine.

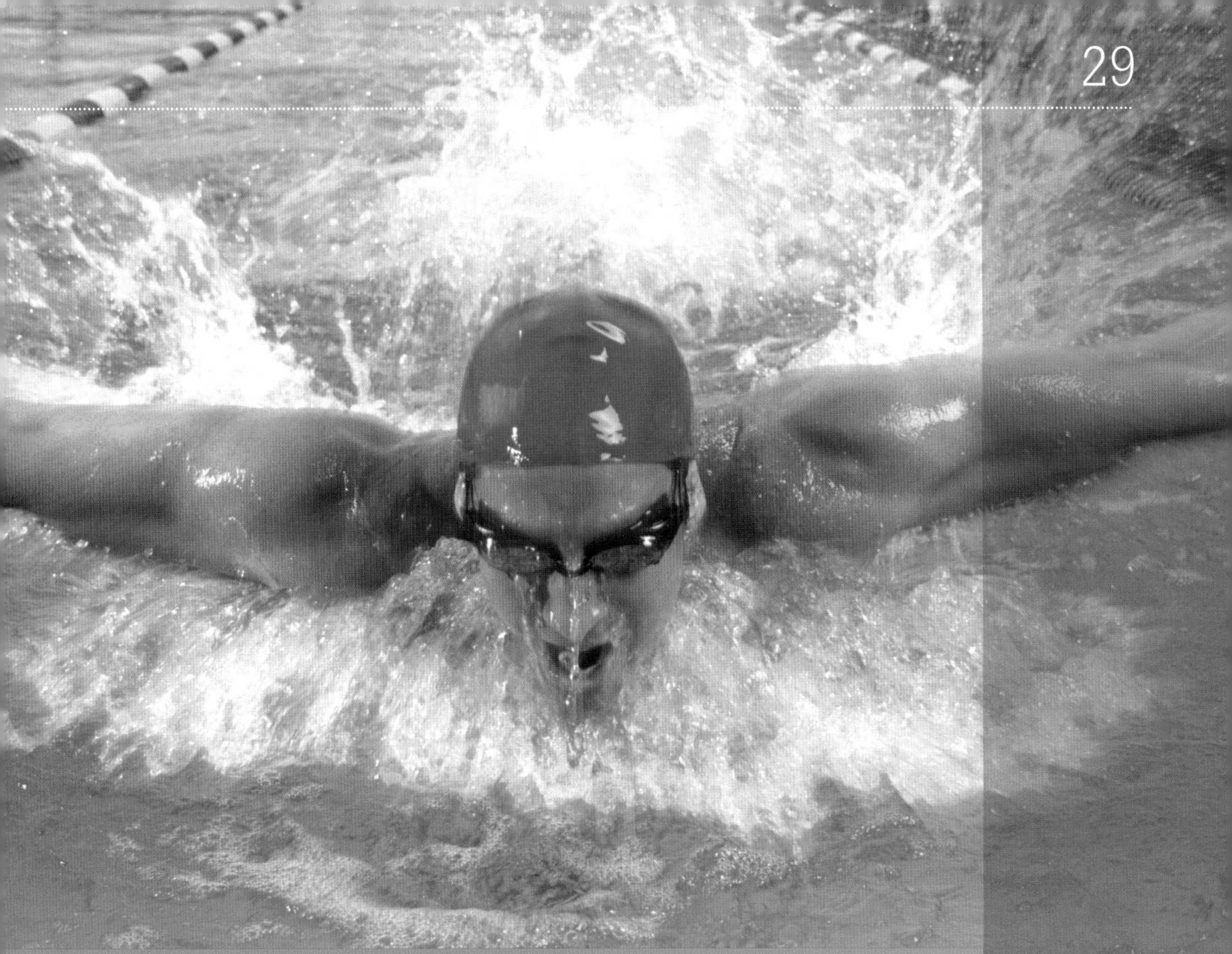

ExpertView

HEALING STROKES

How swimming helped a hip-replacement patient get back on his feet

Steven Shaw, whose Shaw Method, based on the Alexander Technique of body alignment, promotes healing through swimming, describes how hydrotherapy sessions benefited one arthritis patient.

“One of my clients is a man in his 50s who was told he needed a hip replacement and came to us to learn butterfly before the op. Breast stroke, which he used to swim, is not recommended after hip replacement because you cannot turn the foot out fully.

He was back in the water within a few days of being discharged from hospital and was soon doing length after length of butterfly. It's a great stroke because it opens up and strengthens the whole back. The doctors were amazed at how quickly he got rid of the crutches. They had never seen anything like it.”

4: Sleep

Few things refresh body and mind like a sound night's sleep. And we now know that this is largely due to the relationship between physiological processes that take place in the body during sleep and the immune system.

THE HEALING POWER OF SLEEP

We have all had the experience of going to bed feeling ill, and waking in the morning feeling a hundred times better. This is not simply the result of rest; it is now known that while we are asleep, the body's immune system is hard at work fighting germs, and hormones are released that repair damaged tissue. The relationship between the immune system and sleep may work both ways: while lack of sleep interferes with immune function, an immune system under attack interferes with sleep. Breaking this cycle may be an important component in recovery.

HOW MUCH DO WE NEED?

There is a huge variation in the amount of sleep that people need. Some seem to function perfectly well on 5 hours a night, whereas others find they need 8 hours or more. Professor Colin Espie, director of the University of Glasgow Sleep Research Laboratory, estimates that on average adults need 7 to 8 hours of sleep a night, falling to around

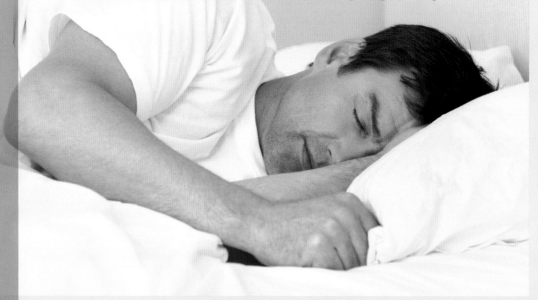

Relaxation exercise

Too much stress during the day can affect sleep. If you are feeling tense try this technique, taught at the Benson-Henry Institute at the Massachusetts General Hospital, a world leader in mind-body medicine research:

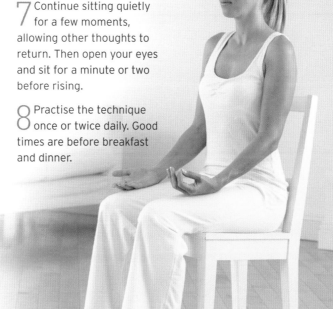

1 Pick a focus word, short phrase, sound or prayer that means something to you.

2 Sit quietly in a comfortable position and close your eyes.

3 Relax your muscles, progressing from your feet to your calves, thighs, abdomen, shoulders, head and neck.

4 Breathe slowly and naturally, saying your focus word silently to yourself as you exhale.

5 When other thoughts come to mind, gently return to your repetition.

6 Continue for 10 to 20 minutes.

7 Continue sitting quietly for a few moments, allowing other thoughts to return. Then open your eyes and sit for a minute or two before rising.

8 Practise the technique once or twice daily. Good times are before breakfast and dinner.

6 hours in later life, although some people need more or less than this. He says that 'One of the purposes of sleep is to ensure good-quality daytime functioning – physical, mental and emotional.' If you wake feeling refreshed and are able to perform your daily activities without losing concentration through tiredness, you are probably getting enough sleep.

STRESS AND SLEEP

Insomnia can be the result of stress in your daily life. It's hard to sleep when you are overwhelmed by worry – whether about your job or your personal relationships, for example. All of us have suffered from nights of sleeplessness when it seems impossible to prevent our thoughts repeatedly going over the day's incidents or anticipating events in the days to come. If this sounds like you, make it a priority to deal with ongoing problems.

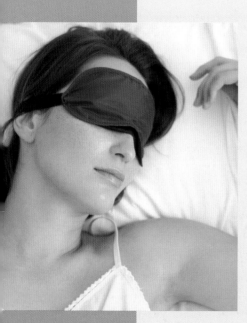

In the meantime, there is plenty you can do to reduce the effects of stress and prepare your body and mind for a good night's sleep. Practising a variety of relaxation techniques both during the day and in the evening before going to bed can help. For example, try the relaxation routine on page 31 on a chair, as shown, or while lying down in bed at night. The breathing exercise on page 250 is also a useful way to dispel feelings of tension. Many people develop a favourite visualisation to help take their minds off daily worries and promote feelings of tranquillity. This involves imagining you are in a place far away from all sources of worry – perhaps a favourite holiday destination. See also *Visualise it*, page 223.

DOS AND DON'TS FOR GETTING A GOOD NIGHT'S SLEEP

'Sleep hygiene' is a term often used to describe the optimum conditions to promote sleep, including the avoidance of stimulants, the creation of a sleep-friendly environment and putting into place a bedtime routine. Experts recommend the following measures to help you get to sleep and stay asleep for as long as you need:

Do get plenty of exercise during the day. People who are both physically fit and physically tired sleep better.

Do let some fresh air into the room during the evening.

Do consider changing your bed and pillows. If you find it easier to sleep away from home, the bed could be a factor.

Do avoid taking a hot bath within an hour of your bedtime.

Do identify what may disturb your sleeping patterns – for example, watching television or surfing the internet just before bedtime. Try keeping a note of what you do in the evenings and how you sleep later.

Do block out as much noise and light as you can. Use earplugs and an eyemask if they help.

Do develop a bedtime routine – for instance, doing 'winding-down' tasks, reading or listening to music, and finally brushing your teeth and putting on your nightclothes.

Do get out of bed if you're not asleep within 15 minutes and do something relaxing in another room.

Do stick to a regular waking time – even after a poor night's sleep – to establish a healthy sleep pattern.

Don't have any caffeine (coffee, tea and cola), nicotine, or spicy or sugary food in the 4 to 6 hours before bed. Some people need to cut out caffeine even earlier in the day.

ExpertView

RELAXATION FOR PEACE OF MIND

How learning relaxation techniques leading to
better sleep helped a cancer victim cope

Clinical psychologist Dr Ray Owen has found that teaching patients ways to relax can bring them big physical and psychological benefits. He tells the story of one of his patients:

66 One cancer patient was kept awake by her fear of the cancer returning, which seemed even more real in the early hours of the morning. She was also spending a lot of time in the day worrying. This made her tense – leading to muscle aches – and more likely to shout at her kids.

Her GP suggested a simple form of relaxation, involving tensing then relaxing each muscle of the body in turn, and then concentrating on her breathing. She was to try it once each day for about 20 minutes, and could also use it at night if she was awake worrying.

At first she found that her mind wandered. With practice, though, she noticed that she felt calmer, learned how to 'let go' if the tension built up, and could use the relaxation to help herself get back to sleep if she started worrying.

Better rested, she had more energy during the day and achieved more. Being more relaxed, her muscles also ached less and she found she could cope better with the normal stresses of daily life. 99

Don't drink alcohol less than 4 hours before bedtime. You'll drop off quickly but the chances are that you'll wake up in the night as the alcohol's sedative effects wear off.

Don't go to bed hungry – or too full. Have a light snack before bedtime, but avoid heavy late-night meals.

Don't take vigorous exercise for at least 2 hours before bedtime.

Don't let your bedroom become too hot or too cold. Aim for a temperature of about 18°C.

Don't keep a clock right next to your bed. Put it out of view, so you can't see the hours ticking away.

Don't stay in bed tossing and turning for hours if you can't sleep. Get up, have a hot, milky drink (milk contains tryptophan, which helps to promote relaxation). Then try going back to bed.

SLEEP

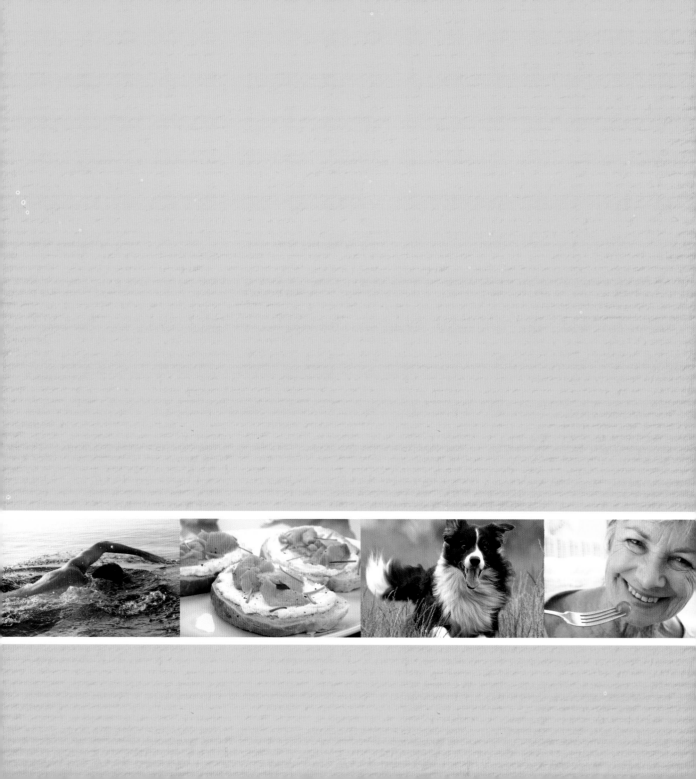

part 2

the
road to
recovery

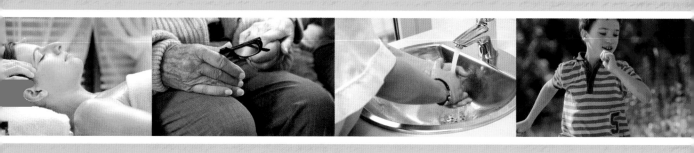

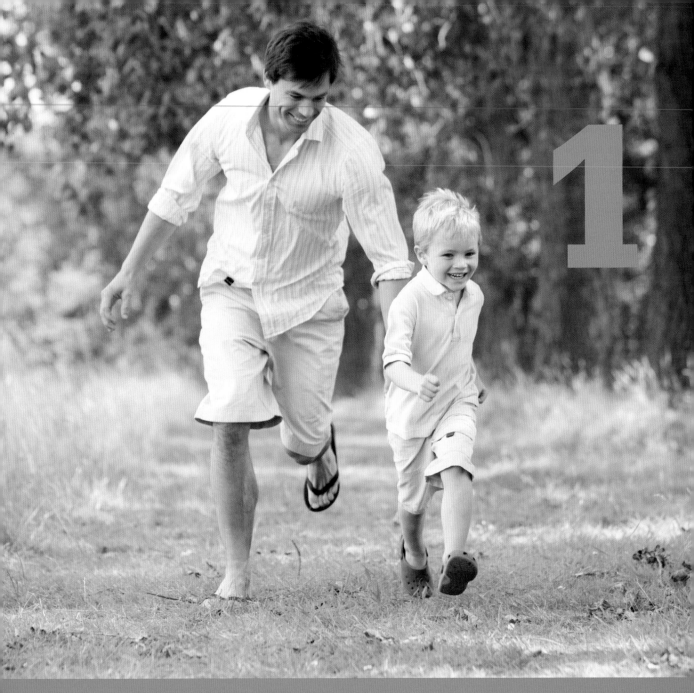

Bouncing back from everyday ailments

Minor ills can still make you feel miserable. Here are some simple ways to get over them as quickly as possible

Deciding what to do

Your body has an enormous capacity for healing and repair, which means that most ordinary ailments resolve themselves within a couple of weeks. In some cases you can speed the recovery process with the help of simple home remedies or over-the-counter medications. But, it is vital to know which conditions you can treat yourself and when you should call your doctor or, in more serious cases, seek emergency medical attention. This chapter will give you all the information you need to cope with a variety of common disorders. It will also help you decide when you need to call in outside help.

While there are many minor ailments that do not require expert medical attention, you should always seek help if symptoms are exceptionally severe or if the person affected is especially vulnerable – people in this group include babies and small children, elderly people and anyone who is suffering from another medical condition. There are also combinations of symptoms that require initial diagnosis or treatment, such as those produced by asthma, eczema, irritable bowel syndrome and urinary tract infections such as cystitis. But there are still measures you can take to help ease discomfort, hasten recovery and prevent repeat attacks.

ASSESSING TRADITIONAL KNOWLEDGE

Many of us are aware of traditional remedies that are reputed to help relieve everyday ailments such as constipation, heartburn or wasp stings, but do these really work? Perhaps surprisingly, there's scientific backing for many such folk remedies. But how can you tell what's likely to work and what will not? Does the saying 'feed a cold and starve a fever' actually hold true? Can you really use yoghurt to help relieve thrush? Will honey help a cough? Does echinacea boost your immune system? This chapter offers the answers to all these questions, and many more as well.

WHEN TO GET MEDICAL HELP

For your own health and that of your family, it's crucial to know when expert help should be sought – whether at the outset or if home treatment hasn't quite worked. Generally, it's wise to take advice if any symptom fails to improve after a reasonable period of home treatment, if symptoms become significantly worse or if new symptoms appear. Trust your instincts, and if you are concerned, always seek your doctor's opinion.

Ailments to treat at home

You can normally treat the following ailments and symptoms at home, at least in the first instance:

- bites and stings
- constipation
- allergic or irritant skin rash
- cough
- diarrhoea
- indigestion
- fever (raised temperature)
- hay fever
- headache
- heartburn
- minor wounds
- mouth ulcers
- nasal symptoms (blocked or runny nose)
- sore throat
- sunburn
- thrush (vaginal yeast infection)
- upper respiratory tract infection (colds and flu)
- vomiting.

WHEN TO CALL THE DOCTOR OR EMERGENCY SERVICES

A medical emergency is an acute condition, either an injury or an illness, that places a person's life or long-term health at immediate risk, and for which immediate medical attention is urgently required.

Emergencies that require urgent medical advice and treatment include:

- difficulty breathing or shortness of breath that interferes with speech
- sudden confusion, unnatural drowsiness or difficulty in rousing someone from sleep
- inability to swallow
- chest pain, especially if it spreads to the neck, jaw or arms or is accompanied by sweating, shortness of breath, dizziness or vomiting
- paralysis or weakness, especially of one side of the face or body
- an asthma attack that lasts for more than 10 minutes despite the use of your regular medication
- pain in the calf accompanied by chest pain, shortness of breath or coughing up blood
- sudden intensely severe headache
- sudden loss of vision or visual disturbances.

In any of the above cases, dial 000 (in Australia) or use other means to get the person to the nearest hospital emergency department (ED) as quickly as possible.

You need a doctor's advice within a day for:

- dramatic worsening of any symptom not listed as emergencies (left)
- increasing pain
- high fever
- vomiting for more than 24 hours
- unexplained bleeding from any orifice, or blood appearing in urine, faeces, sputum or vomit
- a skin infection or wound that becomes hot, red and throbbing, is painful or leaks pus
- inability to pass urine
- constipation that is severe or sudden, especially if you are aged over 50, or if there is any blood in the faeces or any accompanying abdominal pain
- significant unexplained weight loss over two months or longer
- hoarseness that lasts for more than two weeks
- sore throat with a raised temperature, swollen lymph nodes in the neck and pain on swallowing.

YOU DON'T ALWAYS HAVE TO SEE A DOCTOR

Sometimes you'll need to seek formal medical attention, either through a visit to your GP or to your local hospital accident and emergency department, or by dialling 000 (in Australia), depending on the degree of urgency. But there are other excellent sources of help and advice for non-emergencies that you can usually access quickly.

After Hours GP Helpline This Australian government-run helpline can be accessed by calling 1800 022 222. It is available Monday to Friday from 6 pm to 8 am; from 6 pm Friday to 8 am Saturday; and from 12 noon Saturday to 8 am Monday, and all day on public holidays. Your call will be answered by a registered nurse.

Your practice nurse Most GP practices now have a team of nurses and other health-care professionals – either on staff or as visiting specialists – including physiotherapists, midwives and health visitors. They are often able to undertake basic health assessments and advise you on treatment for minor ailments or suggest that you should seek advice from your GP.

The pharmacist Pharmacists are often able to offer valuable advice. They can usually suggest appropriate over-the-counter (OTC) remedies or, if necessary, advise you to seek further help from a doctor or other health professional. They can tell you about any common side effects of OTC or prescribed medications and suggest ways to minimise or counteract them. A pharmacist will also warn you about a medication's potential interactions with other medications, foods and drink, herbal preparations or vitamin and mineral supplements.

Your local pharmacist can be a useful source of advice on treating minor ailments

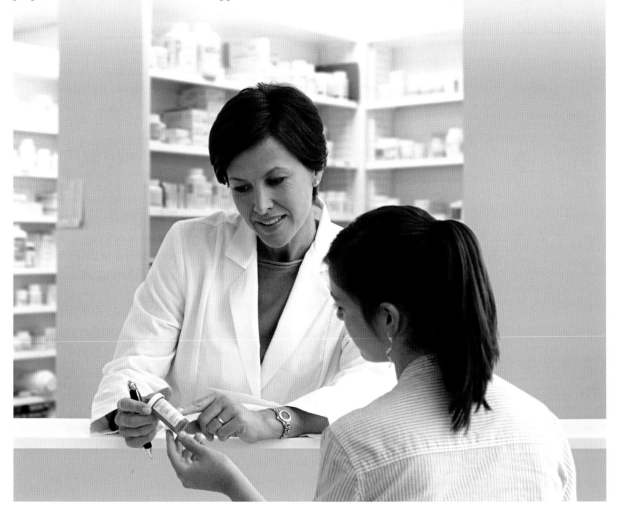

Respiratory problems

We've all experienced respiratory tract problems in the form of colds and flu; the average adult gets approximately two or three such infections each year. Conditions such as asthma and hay fever are also common. In all cases sensible home treatments can speed recovery.

Curbing colds and flu

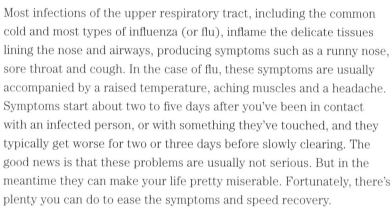

Sneeze into a tissue to reduce the spread of cold viruses via your hands or objects you've touched

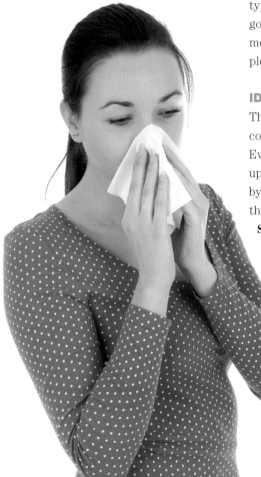

Most infections of the upper respiratory tract, including the common cold and most types of influenza (or flu), inflame the delicate tissues lining the nose and airways, producing symptoms such as a runny nose, sore throat and cough. In the case of flu, these symptoms are usually accompanied by a raised temperature, aching muscles and a headache. Symptoms start about two to five days after you've been in contact with an infected person, or with something they've touched, and they typically get worse for two or three days before slowly clearing. The good news is that these problems are usually not serious. But in the meantime they can make your life pretty miserable. Fortunately, there's plenty you can do to ease the symptoms and speed recovery.

IDENTIFYING THE PROBLEM

The majority of us can easily recognise a common cold but are less confident in identifying the difference between a severe cold and flu. Even doctors can sometimes find it hard to tell the difference. Both are upper respiratory infections with similar features and both are caused by viruses, so antibiotics won't help. It's tricky to distinguish between them, but some clues are:

Sneezing Usual with a cold, but sometimes triggered in flu too.

Cough Common with both colds and flu. With a cold the cough is often accompanied by mucus (phlegm), whereas with flu it is usually a dry cough and may be severe.

Sore throat Often precedes or accompanies a cold, sometimes present with flu.

Runny nose Usually prominent with colds, not usually with flu; a blocked nose from nasal congestion is also more common with a cold.

Feeling shivery Common with a fever caused by flu, but rare with a cold.

Fever Temperature is almost always raised with flu, when it can be quite high (more than 38°C) and remain raised for two or three days. Fever is less common with a cold and tends to be less severe.

Aching muscles If you feel extremely unwell and can barely get out of bed, it's quite likely to be flu. Colds can cause general aches and pains, but these are less common and less severe.

Headache Frequent with flu, rare with a cold.

Feeling generally ill, weak and exhausted The hallmark of flu, but can also occur with a cold. With flu, you may feel severely ill and this may last for many days or even weeks.

In most cases, the only practical difference between a cold or flu is that a dose of flu is likely to make you feel a lot worse for longer. However, it is important to be able to recognise the warning signs that the infection may have spread to the airways in your lungs or that a cold or flu has been disguising a more serious underlying problem (see *What if I start to feel worse?*, page 44).

Cold or flu symptoms usually disappear within a week, although a cough may persist for two or three weeks. On the following pages, you'll find advice on how you can relieve the symptoms.

LOOK AFTER YOURSELF

Your recovery will be speedier if you take care of yourself rather than trying to tough it out. Don't struggle into work feeling dreadful. Instead take it easy for a day or two, especially if you have a fever or a bad cough – you'll get better faster and reduce the risk of spreading your germs to colleagues. Keep warm and stay in bed if you feel exhausted – sleep helps your immune system to combat infection. Eat a healthy diet, rich in infection-fighting nutrients (see *Top tips*, page 44), and avoid dusty or smoky atmospheres, which will aggravate your symptoms.

While adequate rest and sleep are important, research shows that when you have a respiratory infection, taking some gentle exercise can boost your immune system and help to fight off the bugs. Gentle stretching exercises or yoga for 20 to 30 minutes a day are ideal. But, avoid doing anything too strenuous – vigorous exercise, especially if you're not used to it, can set back your recovery.

NURSING KNOW-HOW

Humidify the air

One of the best ways to relieve a stuffy nose is to add water vapour to the air. You can do this by means of a humidifier or by placing bowls of water on the tops of radiators. Alternatively, try sitting in a steamy bathroom for a while. Adding moisture to the air helps to reduce irritation and makes it easier for you to sleep. Dry air not only dries out mucous membranes, which makes nasal congestion, sore throat and coughing more likely, but also helps flu viruses to survive. If you use a humidifier, make sure you change the water daily and clean it thoroughly, according to the manufacturer's instructions, to avoid spreading germs or mould spores.

True or False?

Feed a cold and starve a fever

Partly true According to Dutch researchers, this traditional advice can be misleading, depending on the cause of the fever. Six volunteers fasted overnight, then were given either a liquid meal or water. Blood samples taken 6 hours later revealed that a meal stimulates the body's antiviral response. But after water alone, the antiviral response dropped, while the immune response to bacterial infections, which are often responsible for fevers, improved. As both colds and flu are due to viral infections, it may make sense to eat, whether or not you also have a raised temperature.

When you have a cold or flu, drinking extra fluid may help to keep mucus loose and avoid dehydration. Drinking plenty will also ease congestion and makes up for moisture lost in mucus production and by fever. Water, juices and soups are ideal, but avoid alcohol and caffeinated drinks as these cause dehydration.

SUPPLEMENTS CAN HELP

At the first sign of a cold or flu, take an echinacea supplement. This herb, widely available in tablet or tincture form, could cut the duration of cold symptoms, according to research published in the journal *The Lancet Infectious Diseases*. Taking echinacea regularly could more than halve your chances of catching a cold in the first place. Researchers combined the results of 14 studies involving more than 2,900 people and found that on average those taking echinacea, whether on its own or in combination with other remedies, reduced their risk of infection by 58 per cent and cut the average duration of cold symptoms by 1.4 days. Because it stimulates the immune system, echinacea is not recommended for people with autoimmune disorders such as multiple sclerosis (MS) and rheumatoid arthritis.

Some studies suggest that zinc taken within a day of the onset of symptoms may also help to shorten the duration of a cold. Use a supplement or lozenges, but avoid zinc nasal sprays, as these may occasionally damage your sense of smell, sometimes permanently. Taking zinc combined with high dose (2 g) vitamin C is even more effective, various studies conclude. According to a review at the Alfa Institute of Biomedical Sciences in Athens, Greece, studies show that supplements of 'friendly bacteria' may reduce the severity and duration of cold and flu symptoms (although not the likelihood of infection). Look out for products containing *Lactobacillus* strains of bacteria, which are thought to be particularly effective against colds and flu.

SIPPING AND GARGLING

There's science behind the traditional advice to sip a hot lemon drink. Lemons are rich in vitamin C, which improves the function of macrophages – the white blood cells that destroy viruses once they've been flagged with markers called antibodies. Lemon also reduces mucus production. Add some honey to the drink to coat your throat and help ease soreness and reduce coughing. Another

Echinacea is a herbal remedy that could cut the duration of a cold

Q&A

I have a stuffy nose. Is it true that I should avoid dairy products?

There is now evidence that the widely held belief that milk products produce mucus is without scientific foundation. Researchers at the University of Adelaide and the Royal Adelaide Hospital in Australia tested 60 volunteers, who were deliberately infected with a cold virus and followed for ten days while consuming varying amounts of milk from nil to 11 glasses daily. Although more than a quarter of them believed milk and other dairy products to be mucus-forming and bad for colds, in fact there was no association between milk intake and cold symptoms or the amount of nasal secretions.

time-honoured remedy to ease a sore throat is a warm salt water gargle. Dissolve about half a teaspoon of salt in half a glass of warm water and gargle for 1 or 2 minutes, then spit out. Be careful not to swallow. A salt water gargle soothes soreness and may also help to clear mucus.

POP A PILL FOR FAST FEVER RELIEF

Debate still rages as to whether it's a good idea to damp down a fever or let it do its job of fighting off germs. But if you're feeling wretched, an over-the-counter painkiller such as paracetamol, aspirin or ibuprofen will help to lower your temperature and combat headache or general aches and pains. Remember that babies under 3 months should not be given ibuprofen, and that children under 16 should not be given aspirin. Take care not to exceed the maximum recommended daily intake of paracetamol (for adults 4,000 mg or eight 500 mg tablets). Overdose of this drug can cause permanent liver damage. Be sure to include all possible sources in your calculations – it is often present in over-the-counter cold remedies as well as in single-ingredient products.

THE PROS AND CONS OF COUGH MEDICINES

It's important to remember that coughing has a purpose – helping to clear mucus from the airways – so with a 'wet' cough it's often better to 'cough it out'. However, if persistent coughing is keeping you awake

Garlic and onions

Folklore has it that eating a whole raw onion at the first hint of a cold will stop infection in its tracks. Although there's no research evidence for this claim, the suggestion makes some scientific sense. Both onions and garlic contain allicin, which can boost immunity and reduce the severity of cold and flu symptoms. Onions also contain sulphur compounds with antimicrobial properties, and quercetin, a powerful immune-system stimulant. What's more, the highly volatile vapour released when you chop onions contains irritant chemicals, which make your eyes stream. As this invariably makes your nose run too, this could flush out virus particles before they take hold, and would certainly help to loosen mucus and ease congestion. You can eat garlic raw, add it to cooking or, if you want to avoid 'garlic breath', take garlic capsules.

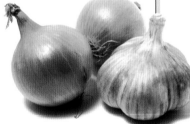

Top Tips

Boost your immune system

Kick-start your natural recovery process by including plenty of the following infection-fighting nutrients in your diet:

- **Protein** Rebuilds strength and many sources also supply B vitamins, zinc and selenium, which are vital for a healthy immune system. Try to eat at least 50 g of protein daily from lean meat, poultry, fish, eggs, legumes, nuts and seeds.

- **Antioxidants** Health-boosting compounds, such as vitamins C, E and beta carotene, found in many plant foods. Try to eat at least seven portions of fruit and vegetables every day. Lightly steam, rather than boil, vegetables when possible, to minimise the loss of their nutrients during cooking.

- **Glutathione** An antioxidant that strengthens the immune system to fight infection. Watermelon can provide glutathione, which is also found in vegetables of the brassica family, such as kale, broccoli, Brussels sprouts, spinach and cabbage.

- **Bioflavonoids** Nutrients that boost immune responses and help speed recovery from infections. Found especially in citrus fruits, such as oranges, lemons and grapefruit, which also contain the powerful immune-boosting nutrient vitamin C.

- **Quercetin** A type of bioflavonoid with the ability to stimulate the immune system. Quercetin-rich foods include broccoli, citrus fruits and onions.

- **Zinc** Important for healthy immune-system function and resistance to infections. Foods rich in zinc include oysters, eggs, seeds, nuts and wholegrain cereals.

at night, try taking 1 tablespoon of honey at bedtime (but note that babies younger than 12 months old should not be given honey). A 2010 review of studies found no evidence to support the claim that over-the-counter cough medicines are effective. And since they carry a risk of side effects, it's best to avoid them. However, expectorant cough medicines, which contain the ingredient guaiphenesin, make it easier to bring up phlegm. It's a good idea to ask the pharmacist's advice when choosing a cough medicine.

WHAT IF I START TO FEEL WORSE?

If any respiratory infection makes it difficult for you to breathe or you feel unusually drowsy, or if you have difficulty rousing someone else, seek immediate medical help. Also talk to your doctor if the symptoms worsen or don't improve within a week or so. Cold and flu viruses can sometimes attack sites other than your nose and throat. Seek help for:

- Prolonged hoarseness that persists for longer than two weeks.
- Pain or pressure in the region of the nose, eyes or forehead that persists for more than two weeks (possible indications of sinusitis).
- A worsening sore throat accompanied by fever, swollen lymph nodes in the neck, hoarseness and painful swallowing.
- Increased coughing with grey-green sputum and perhaps accompanied by fever, wheezing, shortness of breath and chest discomfort (possible indications of bronchitis).
- Suddenly feeling very ill, perhaps occurring with persistent cough, shortness of breath, high fever accompanied by sweating or chills, chest pain, muscle aches and headaches (possible indications of pneumonia).

WHICH BUG?

Both bacteria and viruses may cause respiratory infections and it's difficult to tell them apart just from the symptoms. However, the difference is important, since antibiotics don't work against viruses, which cause the vast majority of everyday coughs and colds. Inappropriate use of antibiotics for viral respiratory infections is one factor that has contributed to bacterial resistance to common antibiotics.

Sometimes a viral infection may be complicated by a more serious bacterial infection, while some potentially very serious problems, such as pneumonia, may be caused by either viruses or bacteria. Generally, if an upper respiratory tract infection persists for longer than seven to ten days, the likelihood of its being bacterial is higher.

Without diagnostic tests, such as a throat swab or a sputum sample, it's impossible to determine with certainty whether an infection is due to a virus or a bacterium, but some of the differences between them are listed below:

Viral infection	Bacterial infection
Much more common in winter	Occurs with equal frequency at all times of the year
Usually resolves itself on its own within a week	May not get better without antibiotics
May or may not cause a fever	Often causes a fever

Getting the better of asthma

Increasingly common in the developed world, asthma is a potentially dangerous condition, but one that can be effectively managed by medication and lifestyle adaptation. It is often triggered by an allergic reaction that leads to a narrowing of the airways, and is characterised by intermittent attacks of wheezing, coughing, and feeling short of breath and 'tight-chested'. It is important to make sure that you have appropriate medication (usually in the form of inhalers) to use in case of an attack and to seek medical advice if you notice an increase in the frequency of asthma attacks. The self-help advice in this chapter is intended to supplement any treatment advised by your doctor.

EAT TO BREATHE

If you have asthma, healthy eating is very important. Typical Western diets – with too many unhealthy fats and too much sugar, salt and processed carbohydrates, but inadequate amounts of fresh fruit, vegetables and fish – are associated with a higher risk of developing asthma, worse symptoms and more attacks. What's more, such a diet

! ALERT

When to call for help

Seek emergency medical attention for your asthma if:

- An acute attack does not subside within 10 minutes despite treatment (see page 48).

- An attack prevents you from speaking more than a few words at a time.

- Your chest muscles are straining to enable you to breathe.

- You develop unusually severe breathlessness or wheezing, especially at night or early in the morning.

causes obesity, which is itself linked with asthma in both adults and children. Fortunately, it's easy to make small changes to your diet, and losing a little weight can improve lung function, reduce the need for asthma medication and lower the frequency of attacks. Here are some top dietary tips to help you breathe more easily:

Avoid fatty 'junk' foods Researchers at the University of Newcastle, Australia, fed 40 asthma patients either a high-fat, high-kilojoule meal of fast-food burgers and hash browns or a low-fat, low-kilojoule meal of yoghurt. Those who ate the high-fat meal showed marked increases in inflammatory cells in their sputum (they had become more susceptible to an asthma attack) and responded less well to asthma medication.

Reduce your salt intake Evidence suggests that high-salt diets are linked with asthma severity. The majority of salt in our diet comes from processed foods, so remember to check the labels when you are shopping and look out for sodium content (salt is sodium chloride) as well as salt (see page 26).

Eat more fish The omega-3 fatty acids EPA and DHA in oily fish can reduce airway inflammation. In one Cambridge University study of 750 people, asthmatics who regularly ate oily fish were less likely to report wheeziness, breathlessness or waking up with a tight chest. Choose oily fish such as salmon, trout, herring, fresh tuna, sardines and mackerel, and aim to eat two portions per week. If you don't like fish, try a supplement containing 1 to 1.2 g of EPA plus DHA per day.

Have seven servings of fruit and vegetables daily Plant foods are high in protective antioxidants, which may help lung function. One international study of more than 50,000 children showed that those who ate the most fruit were the least likely to wheeze.

Snack on nuts and seeds Eat these healthy snacks to help combat asthma attacks. Instead of cakes, biscuits and chips, keep nuts and seeds to hand for between-meal nibbling (unless you are allergic to them). As well as having a low sugar content, these foods are high in omega-3

Q&A

I have a charity race coming up – can I do anything to reduce the chances of getting an asthma attack?

Cut down on salt. In one study, reducing salt intake for just two weeks helped to reduce symptoms and improve lung function in people whose asthma was usually triggered by sports or physical activity. It may also be of benefit to take regular doses of vitamin C (1 to 2 g daily); high doses of this vitamin may be particularly helpful in exercise-induced asthma.

FOCUS

Allergy action

Although it's possible that some people may be genetically susceptible to respiratory allergies, the triggers that prompt symptoms tend to be allergens in the environment or aspects of lifestyle. As a result, there is much that can be done to counteract or reduce the impact of these factors.

The most common allergic conditions affecting the respiratory system are asthma and hay fever (also known as allergic rhinitis) a minor, often seasonal complaint in which sneezing, runny nose and itchy, inflamed eyes are the main symptoms. If you're allergic to anything you encounter frequently – common triggers include house-dust mites (pictured below), pet fur and dander, pollen and mould spores – life can be miserable. Allergen-avoidance cleaning strategies around the house can make all the difference.

COUNTDOWN TO CLEANING

Floors	● Install easy-to-clean hard floors (tiles, wood or vinyl) where possible and mop them at least weekly. ● Opt for rugs on hard floors rather than fitted carpets. ● Choose short-pile rather than deep-pile carpets. ● Vacuum at least weekly and clean carpets regularly.
Windows	● Choose easy-to-wash blinds rather than curtains (ensure any curtains are made of washable fabrics). ● Close windows during the pollen season. ● Wipe condensation from frames and sills regularly and clean any mould using a bleach-based solution.
Furniture	● Choose leather, wood, metal or plastic and avoid having upholstery where possible. ● Damp-dust at least weekly.
Beds	● Wash all bed linen on a hot setting at least weekly. ● Fit dust mite-proof covers for mattresses and pillows. ● Every few weeks, if practical, place pillows in the freezer overnight to kill dust mites, or replace them regularly.
Kitchen	● Clean sinks, taps and food-preparation surfaces daily using an antibacterial spray. ● Wipe any excess moisture from the fridge and throw away any out-of-date items. Don't allow food to go mouldy.
Bathroom	● Choose tiled walls and clean them twice a week. ● Wipe the bath or shower after use and open a window, or install an extractor fan. Don't allow mould to grow.
Clutter	● Store all dust-collecting objects in cupboards or plastic storage containers. ● Wash children's soft toys on a hot cycle at least weekly.
Pets	● Ideally, don't have any. If you must, keep them outside or at least ban them from bedrooms.

fatty acids, which are thought to help to relieve inflammation and dampen asthma symptoms. Walnuts and linseeds, in particular, are good sources of this nutrient.

EXERCISE AND ASTHMA

In the past, it was believed that people with asthma should avoid strenuous activity, but it is now known that regular exercise improves symptoms in the long term. If physical exertion worsens your asthma, talk to your doctor – it could be a sign that your medication needs to be reviewed. If your asthma is well controlled and you take a few simple precautions, there is no reason why you can't participate in almost any physical

 NURSING KNOW-HOW

Four-point plan...
to deal with asthma attacks

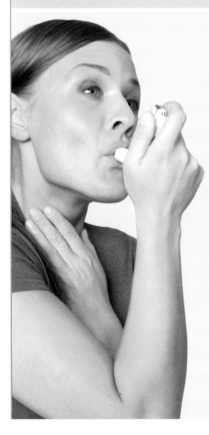

1 **Sit the person upright** Be calm and reassuring. Do not leave them alone.

2 **Give 4 puffs of blue reliever puffer medication** Use a spacer is there is one. Shake puffer. Put 1 puff into spacer. Take 4 breaths from spacer. Repeat until 4 puffs have been taken. Remember: shake, 1 puff, 4 breaths.

3 **Wait 4 minutes** If there is no improvement, give 4 more puffs as above.

4 **If there is still no improvement, call for emergency assistance (dial OOO in Australia)** Say 'ambulance' and that someone is having an asthma attack. Keep giving 4 puffs ever 4 minutes until emergency assistance arrives.

Call emergency assistance immediately (dial OOO in Australia) if:

● The person is not breathing

● The person's asthma suddenly becomes worse, or is not improving

● The person is having an asthma attack and a puffer is not available

● You're not sure if it's asthma

Note: blue reliever medication is unlikely to harm, even if the person does not have asthma.

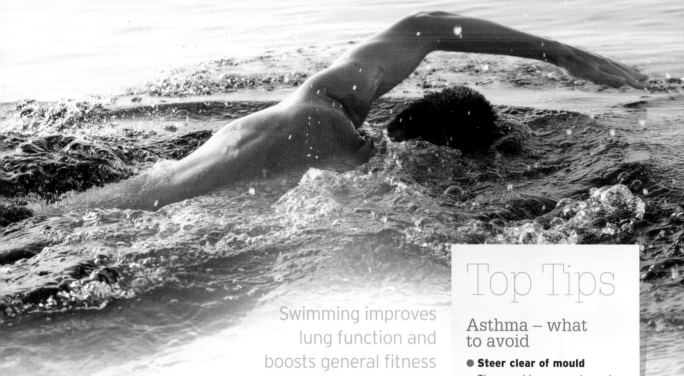

Swimming improves
lung function and
boosts general fitness

activity. If symptoms start, stop exercising, use your 'reliever' inhaler
and wait until you feel better. It may help to use it just before you warm
up. Make sure you take any 'preventer' medications as directed by your
GP. Always use proper warm-up and cool-down routines and avoid
sudden increases in training intensity.

CHOOSE YOUR EXERCISE

While there is some evidence that prolonged exposure to chlorinated
water in pools may increase asthma, swimming is a great exercise for
people with asthma: it expands lung volume, develops good breathing
techniques and improves physical fitness. In a study at Taipei Medical
University, Taiwan, children who took a six-week swimming course while
continuing their regular medication had milder asthma attacks, fewer
breathing problems, fewer trips to hospital and less time off school.

Many other forms of exercise are suitable for asthma sufferers. Yoga,
for example, can improve your breathing technique as well as helping
you relax. Activities such as weightlifting, golf and walking are less likely
to trigger symptoms than aerobic exercise that makes you breathe hard,
such as running or playing football. If you want to undertake aerobic
exercise, team sports such as football or hockey in which the individual
players are generally involved in only brief bursts of intense exertion,
with short breaks in between, are less likely to provoke symptoms than
those involving prolonged intensive effort, such as squash.

Exercise-induced asthma can be triggered or worsened by cold, dry air,
pollen and pollution. If you are affected, take into account the weather
and location when you are deciding what form of exercise to do.

Top Tips

Asthma – what to avoid

● **Steer clear of mould**
Tiny mould spores released
into the air can sometimes
trigger asthma attacks.
Avoid compost heaps, piles
of rotting leaves and damp
woody areas. Make sure your
home is well ventilated, don't
leave piles of damp clothes
or towels lying around, wipe
up condensation quickly and
treat any areas of mould
as soon as you can.

● **Avoid royal jelly**
Supplements containing
the bee product royal jelly
may be dangerous if you
have asthma. Royal jelly can
provoke a serious - even
lethal - respiratory reaction.

● **Keep away from pollution**
A 2007 study in the *New
England Journal of Medicine*
found that 2 hours' exposure
to diesel fumes in a busy
urban street had a marked
adverse effect on lung
function, especially among
asthmatics.

Dealing with digestive upsets

Most of us pay little attention to our digestive tract – until something goes wrong. Whether it's indigestion, a stomach ache, a case of travellers' diarrhoea or an annoying bout of constipation, you can take swift action to make yourself feel better fast.

Indigestion or a heart attack?

Seek immediate medical attention if the pain is different or more severe than usual, comes on with exercise rather than after food, travels to anywhere else in the body, such as your arm or jaw, or is accompanied by shortness of breath, sweating or nausea.

A sudden attack of belching, often with accompanying chest pain, is a common symptom of reduced blood supply to the heart, which occurs during a heart attack, and it requires emergency attention.

If you are in any doubt, seek help at once by dialling 000 (in Australia). Ambulance crews would rather attend a false alarm than miss the opportunity to give prompt and possibly life-saving treatment to a potential heart attack sufferer.

Controlling indigestion

This common digestive problem involves discomfort or pain in the upper abdomen provoked by eating, sometimes accompanied by a burning sensation behind the breastbone, known as heartburn, and often together with feelings of fullness, bloating and nausea along with stomach rumbling, belching and an acidic taste in the mouth. An excess of stomach acid is the main cause and there are a number of lifestyle factors that play a role, including eating too fast or at the wrong times, making poor food choices, being overweight and drinking too much alcohol. Tackling such bad lifestyle habits will help to alleviate the problem, and there are other positive steps you can take.

FINDING RELIEF

There is no universal panacea for indigestion. It is often a question of trying different approaches and finding out what works best for you. For many people, instant relief from discomfort is best provided by medicines that counter acid in the stomach, such as simple antacids (aluminium hydroxide and magnesium carbonate) and proton-pump inhibitors. There are also natural remedies that have some proven benefits.

Ginger A natural remedy that has been used for centuries to combat indigestion, ginger can help to calm intestinal spasm and stimulate digestive secretions. It is best taken as a tea: steep about 0.25 g of powdered ginger, or a few slices of ginger root, in water and sip either warm or cooled following each meal.

Caraway Try making a tea from the seeds or add a couple of drops of the oil to a glass of water. You could also try a tea made from a combination of caraway and peppermint, which may work even better than either ingredient alone.

KEEPING THE PROBLEM AT BAY

If you frequently suffer from indigestion, fear of an attack may start to spoil your enjoyment of meals. Knowing how to control the problem is therefore central to you getting more out of life. Here are some useful tips:

- Eat little and often so that your stomach is never overloaded. And don't have your main meal too close to bedtime.
- Eat slowly and keep your mouth closed while you are chewing – no talking. This prevents you from swallowing air and ensures that food reaches the stomach in smaller pieces, helping the digestive process.
- It may be helpful to avoid drinking with meals.
- Avoid alcohol, fizzy or caffeinated drinks.
- Don't smoke.
- Avoid spicy or greasy foods.
- Don't wear clothes with tight waistbands, which can constrict the stomach and inhibit digestion.
- Avoid aspirin and anti-inflammatory drugs that could irritate the stomach lining.
- Don't do anything energetic for an hour after a meal.
- Watch your weight. If you are overweight, try to shed a few kilograms as this will lessen pressure on the stomach and may reduce regurgitation and acid reflux.

ASK YOUR DOCTOR

If simple measures don't solve the problem, see your doctor in case there's an underlying condition that needs treatment. Your doctor may want to check whether you have a peptic ulcer (see page 239); peptic ulcers have some symptoms in common with indigestion. Seek prompt medical advice if you also develop symptoms such as persistent vomiting, blood in your vomit, black tarry faeces, difficulty swallowing, unexplained weight loss or extreme fatigue.

Your doctor may prescribe antacids or other medication to relieve irritation of the stomach lining. If it seems possible that there is an underlying cause for your indigestion, such as a hiatus hernia (in which the upper part of the stomach is squeezed upwards into the chest through the gap in the muscle of the diaphragm), you may be referred to a hospital specialist for further investigations and, if necessary, surgery to correct the problem.

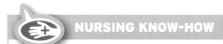

NURSING KNOW-HOW

Pillow talk

If you tend to get symptoms of reflux – acid from stomach contents passing back up the oesophagus – then raising your bedhead slightly or using an extra pillow can often prevent or ease symptoms.

After dinner relief

There's a sound reason for traditional 'after-dinner mints'. The menthol in peppermint helps to ease the pain and bloating of indigestion and dispel intestinal gas. When indigestion strikes, try sucking a peppermint or slowly sipping peppermint tea. However, if you have heartburn due to reflux of stomach acid, peppermint may make it worse, so be sure to test it out cautiously.

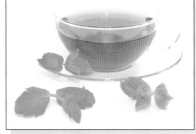

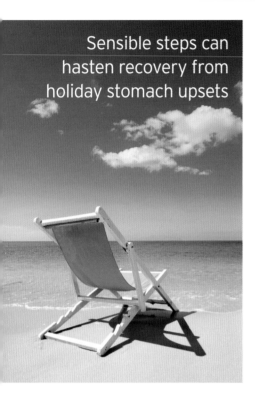

Sensible steps can hasten recovery from holiday stomach upsets

Coping with an upset stomach

The combination, familiar to most of us, of nausea, vomiting, diarrhoea and sometimes abdominal pain or cramping is a classic indication of gastrointestinal infections ('tummy bugs') or food poisoning from contaminated food or drink (travellers' diarrhoea). In most cases, home treatment quickly clears up the problem.

Although cases of diarrhoea tend to last only a day or two and require no specific medication, moderate to severe diarrhoea is often best treated with over-the-counter remedies. Products that contain loperamide will bring immediate relief from diarrhoea, but make sure you seek medical advice if symptoms aren't better within two days, get worse or if other problems develop. The following measures will help you recover quickly:

Drink plenty of water Even if you're feeling sick, try to take frequent sips of plain water, herb teas, diluted juice or clear soups. This is important for everyone but especially for babies and young children, older people and those with existing illnesses, who are more susceptible to dehydration and its effects. Those who are vulnerable should take a sip every 10 minutes or so. Specific rehydration fluids, available from pharmacies, that replace the correct balance of salts (electrolytes) in the blood are best. You should encourage a baby to carry on feeding from the breast or bottle as usual.

Keep it bland As symptoms improve, eat only soft, bland foods to maintain nutrition and reduce symptoms until you're feeling better.

Avoid fatty foods When you begin to feel like eating normally, be sure to steer clear of fatty and fried foods, which can make you feel nauseous and worsen diarrhoea. Also avoid milk and milk products, such as cheese and ice cream; citrus fruits; and beware of sugar-laden foods or drinks (cakes, biscuits and cola-style drinks). Continue to base meals around bland, starchy foods. Try bananas, rice, boiled potatoes, toast, pasta and crackers. Skinless baked chicken breast is a good choice if you feel like some protein.

FOOD POISONING

Food poisoning is the result of eating food that has become contaminated by germs or other harmful substances. The symptoms are very similar to those of a non-food-related gastrointestinal infection, but often come on more suddenly. It most commonly occurs as a result of poor hygiene

Signs of dehydration

If you or an adult member of your family is suffering from diarrhoea and/or vomiting, look out for the signs of dehydration listed below. Dehydration in babies and young children is discussed under *When to seek medical help*, page 54.

- thirst
- dry mouth and lips
- reduced urine output
- dark-coloured urine
- dry skin
- feeling tired
- feeling giddy or fainting.

in the preparation of food or the consumption of food that has been kept for too long or in the wrong conditions. You can easily prevent food poisoning at home by paying scrupulous attention to hygiene precautions, and food storage and preparation.

Avoiding holiday hell 'Montezuma's revenge', 'Delhi belly' and other varieties of travellers' diarrhoea can ruin the most perfect holiday or the most vital business trip. The usual cause is the consumption of contaminated food or drinking water. Visitors to Africa, the Middle East, Asia and South America are especially at risk and, because they have no immunity to local bugs, they may develop symptoms even if residents can eat and drink the same fare with no adverse effects. Fortunately, you can usually resist these infections with a little knowledge and forethought. Do not drink non-bottled water or drinks containing ice cubes, and use bottled water for cleaning teeth. Avoid seafood, reheated or merely warmed foods and uncooked foods that may have been washed in contaminated water, such as salads. Always peel fruit before eating.

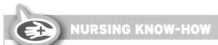

NURSING KNOW-HOW

Wash it away

If you or someone else in the family has diarrhoea and/or vomiting, it's important to take strict hygiene measures to prevent the spread of infection. This includes washing hands thoroughly after using the toilet, changing nappies or cleaning up after the affected person and before preparing food or drink. Disinfect all surfaces and items that have come into contact with the person or their body fluids. Someone recovering from a gastrointestinal infection should stay away from work or school for 48 hours after the symptoms have cleared, to avoid spreading the bug.

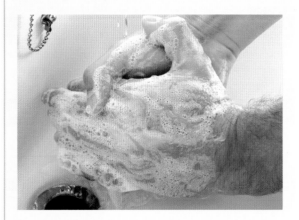

Controlling constipation

Although this complaint is not usually a serious risk to health, it is very common, particularly among older, less active people, and among those whose diet does not contain sufficient fibre. The normal frequency of bowel movements ranges from three times a day to three times a week. Some people on the less frequent end of this range may think they have constipation when they don't. As well as infrequent bowel movements, constipation means having hard stools that are difficult to pass, leading to straining during bowel movements, and the feeling that you have not emptied your bowel completely.

Fortunately, constipation is often temporary – for example, due to medication, illness, the absence of a private toilet, pregnancy or just a change of daily routine, diet or time zone – and there are many simple ways to tackle the problem.

! ALERT

When to seek medical help

If you are an otherwise healthy adult, talk to your doctor if your digestive upset gets worse despite treatment or has not improved within 48 hours. Also seek medical help if you have these additional symptoms:

- severe pain in your abdomen or rectum
- fever
- blood in your faeces or black, tarry motions
- signs of dehydration (page 52).

If the person affected is a child under five, an older person or someone with other medical problems, seek help if: symptoms do not improve within 12 hours, fluids cannot be kept down, signs of dehydration develop, or you are worried about the person's condition. Seek immediate medical attention if there is blood in the vomit or faeces, or if any of the following signs of severe dehydration develop:

- sunken eyes
- rapid pulse rate
- pale or mottled skin
- increasing drowsiness.

FILL UP ON FIBRE

It's important for constipation sufferers to eat more fibre than usual. The indigestible, fibrous parts of plants add bulk to your stools, both softening them and stimulating the urge to defecate. Aim to eat between seven and nine portions of fruit, vegetables and beans daily and choose wholemeal (made from whole grains) bread and pasta and brown rice over the white alternatives. If you can't manage this, take a supplement such as ispaghula husk (psyllium). Try to drink more as adding fluid to your digestive contents softens the stool and makes it easier to pass. Aim to drink at least six to eight glasses of fluids a day. Most constipation sufferers find that their bowel habits improve by following these simple dietary measures.

A MATTER OF HABIT

Your body becomes used to you opening your bowels at a particular time each day, so it's important to get into a regular habit. In the morning, just after breakfast, is often the best time, and at other times go when you feel the urge. But don't strain to defecate if you don't feel the need to do so; this can lead to the development of haemorrhoids (piles). When you feel the need, don't delay opening your bowels, and leave yourself enough time to do so without straining. It's important to try to make sure you are undisturbed. If you can, become more active, since even gentle physical activity promotes bowel health and encourages intestinal contractions.

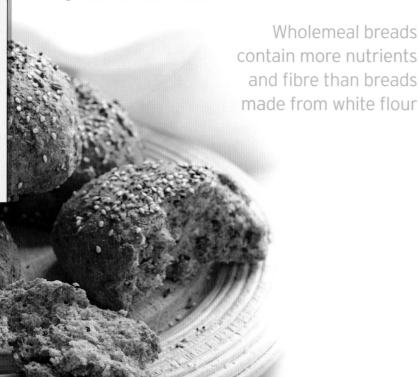

Wholemeal breads contain more nutrients and fibre than breads made from white flour

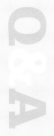

I don't do a lot of cooking and often eat convenience foods. When I suffer from constipation, I simply take laxatives – does that matter?

Don't be tempted by 'easy' solutions such as laxatives other than for occasional use. Some of these remedies simply get your bowel out of the habit of contracting by itself, so persistent use may make your constipation worse. Eating a high-fibre diet with plenty of fresh fruit, vegetables and whole grains is far more effective in the long term.

Calming an irritable bowel

This common problem, which affects the large intestine, isn't serious but does cause distressing symptoms such as abdominal cramps, bloating, flatulence and a change in bowel habits – diarrhoea, constipation or alternation between the two. Most people with irritable bowel syndrome (IBS) find that they can learn to control their condition and improve their symptoms greatly just by taking a few simple measures.

KEEP A FOOD DIARY

Many people find that certain foods make their symptoms worse, so it's a good idea to log everything you eat and drink, along with your symptoms, for three weeks to try to spot any links. You can then avoid suspect items. Common culprits include alcohol, tea, coffee, chocolate, dairy products and sugar-free sweeteners such as sorbitol. If dairy products tend to provoke symptoms, you may be lactose-intolerant and need to avoid them altogether.

MONITOR YOUR FIBRE INTAKE

Increasing the fibre in your diet may relieve your IBS, but some people find that it makes symptoms worse because the extra fibre treats their constipation effectively but exacerbates their bloating and wind. Foods with plenty of fibre include fruit and vegetables, whole grains and beans. A fibre supplement such as ispaghula husk (psyllium) can be taken, but it may also make bloating worse.

TURN OFF THE GAS

If bloating and intestinal gas are prominent symptoms, try cutting down or reducing your intake of gas-producing foods such as beans, cabbages, broccoli, cauliflower. Some

Magic mint

Several formal randomised trials have shown peppermint to be effective in reducing the symptoms of IBS. Drink peppermint tea after meals – and at other times. Peppermint is also available in capsule form.

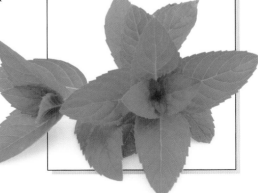

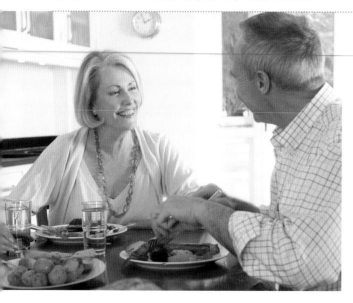

Make relaxed and
regular meals the
centre of your IBS
recovery plan

raw fruits and vegetables should also be avoided.
Frequent consumption of fizzy drinks, chewing gum
or drinking through straws can increase the amount
of air passing into the intestines, producing gas.

EAT AND DRINK REGULARLY

Hurried and irregular meals can contribute to IBS.
It's therefore important to have regular mealtimes
and allow yourself the time to eat in a relaxed
fashion. Your bowel gets into the habit of being
'fed' at consistent intervals, so try to eat at roughly
the same time each day. Eating small, frequent
meals tends to help those for whom diarrhoea is a
troublesome symptom, while fewer, larger fibre-rich meals may be of
benefit to people whose main symptom is constipation.

It's a good idea to increase the amount you drink because consuming
more fluid, especially water, helps to relieve constipation. But be aware
that alcoholic drinks or tea, coffee and other beverages containing
caffeine may worsen diarrhoea.

THINK ABOUT YOUR LIFESTYLE

IBS is a complicated condition in which both physiological and
psychological factors play a role. Most doctors recommend taking more
exercise – not only will this help to counteract stress and depression,
but it also encourages regular intestinal movements and keeps your
bowels running smoothly.

If you suffer from stress, it's a good idea to learn to manage it. Although
stress and tension don't cause IBS, they can worsen your symptoms. Get
plenty of fresh air – in a calming leafy green setting, if possible – and make
some time to relax every day. You could also book a massage, try stress-
busting activities such as yoga or tai chi, or learn to meditate.

SUPPLEMENTARY ADVICE

A probiotic supplement can be helpful for the relief of abdominal pain
and bloating. 'Friendly' bacteria found naturally in your gut may be
disturbed in IBS, and some studies suggest that foods such as yoghurt
containing live probiotic organisms, or probiotic supplements, help to
restore your bowel to health.

If you want to try an alternative therapy, acupuncture may be a good
option. Although it's not proven to counteract IBS symptoms, some
people find it relieves intestinal cramps and improves bowel regularity.

! ALERT

Beware of change

If you suddenly experience a
change in bowel habit for no
apparent reason, or you have
constipation or diarrhoea
accompanied by abdominal
pain, weight loss or blood in
your faeces, see your doctor
in case there is an underlying
problem that requires medical
diagnosis and treatment.

Urinary and vaginal infections

Varying from an irritating minor annoyance to a more serious long-term problem, urinary tract infections (UTIs) and vaginal infections are among the most common ailments affecting women. Luckily, there is plenty you can do to complement any treatment prescribed by your doctor, ensure a rapid recovery and prevent a recurrence.

UTI guidelines

If you've ever had a urinary tract infection (UTI), you will know how painful they can be. The good news is that treatment usually brings about speedy relief. Symptoms of UTI include an urgent need to pass urine and an intense, painful, burning sensation when you do – it has been likened to passing razor blades. You'll probably also find you want to urinate frequently but pass only small amounts when you do, and your urine may be cloudy, strong-smelling or even contain blood. Sometimes a UTI is accompanied by a raised temperature, nausea or sensations of pressure or pain in the lower abdomen or back.

Women are more likely to get UTIs than men because they have a short urethra – the tube leading from the bladder to the outside – making it easier for germs to enter. The opening of the urethra is also closer to the anus in women than in men. The infection usually starts in the urethra (urethritis) and may then ascend to the bladder (cystitis).

It's important to see your doctor if you suspect a UTI, because untreated infections can spread further up the urinary tract to the kidneys, leading to a more serious problem. If a UTI is confirmed, you'll probably be given antibiotics, which usually produce rapid and effective relief. Be sure to take the full course to clear the infection completely.

FLUSH OUT THE PROBLEM

Here are some things you can do to ease symptoms and reduce the chance of a recurrence while you're waiting for the antibiotics to work (see also the advice for relieving the pain of cystitis on page 237):

Drink more water Increasing your fluid intake dilutes urine and helps to flush out bacteria. Aim to drink six to eight glasses of fluid a day.

> **! ALERT**
>
> ### Kidney trouble
> Get help fast if you have a high temperature, shaking or chills, nausea and vomiting, or pain spreading to the upper back and sides. These symptoms could indicate a kidney infection.

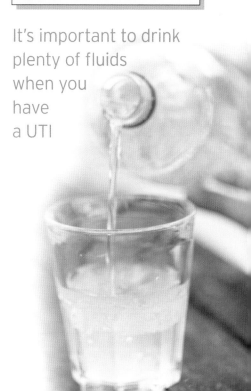

It's important to drink plenty of fluids when you have a UTI

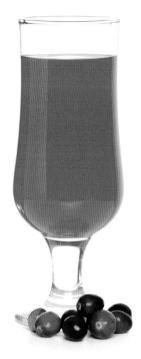

Cranberry juice can be a delicious addition to a cystitis prevention program

Avoid drinking alcohol, fruit juices (other than cranberry juice), coffee, tea and other caffeine-containing drinks, which can further irritate the bladder and increase frequency or urgency of urination.

Drink cranberry juice While early studies suggested cranberry products could help treat and prevent UTIs because they contain substances that discourage bacteria from sticking to the bladder wall, overall the results are unimpressive. If you do want to give cranberry a try, go for the berries, unsweetened cranberry juice or cranberry supplements (400 mg twice a day). But if you take the anticoagulant warfarin, check with your doctor first, as cranberries may interact dangerously with this medication.

Urinate frequently Don't put it off because you know it might hurt – go as soon as you feel the urge because bacteria are more likely to grow if urine sits in the bladder for too long. If it's very painful, passing urine while sitting in a warm bath can lessen the burning sensation.

Wipe from front to back To avoid introducing germs from the intestines into the urethra, women should always wipe from front to back after a bowel movement, or wipe each area separately. Parents are advised to teach daughters this technique as early as possible.

Urinate after sex In women especially, bacteria may enter the urethra during sex. Passing urine immediately afterwards helps to flush them out. Some women find that using a diaphragm promotes infection. If this is the case, it may help to change your method of contraception. Unlubricated condoms can also cause problems – use the lubricated type.

Wear cotton underwear and loose clothes Keeping the air circulating helps to counter infection, which thrives in moist, sweaty conditions. Avoid nylon underwear and tight jeans.

Avoid irritant toiletries The use of talcum powder, deodorant sprays, douches and similar products around the genital area can further irritate an already inflamed urethra.

Contraceptive care
Creams or suppositories used to treat thrush can weaken the latex used to make condoms and diaphragms. It is sensible to avoid sex or switch to an alternative form of contraception until you have finished the treatment.

Vaginal infections

Most women experience a vaginal infection at least once in their life. Symptoms vary according to the type of infection, but vaginal discharge, itching and discomfort are common signs of many infections. The problem is usually easy to recognise and generally simple to treat, and with the right treatment usually clears up quite quickly. However, if you're prone to such problems, they may recur.

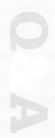

I suffer from repeated bouts of thrush. Is it true that this could be a sign of diabetes?

Partly true While thrush can take hold for a variety of reasons, women who have high blood glucose levels resulting from untreated diabetes are especially vulnerable. This is because the elevated glucose level provides food for the fungus, encouraging its overgrowth. If you have more than four thrush attacks in a year, ask your doctor to check your blood glucose levels.

BE STI AWARE

Some vaginal infections are sexually transmitted and are most effectively prevented by the use of condoms. If you suspect that you may have contracted a sexually transmissable infection, consult your doctor for treatment.

CANDIDA ADVICE

The most common infection, known as candidiasis or 'thrush', is caused by a fungus or yeast called *Candida albicans* and will affect most women at some time in their lives. It causes a thick white discharge that is often described as looking like cottage cheese, along with intense itching and sometimes pain in the vulval area.

If you've had it before and you recognise the symptoms, you can buy an antifungal treatment over the counter that will sort it out rapidly. If you're not sure, or if symptoms are slightly different from those you've had before, if they persist or recur despite treatment, or if you have had a recent new sexual partner or are pregnant, see your doctor for a proper diagnosis and treatment. Meanwhile, here are some other actions that can ease the symptoms, help clear the infection and prevent a recurrence.

Wear cotton underwear Underwear made of cotton rather than synthetic fabrics such as nylon reduces sweating and allows the genital region to 'breathe', so that it stays drier, which helps to counteract yeast infections. For the same reason, avoid wearing tights or close-fitting jeans, and don't lounge around in a wet swimsuit: after swimming, dry yourself thoroughly and put on clean, dry underclothes as soon as possible.

Avoid products containing chemicals and perfumes Anything that potentially irritates the delicate skin and membranes of the vulva and vagina can encourage infections to take hold, so avoid talc, deodorant sprays, bubble baths and coloured or scented toilet paper. Choose plain,

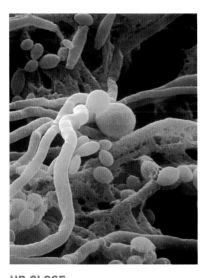

UP CLOSE
The Candida albicans *fungus, seen here many times enlarged, is the organism responsible for thrush infections.*

Male sexual partners always need treatment, too, if you have thrush

False Thrush is not considered a sexually transmissable infection, as sexual contact isn't needed for the infection to take hold. However, it can be passed on during oral and genital sexual contact and can occasionally cause inflammation of the tip of the penis in men – symptoms include redness, itching and soreness, and in this case treatment is necessary.

unperfumed soap or select a pH-balanced wash specially formulated for the genital area. A flannel soaked in cool water laid over the area can provide temporary relief of external itching.

Take a probiotic Some women maintain that inserting 'live' yoghurt into the vagina will alleviate thrush symptoms. The theory is that the 'friendly bacteria' in yoghurt help to restore the natural balance in the vagina and drive out the *Candida* fungus. Although too few formal tests have been carried out to confirm that this works, some small studies found that *Lactobacillus*, a bacterium normally found in the vagina as well as in yoghurt, successfully reduced yeast in the vagina and relieved symptoms whether taken by mouth or inserted into the vagina. One study showed that eating 225 g of live yoghurt daily reduced recurrent thrush infections three-fold among women prone to them. So a probiotic containing *Lactobacillus*, either as yoghurt or supplements, may help. If you use yoghurt in the vagina, it should be plain and unsweetened and should specify that it contains live *Lactobacillus*. Insert by covering a tampon or using a plastic vaginal applicator.

Unperfumed soaps are best for those who suffer from thrush

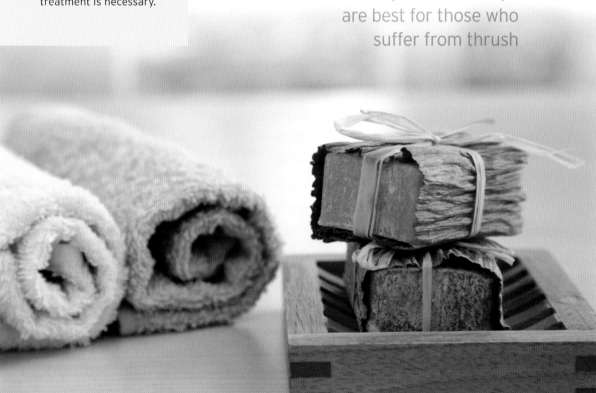

Saving your skin

Most skin problems aren't serious, but they can be irritating, or even painful, and may make you feel self-conscious about your appearance. Fortunately, there's plenty you can do to ease troublesome symptoms and help your skin to look and feel great again.

Easing eczema

The classic signs of eczema are red, itchy patches that scale or weep and crust, most often on the arms and behind the knees. This annoying, but generally harmless, condition is a form of dermatitis, which just means inflammation of the skin. It tends to run in families, along with asthma and hay fever, and to come in bouts, flaring up and then subsiding again. Eczema usually starts in early childhood and often improves or disappears altogether with age.

Here's what to do to speed healing when you get an outbreak of eczema:

Try not to scratch This is hard because eczema can be intensely itchy, but scratching releases chemicals in the skin that actually make the itching worse. And for many people – especially young children – the scratching causes more problems than the eczema, especially if skin becomes infected. It helps to keep nails well trimmed, and to put on a pair of thin cotton gloves at night, when the irritation, and therefore scratching, may be worse.

Use a soothing cream Choose a simple moisturising cream (your pharmacist will advise you). Moisturisers are important in both preventing and treating flare-ups, so use them liberally every day. Steroid creams are a vital part of the treatment of a flare-up. Ask your doctor which is the best product for you and how much to use.

Keep irritated, dry skin well moisturised with a simple emollient cream

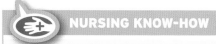

NURSING KNOW-HOW

Cool bathing

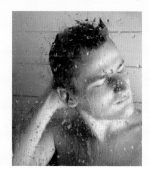

Use warm – not hot – water when you bathe or shower; hot water can intensify itching, as can sweating and rapid changes of temperature.

Top Tips

Coping with dry skin

Deal with this common problem by adopting the following strategies:

- **Moisturise** You can't moisturise too much or too often. Apply a moisturiser at night, in the morning and every time you wash, while your skin is still damp. You don't need expensive brands; cheaper moisturisers are just as effective.

- **Bathe less** Taking a shower or bath depletes your skin of nourishing oils, which is why it's important to moisturise afterwards. You may find it acceptable to flannel-wash critical areas, such as armpits, groin and feet, daily, and save a full bath or shower for every few days. Avoid long soaks – allow yourself 15 minutes maximum – and keep the water warm rather than hot.

- **Avoid harsh soaps** Try to do without soap altogether, and wash most areas simply with warm water, or use a proprietary wash specially designed for dry skin.

- **Humidify indoor air** Use a humidifier or place bowls of water on radiators to avoid dry air sucking more moisture from your skin.

- **Avoid too much sun** Heat and ultraviolet (UV) radiation, even when you've applied sunscreens, accelerate skin drying and ageing. Limiting your exposure is the best policy.

- **Choose fabrics with care** Where possible choose natural fibres such as cotton and silk, which allow your skin to breathe – but avoid wool, which can scratch and irritate. Use non-biological, unperfumed detergents when washing clothes, towels and bed linen.

Consider an oral antihistamine This remedy may help relieve night-time itching. Older antihistamines can make you drowsy, which can be helpful if the itch is keeping you awake. However, don't take these medicines during the day if you intend to drive or operate potentially dangerous machinery and watch out for possible 'hangover' effects the next morning.

PREVENTING FLARE-UPS

To prevent flare-ups of eczema, do your best to avoid any soaps, creams, shampoos and detergents that irritate your skin. You may find it helpful to keep a diary of your symptoms and product use. Where possible, choose unperfumed products and those designed for people with sensitive skin or allergies. It's also a good idea to stick to non-biological washing powder. Avoid wearing wool and synthetic fabrics next to the skin; choose cotton or a fabric that is fine and non-scratchy to avoid irritating sensitive skin.

For some people, certain foods seem to provoke outbreaks of eczema. The most common culprits are dairy products such as milk and eggs, wheat, fish and foods that contain soy. If you are able to identify your food triggers, do your best to avoid them.

It's important to stay cool. At night, sleep under a cotton sheet rather than a doona or blankets during hot weather. Keep your skin well moisturised, as dry skin exacerbates eczema. You might find it helpful to use an emollient bath oil (your pharmacist will be able to recommend a suitable product) or sprinkle bicarbonate or oatmeal into the bathwater to soothe irritated skin.

Some people with eczema have a reaction to house-dust mites, so keep your home as dust-free as possible (see *Allergy action*, page 47). Also, try to keep calm in stressful situations, as stress can provoke a flare-up. It's important to be able to relax and to create a soothing environment at home. If these measures don't control your symptoms, talk to your doctor, who may prescribe stronger creams or oral medication. See your doctor if you think your skin is infected.

Dealing with psoriasis

This recurrent condition causes the formation of thick, scaly patches on the skin, typically on elbows, knees, scalp and lower back, usually starting in young adults. Psoriasis is due to accelerated production of skin cells, leading to thickening and inflammation of the outer layer of skin. For some sufferers the extent of the condition leads to considerable social embarrassment. There is at present no cure, but there are many steps you can take to minimise symptoms and promote skin healing.

SYMPTOM RELIEF

As no two people respond in the same way to treatment, it's important to try a variety of approaches until you find the measures that work best for you. Here are some self-help ideas that psoriasis sufferers have found to be of benefit:

Bathing A daily warm – not hot – bath can soothe sore skin and helps remove dead skin cells. Add some emollient bath oil, oatmeal or Epsom salts to the water, and avoid harsh or perfumed soaps that can irritate the skin. Pat yourself dry and use moisturiser liberally.

Sunlight Sun exposure for short periods – about 20 minutes three or four times a week – can help keep psoriasis under control. But be careful not to overdo it, as prolonged or intensive sunlight can make psoriasis worse or even trigger a flare-up.

Use clingfilm Apply an emollient ointment to patches of psoriasis and cover with clingfilm overnight. In the morning, wash scales away under a lukewarm shower.

Fish oil Although not all studies have shown benefits, many have reported improvements in itching and scaling following a course of fish oil supplements. The omega-3 fatty acids in fish oils reduce inflammation and dampen immune responses thought to underlie skin-thickening in psoriasis. Try 1 to 3 g of fish oil daily, but no more, as high doses can interfere with the normal blood-clotting mechanism.

Stop smoking Try to give up smoking, which is known to trigger more frequent and more severe episodes of psoriasis.

True or False?

A 'psoriasis diet' can help alleviate this condition

False Although some people notice that certain foods worsen or improve their psoriasis, there is no specific diet that deals with the underlying problem. A healthy diet helps to maintain healthy skin, though, so make sure that yours includes plenty of fruit and vegetables along with fish, lean meat and whole grains.

Fish oil supplements can often improve psoriasis symptoms

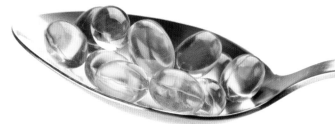

Sunburn and stings

Your skin is your first line of protection against damage from the environment and attack from other creatures. Here you'll find advice to help speed your recovery from minor skin damage. Note: recommendations for action on burns, cuts and wounds are discussed on pages 80–83.

MINOR SUNBURN

Always seek medical attention for severe (with blistering) or extensive sunburn. For more minor redness (without blistering), try one or more of the following fast-relief measures:

● Take a cool (not cold) shower, then apply pure aloe vera gel, which is instantly cooling.
● Soak a towel in strong, tepid tea and apply as a compress. Alternatively, aromatherapists suggest a compress dampened by water with a few drops of lavender oil added.

BEE OR WASP STINGS

● Dab vinegar or lemon juice (acid) to counteract wasp stings, which are alkaline.
● Apply bicarbonate of soda (alkali) to bee stings, which are acidic.
● If the sting remains in the skin remove it as soon as possible. Scrape it out with a clean fingernail or a flat, smooth edge, such as a credit card – don't try to pull it out with tweezers as this is likely to squeeze more poison into the skin.

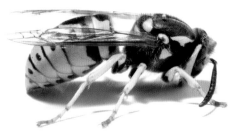

Wasp stings can be painful, but they are easy to treat with home remedies

Jellyfish stings

These are strongly alkaline, which explains why washing with an acidic solution is the best approach.

● Pour an acid liquid such as vinegar or lemon juice into the area to reduce pain. If these are not available, urine may also be effective.

● Remove any tentacles by rinsing or peeling off with a gloved hand and seek medical advice promptly.

Cold sore sense

These painful and unsightly blisters around the lips and sometimes nostrils are caused by a herpes virus, usually *Herpes simplex* type 1. This is not the same as the type 2 virus, which causes genital herpes, although occasionally the two can cross over. Cold sores are not dangerous, but they can make life a misery. Luckily there's plenty you can do to ease symptoms and speed healing.

WHY DO COLD SORES RECUR?

Once you have contracted the virus, cold sores tend to recur, frequently affecting the same sites at each recurrence. The virus is thought to 'hide away' in nerve cells in between attacks until something reactivates it. Stress, illness or even sunlight are among the common triggers. Each flare-up usually consists of the appearance of a blister, which crusts over within a few days and then gradually gets better. A cold sore outbreak generally heals within a couple of weeks.

STOPPING A COLD SORE BEFORE IT STARTS

Cold sores typically start with a tingling or burning sensation in the area before the blister appears. Now is the time to act. Wash the area gently with soap and water then apply ice. Don't use ice directly on your skin, wrap it in a towel or use a cold pack, and don't leave it in place for longer than 10 minutes at a time. Alternate ice with heat – carefully – either from a heat pack or using a hairdryer on a low setting for no more than 2 minutes at a time. Do this two or three times a day.

Creams that contain the antiviral medication aciclovir (see *Get the most from your medicine*, pages 312–339) are available without prescription. Apply them at the first sign of a sore – any later and the virus will have spread, so they are unlikely to be as effective. If you're prone to cold sores, keep a supply on hand.

ONCE A COLD SORE HAS DEVELOPED

Take a painkiller such as paracetamol or ibuprofen, if necessary. Never pick at a sore – you risk spreading the virus, slowing healing and leaving a scar. Cold sores are highly contagious. During an outbreak take the following precautions to avoid spreading the infection elsewhere on your body or to others:

- Throw away any cotton buds, cotton wool or tissues that have touched the sore, sterilise any make-up brushes or pads and wash towels and flannels in hot water.
- Don't share crockery and cutlery (unless washed between users) or towels, flannels, toothbrushes or make-up.
- Avoid kissing anyone.
- Try not to touch the sore; you could transfer the virus to other sites on your body (the eyes and genital area are especially vulnerable) or to others.
- If you do touch a sore, wash your hands thoroughly in warm water with soap.
- Change your toothbrush once the sore has healed.

Should I see my doctor?

If you are not sure whether it's a cold sore, or if you get frequent attacks, talk to your GP. Also seek medical advice if you have a condition causing reduced immunity or if a cold sore appears anywhere near your eyes.

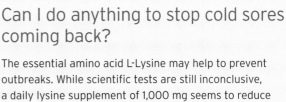

Can I do anything to stop cold sores coming back?

The essential amino acid L-Lysine may help to prevent outbreaks. While scientific tests are still inconclusive, a daily lysine supplement of 1,000 mg seems to reduce frequent outbreaks for some people. Foods containing lysine include corn, poultry and avocados.

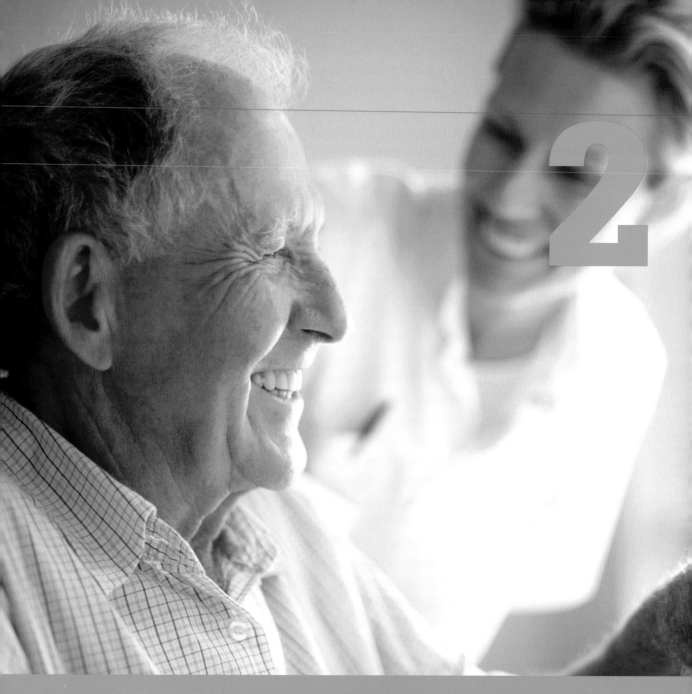

2

Repairing damage

Strains, sprains, burns and fractures can happen in an instant but can be slow to heal. To speed recovery, immediate treatment and expert after-care are essential

Accidents and injuries

The unexpected can strike, any time, anywhere – an inadvertent trip, falls, burns, cuts or, more seriously, a road accident. Some may give you no more than a nasty jolt, but others can result in injuries such as fractures, sprains (ligament damage), strained muscles or tendons, cuts and bruises. Although these can be painful and temporarily disabling, and may require hospital treatment initially, most people will make a full recovery. The healthy body has a remarkable capacity for healing. But everyday accidents can, of course, have more serious consequences for the frail and elderly. Whatever the incident, immediate first-aid treatment is important, but continued care and rehabilitation may also be necessary to ensure that the injury is fully healed. In this chapter you'll find plenty of advice to help you get over both minor and more major accidents in the minimum amount of time.

GENERAL ADVICE

Getting better after a major accident or fall requires patience. Allow yourself time to heal and to get over the physical and emotional effects of the trauma but remember that there is a great deal that you can do to help the healing process. Whatever the type of injury, essential components of your recovery program should include:

Rest The body heals itself while you sleep so make sure you get plenty of rest, and ensure that you sleep well, whether that means taking painkillers or learning relaxation techniques.

Exercises A physiotherapist or specialist may prescribe exercises that can speed up repair of the damaged part of the body. You should also exercise the joints and muscles on the non-affected side of the body.

A nutritious diet Your diet should be rich in the foods and nutrients that promote healing (see page 72).

Self-help treatments These range from relaxation techniques, meditation and self-massage, through herbal teas, flower essences and aromatherapy oils, to consulting relevant therapists and practitioners. They can all help as you recover, making you feel better while your body and the treatments prescribed by your doctor or nurse take care of the healing process.

Preventing recurrence It is important to examine the causes and find ways to ensure that you do not suffer a similar accident in the future as subsequent injury could be doubly damaging.

The following pages explain what you can do to give yourself the best chance of a full recovery from the most common types of injury.

Getting help

If an ambulance is needed, call 000, the emergency number in Australia. If you suspect a spine or neck injury, always call an ambulance.

If the injury is relatively minor, you may be able to save time by transporting the injured person to hospital yourself.

FIRST AID FOR LONG-TERM RECOVERY

More accidents happen in the home than anywhere else. A basic knowledge of first aid in an emergency situation can turn a potentially permanent injury into a temporary one, as well as ensuring a rapid recovery rather than a prolonged period of disability. Knowing some first aid also helps in a non-emergency situation. Dealing with minor injuries such as burns and cuts (see page 80) or stings (see page 64) in the correct way can avoid complications and help to make healing quicker and more straightforward. Basic first-aid courses for non-professionals are run regularly across the country by the Red Cross (www.redcross.org.au) and St John's Ambulance (www.stjohn.org.au).

REACTING TO AN ACCIDENT

If you are at the scene of an accident or are with someone who has been injured, it's important that you stay calm and reassure the casualty that he or she is going to be fine, to ease their anxiety and pain. Call the emergency services, and request aid from other people in the vicinity. Don't move the casualty, but do take steps to stop any heavy bleeding. If you have some first-aid training, be prepared to resuscitate and follow any other procedures you have learned. Keep the patient comfortably warm and watch out for signs of medical shock – a potentially life-threatening drop in blood pressure. Possible symptoms of shock include:

- pale, cold, clammy skin
- a rapid, then weak pulse
- fast, shallow breathing
- sweating
- complaints of nausea and thirst
- agitation and aggression
- if untreated, loss of consciousness.

See *Preventing and treating shock* (left) for advice on what to do in this situation.

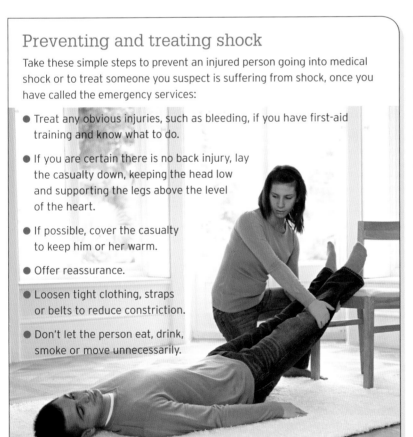

Preventing and treating shock

Take these simple steps to prevent an injured person going into medical shock or to treat someone you suspect is suffering from shock, once you have called the emergency services:

- Treat any obvious injuries, such as bleeding, if you have first-aid training and know what to do.
- If you are certain there is no back injury, lay the casualty down, keeping the head low and supporting the legs above the level of the heart.
- If possible, cover the casualty to keep him or her warm.
- Offer reassurance.
- Loosen tight clothing, straps or belts to reduce constriction.
- Don't let the person eat, drink, smoke or move unnecessarily.

FOCUS

Breezing through casualty

In Australia, there are around 6 million visits a year to hospital emergency departments (ED). By planning ahead and understanding the options available in an emergency, you will get the best care as quickly as possible.

Emergency departments are committed to ensuring patients are seen, treated and admitted or discharged as quickly as possible. To get the best emergency treatment in the shortest time possible, it helps to stay calm and explain clearly and concisely to the medical staff what has happened.

It is also a good idea to make sure you have all the relevant information and documentation about your own medical history, if you are the patient, or that of the patient with you. You should be able to describe:

- any medication(s) being taken by the injured person
- any allergies suffered
- whether the patient has a rare blood group
- if the person could be pregnant
- any immediate symptoms that have now passed, for example, nausea
- any pain relief taken since the accident
- GP details.

WHAT COMES NEXT?

Speak to the medical staff about what happens after treatment at the emergency department. You may need to return for an outpatient appointment or there may be things to do at home to aid recovery.

DO I NEED TO BE HERE?

Emergency departments are busy places, especially on Friday or Saturday nights. You might be able to avoid a long wait by choosing one of the other services that deal with minor emergencies:

- Some emergency departments offer Fast Track Units during busy times to assess and treat non-life threatening conditions such as sprains and strains.
- An out-of-hours GP is always available during the evening/night and at weekends and public holidays. Check with your local surgery.
- An after-hours GP helpline offers 24-hour advice to help you make treatment decisions and to decide whether or not you need to go to the emergency department. Call 1800 022 222.

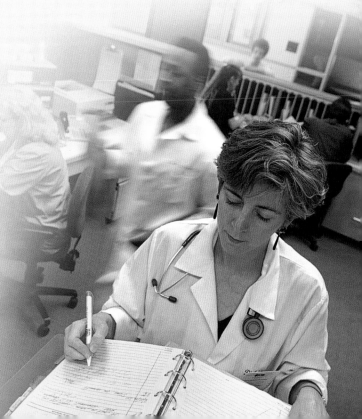

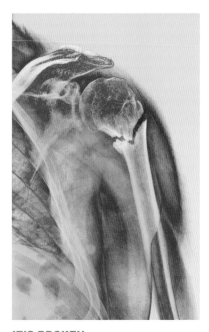

IT'S BROKEN

This false-colour X-ray clearly shows a break (fracture) in the bone of the upper arm, near the shoulder joint. While this injury is likely to be painful and disabling in the short term, with appropriate care, the prospects for a complete recovery are good.

Breaks and strains

In the immediate aftermath of an accident, fall or injury, it may be difficult to know whether you have suffered a broken bone (fracture), a joint injury or a muscle injury. As a general rule of thumb, if you're in doubt, treat the injury as a broken bone.

In fact, healthy bones are extremely strong and are usually able to withstand strong forces. Most people sustain a fracture only as a result of a bad fall or another type of impact, such as a car crash. The bones of older people and those suffering from osteoporosis, however, are more fragile, making fractures more likely as a consequence of minor falls.

The PRICE procedure

After a sprain or strain, you can aid recovery by following the PRICE (Protection, Rest, Ice, Compression, Elevation) procedure as soon as possible:

Protect the area from further strain or damage.

Rest the injured joint or muscle for the first 48-72 hours.

Ice Apply cold for the first 48-72 hours. Wrap crushed ice or a packet of frozen vegetables in a damp towel and place on the injured area for 15-20 minutes every 2 to 3 hours. Never place ice directly on the skin as this could cause a cold burn.

Compress or bandage the injured area to limit swelling and movement (crêpe, elastic or tubular bandages are ideal), but remember to remove the bandage before you go to bed. It should be snug but not too tight, or you risk restricting the circulation of blood.

Elevate the injured area, supported by a pillow if possible.

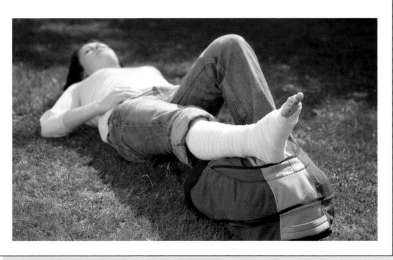

RECOGNISING A FRACTURE

When trying to decide if a bone is broken, look for the following signs:

- severe pain and swelling
- bruising or discoloration around the bone or joint
- inability to bear weight on or move the injured limb/part of the body
- a bend or unusual angle (angulation) in the limb or part of the body affected
- a grating sensation or sound in the bone or joint.

If you suspect a broken bone, secure and support the injured part and go straight to hospital to prevent further injury. Most bones heal successfully and speedily once they have been aligned correctly and immobilised.

AFTER THE BREAK

It can take anywhere from several weeks to several months for a fracture to heal, depending on the extent of the injury. While you're in plaster, your physiotherapist or nurse at the fracture clinic may show you some exercises to keep joints above and below the plaster moving. For a fractured wrist, for example, you may be encouraged to make a fist and stretch out your fingers so that they do not become stiff, or to bend and straighten your elbow and move your shoulder joint frequently to retain mobility.

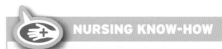

NURSING KNOW-HOW

Keep cool

For the first 72 hours after a sprain or muscle strain, you should avoid hot baths, saunas and heat packs. Also avoid massage and alcohol as they can increase bleeding and swelling, and delay healing.

COUNTDOWN AFTER A FRACTURE

Waiting for a broken bone to heal requires patience. It takes weeks for a basic fracture to mend and a complicated break will take longer. At each stage in recovery, progress is being made, although it can be hard to tell. The typical stages to expect are:

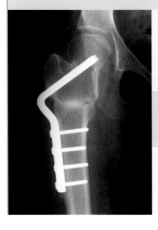

0-3 weeks	Immobilisation with a plaster cast or plastic brace. Metal plates, rods and screws (shown in the X-ray of a broken leg, left) may be used to align and hold the bone in place so that it heals correctly.
3-10 weeks	Immobilisation continues for a variable period dependent on the severity of the break and any complications, such as infection.
3 weeks- 4 months or longer	Following immobilisation, physiotherapy or exercises may be prescribed to rebuild muscle strength and restore mobility to the injured area.

WHEN THE PLASTER COMES OFF

Once the plaster is removed and you are given the all clear to move the affected part normally, you need to work hard to regain flexibility and strength. Here are some ideas for mobilising a wrist following a fracture:

- Start by moving your wrist in all directions in warm water. This also helps your skin if it has been encased in plaster.
- Hold a ball or similar small, soft object. Squeeze it gently and relax. Squeeze the ball harder and hold the contraction for a few seconds longer each day.
- Put your forearms flat on a table in front of you with your palms facing down. Lift your fingers and palms off the table. Compare the movement in the fingers and hands of your affected arm with those of your good arm to see how far you are progressing each day.
- With your forearm supported, make large circles with your thumb.
- Move your thumb across to the base of your little finger. You may find that you cannot touch at first, but this should improve with practice.

Repeat each exercise 10 times, and repeat the sequence 3 times a day.

Warning: If you experience any increase in pain, redness, swelling or other symptoms, seek a medical opinion before continuing.

SUPPLEMENTARY TREATMENTS

After a fracture, the healing process can be accelerated by the use of treatments such as electromagnetic and pulsed laser therapy from a physiotherapist. These low-energy treatments work by 'tickling' the cells to stimulate them into higher activity, using the natural resources of the body to heal itself. The 'excited' cells work faster and harder than normal, thus accelerating recovery. These forms of treatment are also known to aid tissue repair, so they are useful in speeding recovery after a sprain or strain too.

FOOD CHOICES FOR BONE AND MUSCLE REPAIR

What you eat obviously affects your day-to-day health, but it can also determine the rate at which you recover following a bone or muscle injury. Research shows that good nutrition reduces the length of hospital stays and improves a patient's overall recovery.

Meals packed full of vitamins, minerals – especially calcium – and protein may aid the healing process. You should find out from the ward staff what kinds of foods are both suitable and practical for visitors to bring in (in some cases this will depend on what fridge facilities are available). Chocolates are lovely to share with other visitors, but where possible, ask for more nutritious snacks.

Simple exercises such as squeezing a ball to help you regain strength in your wrist can have a big impact

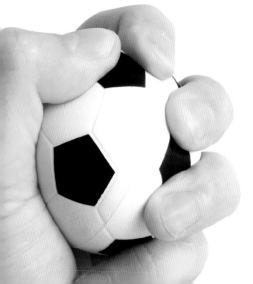

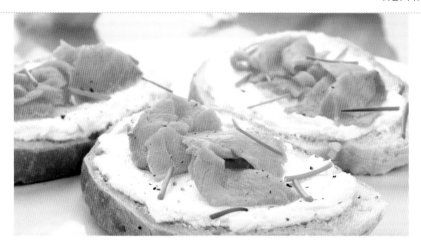

Fish and cheese are high in protein for muscle repair

Once you return home, choose foods rich in the nutrients listed below to support the healing process. Remember that you are probably less active than usual while you're recuperating from an injury, so it's important to limit your intake of fats and sugars if you don't want to pile on the weight.

- Calcium-rich foods such as dairy products, green leafy vegetables, tinned sardines, nuts and legumes help to build bones. Avoid dietary sources of phytic acid, such as bran and brown rice, and oxalic acid such as rhubarb and spinach, as these inhibit calcium absorption.

- A supply of vitamin D is also required for calcium to be deposited in the bones, so eat plenty of oily fish, eggs and vitamin D-fortified foods, such as breakfast cereals. Vitamin D is produced by exposure of the skin to the sun's ultraviolet rays, so get out in the sunshine. Sunscreens inhibit the absorption of vitamin D so expose skin to sunshine, without sun protection for 10–15 minutes per day, at a time of day when the sun is least damaging (before 11 am and after 3 pm). At other times make sure you use a sunscreen. In strong sunlight choose a high SPF (sun protection factor) product.

- Protein helps to repair cells and to build up the strong muscle tissue that you need for good recovery. Sources of high-quality proteins include meat, poultry, fish, eggs and soy beans.

- Vitamin C plays a vital role in producing collagen, a protein needed for healthy skin and bones, which is especially important in healing wounds and burns. Good sources of vitamin C include fresh fruits and vegetables.

- Folate-rich foods, such as offal, legumes and green leafy vegetables, can counter the effects of non-steroidal anti-inflammatory drugs that may be taken to relieve the pain of muscle strains and sprains. Some of these medications contain sulfasalazine, which can reduce the body's absorption of the vitamin folate.

Supplements can speed recovery

False Most nutritionists agree that good nutrition alone should be enough to support the healing process. But if, for any reason, during your recovery you're not eating much or have a restricted choice of diet, vitamin and mineral supplements may help you return to full health faster.

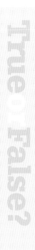

True or False?

Nuts are an excellent source of bone-building calcium

Maintaining mobility

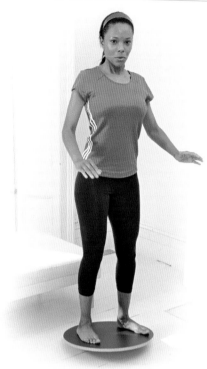

Build balance and strength in an injured ankle using a wobble board

It's hard to estimate how common sprains and strains are, because most people do not report them to their GP. But it is known that the most common types of sprain occur in the ankle, knee, wrist and thumb, while the most common strains affect muscles in the thighs, calf and lower back.

Although painful to move at the time of injury, sprains and strains actually heal more quickly if you don't rest the injured part for too long. If it doesn't cause excessive pain, begin gentle flexibility exercises within 48 to 72 hours of injury. This will also help you to regain the full range of motion in the affected joint.

PREVENTING RECURRENCE

Exercises that improve strength, balance and core strength – for example, Alexander technique, Pilates and tai chi – can help to prevent a repeat injury. Or you could try the following:

On balance Physiotherapists sometimes use wobble boards to retrain the ability to balance. Inexpensive and available to buy on the internet, a wobble board can help you recover faster from injuries, such as a sprained ankle, or a hip replacement. Trying to balance – first with both legs, then alternately on each leg – strengthens the muscles that maintain balance and posture and support the joints. But make sure you consult your physiotherapist before you buy a wobble board and ask when you should start and how you should perform the exercises.

MOBILISE AND STRENGTHEN YOUR SPRAINED ANKLE

If you have no underlying injuries, try these exercises to hasten healing of a sprained ankle once the initial pain has abated. They can be practised from a sitting position at first as on page 98.

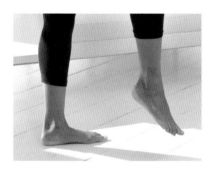

1 *Move your foot up and down as though pressing a pedal.*

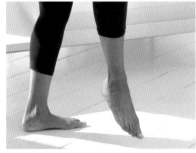

2 *Make circles with your foot in each direction.*

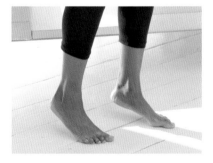

3 *Shift your weight from front to back and from the inside to the outside of your foot.*

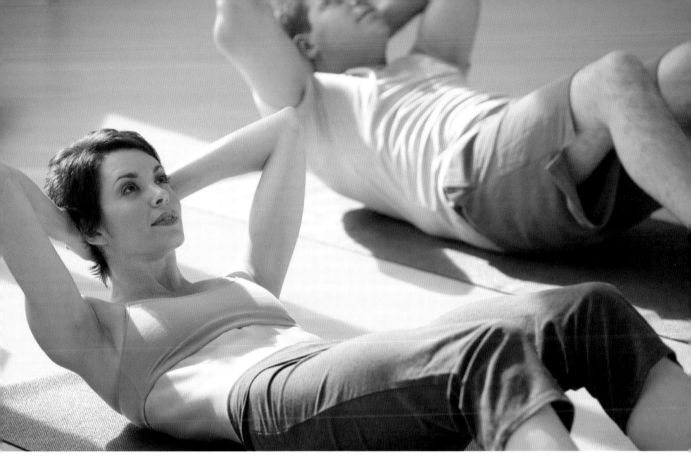

Strengthening the core muscles
of the abdomen can help to protect
your back from injury

Improving core strength The core muscles of
the abdomen stabilise and protect the spine.
Strengthening the core can speed recovery from a
back injury and help you to avoid further injuries.
Contract the abdominal muscles below your navel,
without moving the 'six pack' muscles above, and
hold – building up over time to a count of ten. Repeat
three times, as often as possible (see also *Activities
for back recovery*, page 88).

Building strength Using an exercise ball can help
to prevent recurrent back trouble (see page 88). Sit
with your legs off the ground to work the muscles
that keep your balance and support the spine (those
in the lower back and abdomen). Elderly or frail
people should seek a physiotherapist's advice first
and choose an anti-bounce, 'sitting' type of ball.

Top Tips

Common sports injuries

Most sports injuries benefit from following the
PRICE procedure (see page 70). Later you can
try these tips, but if there is no improvement,
contact your GP or a physiotherapist.

Shin pain (or shin splints)
- Return to running or sport gradually and select
  'forgiving' surfaces such as a running track or
  sprung floor.

Tennis and golf elbow
- Try acupuncture – many health-care practitioners
  use it as part of a treatment plan.

- Ask your physiotherapist to recommend some
  stretching and strengthening exercises.

Pulled hamstring
- Consult a physiotherapist for advice on when to
  start some gentle stretches.

A SPORTSMAN'S STORY

The aggravation of an old sports injury forced Julian to take his recovery into his own hands

After suffering a sports injury, 50-year-old Julian Temple worked hard at home to strengthen the muscles around his knee, with amazing results.

I was playing in a Dads and Lads rugby match at the local club with my young son, when I swerved to avoid a tackle and my knee just gave way completely. I was in agony. I went to the hospital emergency department and was referred to a specialist.

A scan confirmed that I'd aggravated a rugby injury I'd suffered when I was in my mid-twenties. On that occasion, I avoided an operation by strengthening the muscles in the leg around the knee. Although I'm 25 years older, with the consultant's consent, we decided this was what I'd do again, as I didn't fancy having an operation.

Initially, I combined ice treatment with wearing a knee brace. Once I was walking properly, I got a range of physiotherapy exercises to practise at home, which helped me to regain a full range of extension and flexion. To complement these, I returned to cycling to build up muscle strength around the knee.

The biggest problem was that the pain kept me awake at night, and it's so hard to motivate yourself when you're feeling tired and irritable. My wife persuaded me to drink camomile tea before bed and also to put lavender on the pillow, both of which seemed to help. If the pain was too bad, I'd take a painkiller.

Once I was getting a good night's sleep, I was able to resume my rehabilitation and I'm pleased to say that I've managed to avoid the need for an operation, which would have laid me up for months. Two months after the accident, I still do the strength and balance exercises every day and I enjoy cycling. I'm confident that I'll be back to running before long, but I'll give the rugby a miss next time!

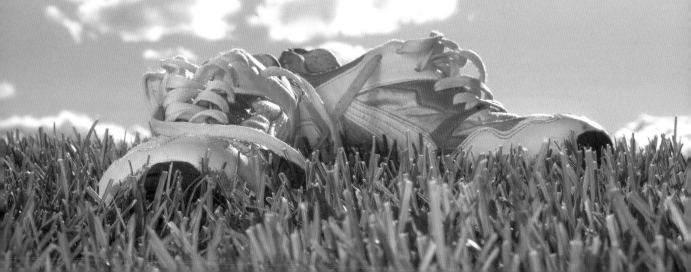

Fall-proofing your life

For the elderly, a fall around the home can mean serious injury that can jeopardise independence. Whether or not you have recently suffered a fall, consider taking some simple precautions to keep yourself safe and active.

According to the Australian and New Zealand Falls Prevention Society, falls are the leading cause of injury-related hospitalisation in persons aged 65 years and over and are responsible for four per cent of all hospital admissions in this age group. The Australian Institute of Health and Welfare says over 80,000 older people are hospitalised because of falls each year and about 70 per cent of these falls happened in the home or an aged care facility. Changes in vision, hearing, coordination, balance and reflexes as we age make the elderly susceptible to falls. As we age, our gait changes – the stride tends to shorten and we lift our feet less, which leads to an increased risk of tripping. And when they do fall, they are more likely to sustain a fracture or serious injury as they have lower bone density than younger people. The two most common injuries from falls in the elderly are wrist fractures or dislocations, and fractures of the femur.

The Royal Australian College of General Practitioners recommends all older people have a falls risk assessment at the family doctor's at least every 12 months.

HELPING YOURSELF

Older people can do a great deal to prevent falls and maintain an active, independent lifestyle for longer. If you may be vulnerable, follow these simple precautions:

- Ask your doctor or pharmacist about the side effects of the medicines you are taking, as some can affect your coordination or balance.
- Have your eyes checked every year as vision problems can cause a slip or trip.

Poor vision can cause falls. Make sure you have regular check-ups

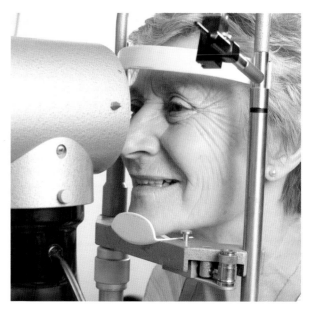

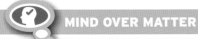

MIND OVER MATTER

Active and confident

While elderly people should take sensible precautions, becoming unduly fearful of falls can reduce their quality of life. If you encourage older loved ones to stay active and involved, so that they remain valued and contributing members of the community, they will be physically fitter and more likely to be confident and independent.

- Visit your GP to make sure you're getting enough vitamin D, as low levels can increase the risk of falls as well as of osteoporosis.
- Don't get up too quickly after eating, sleeping or resting. Your blood pressure may have dropped and could cause dizziness.
- Choose sensible footwear with non-slip soles that are not too thick. Lace-up or Velcro-secured shoes are preferable to slip-ons or slippers.
- Stay as physically active as you can to improve strength and muscle tone, which in turn helps to keep joints, tendons and ligaments flexible so you can move more easily.
- Try exercises to enhance balance and coordination to prevent falls, and mild weight-bearing activity, which can reduce the loss of bone and bone fragility due to osteoporosis. Tai chi and dancing are good as they combine individually paced exercise with a social setting.
- Keep your alcohol intake well below the limits recommended on page 26 as this can adversely affect your balance and reflexes.
- Use a walking stick, walker or other helpful device, if appropriate, and make sure it is the right height. Don't let pride or embarrassment stand in your way.

HOME SAFETY

There are several effective steps you can take to make your home safer and reduce the likelihood of falls and accidents and. Make sure you have:

Good lighting, especially on staircases, in corridors and in bathrooms.

Easy access to light switches, telephones and everyday items such as crockery and pans.

Secure handrails and grab bars on stairs, along corridors and in the bathroom by the toilet, bath and shower.

Electrical cords and wires placed out of the way, and hallways and rooms cleared of obstacles for safe movement.

Level and even floorboards and floor tiles, and rugs and carpets that are non-slip or secured to the floor with tacks, non-skid pads or double-sided tape.

Beds and chairs at the correct height – neither too high nor too low.

Floors are clear of clutter that could trip you up.

Frequently used items stored as close to waist height as possible, not too high to reach easily or too low to risk back strain.

Clear garden paths with no broken or uneven paving stones.

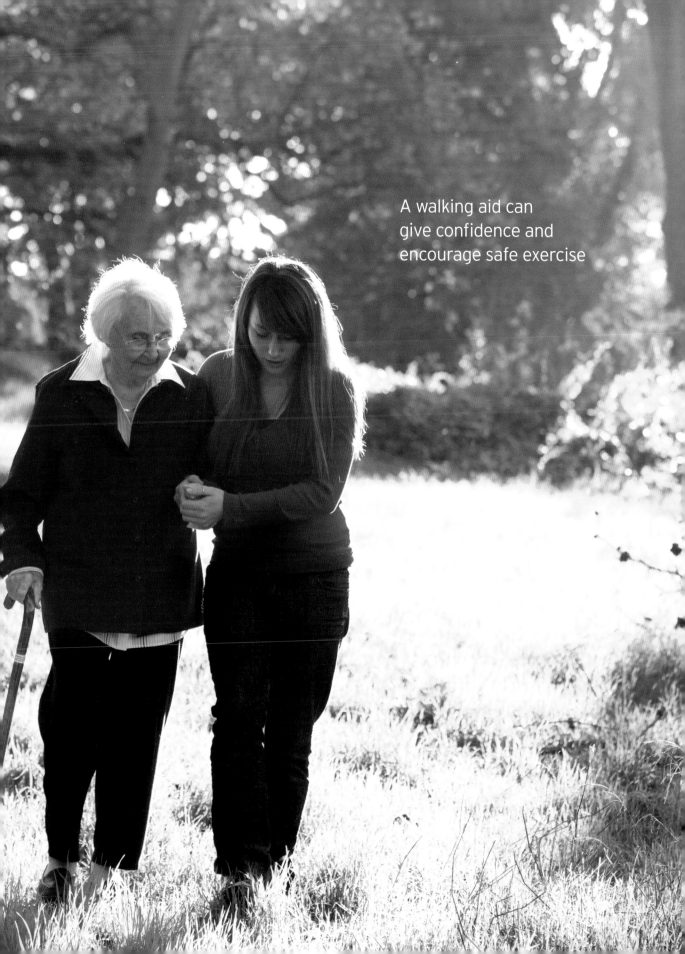

A walking aid can
give confidence and
encourage safe exercise

Skin deep

The skin, the body's first line of defence, is the largest organ in the body and although susceptible to injury due to its size and exposure, it has amazing powers of regeneration.

Immediate action

The skin can scar after a burn or cut, but prompt action at the time of the injury is the key to rapid healing and minimising the risk of scarring. There are also various helpful follow-up steps that will help the skin heal more quickly.

BURNS AND SCALDS

A painful burn or scald needs fast, appropriate first-aid treatment. Never be tempted to put ice directly on a heat injury, as this can produce an additional cold burn. It can also cause the victim's body to cool to a level that is dangerous for other organs. Follow these steps as soon as possible:

- Cool the burn immediately by running cool water onto the area for at least 10 minutes or until the pain is relieved.
- Carefully remove jewellery, watch or clothing from around the burn unless it is sticking to the skin.
- Raise the limb to reduce swelling.
- Cover the area of the burn with a clean, non-fluffy, preferably sterile, dressing, or use clingfilm (see *Keep it clean*, left). Avoid using adhesive dressings and be careful not to burst any blisters that may form.
- If the burn is deep or larger than a postage stamp, seek urgent medical attention.

CUTS AND WOUNDS

Knowing how to treat a cut or wound can help to avoid infection and ensure scar-free healing.
Clean it Wash the area of the burn under running water. Pat dry with a sterile dressing or other clean, lint-free material.

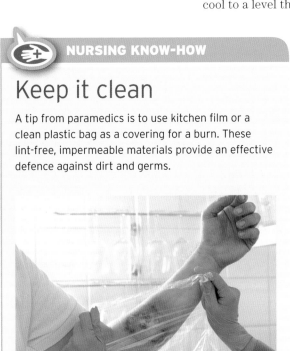

Cover it Clean the surrounding skin with soapy water. Dry and then cover the cut with a plaster or sterile dressing or use steri-strips to close the edges of the wound. A large or deep cut that cannot be easily closed in this way may need to be stitched in hospital.

Apply pressure If bleeding is severe, apply direct pressure to the wound with a clean cloth, pad or even your fingers until a sterile dressing is available. Keep the dressing firmly in place to control bleeding and seek immediate medical attention. Elevate the affected area above the heart, if possible, while waiting for help.

In the longer term

Once you are over the immediate trauma, there are measures you can take to promote fast and scar-free healing. In most cases, burns, scalds and other skin injuries are minor and the scars soon fade. But if the damage to the skin is more severe, visible scars may be upsetting. If you are concerned, talk to your doctor. For deep cuts follow the advice for preventing scarring after surgery on page 208. Several specialist treatments for scars are available and there are also a number of ways in which you can help yourself:

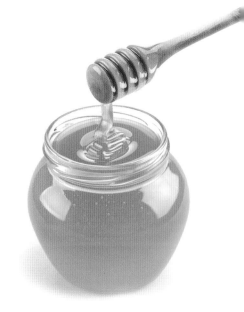

SWEET SUCCESS AGAINST INFECTION
Honey has been used as a wound dressing in traditional medicine for thousands of years. Now, scientific research shows some types of honey, particularly manuka honey, contain antimicrobial factors that can kill a range of antibiotic-resistant bacteria, including MRSA.

- Look into scar therapies (see below) that can help disguise or minimise scarring.
- Remember, a scar always looks worse initially. As it heals and fades, it may no longer seem so problematic.
- Talk to others who have scars or consider counselling.

MINIMISING THE SCAR

While it is not always possible to remove a scar entirely, scar revision treatment can usually improve its appearance and ease any tightness. Much depends on the depth and size of the wound or incision, and its location on your body. Your age, genes, sex and ethnicity can also play a role.

Some scar therapies are carried out by a dermatologist, while others require the skills of a surgeon. Among the available options are: laser therapy (which is suitable for mild scarring); compression therapy, in which pressure is applied to a raised (hypertrophic) scar; cortico-steroid injection; freezing (cryotherapy); and the application of a special silicone sheet (which has to be kept in place for up to a year). A wide scar can in some cases be minimised by further surgery, perhaps involving a skin graft from another part of the body.

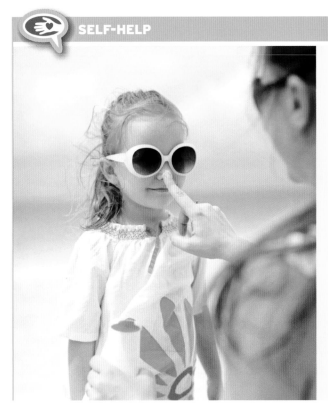

Smart sun protection

If you've suffered serious sunburn, this can double your risk of skin cancer, the most common type of cancer diagnosed in Australia each year. It is important that you take effective steps to avoid suffering sunburn again. Follow these simple guidelines to protect your skin:

- Stay in the shade between 11 am and 3 pm.

- Aim to cover up with T-shirt, hat and sunglasses.

- Never use a sunbed.

- Use sunscreen with an SPF (sun protection factor) of 15 or above.

- Check skin regularly for any new abnormalities that don't go away after 4–6 weeks or existing ones that are getting bigger. See your doctor, if you notice such changes.

For some people whose lives are adversely affected by scarring, a new surgical technique known as tissue expansion may be an option. It is a relatively straightforward procedure that allows the body to 'grow' extra skin for use in reconstructing almost any part of the body. A balloon-like device, called an expander, is inserted under the skin near the area to be repaired and then gradually filled with salt water. Over time, the presence of the expander causes the skin to stretch and grow. The growth of new tissue is permanent, but the skin will retract somewhat when the expander is removed. Tissue expansion is most

Can any foods help protect against sunburn?

Beta-carotene, which is found in many brightly coloured fruit and vegetables, may help to protect against sunburn, but dietary measures are not a substitute for covering up and using sunscreens.

commonly used for breast reconstruction following the removal of a breast (mastectomy), but is also used to repair skin damaged by accidents, surgery and burns.

Another new treatment currently under development involves the injection into the wound area of a synthetic form of a growth factor normally made in the skin. This seems to help prevent scars and trials suggest that in the future this treatment could be found to reduce scars that have already formed.

COSMETIC CAMOUFLAGE

For those who are unsure about reverting to surgery or other forms of treatment for scarring, cosmetic camouflage may be an option. Cosmetic camouflage uses make-up to conceal anything from scarring and broken capillaries, to birthmarks and unwanted tattoos, and can also correct colour mismatches. It can be very effective. Your GP, dermatologist or hospital dermatology department can refer you to a manufacturer, or you can find manufacturers of cosmetics for camouflage online.

Herbal skin soothers

Whether the skin damage is caused by a wound, graze, burn or scald, after you have taken essential first-aid measures, certain herbal preparations, essential oils and creams may help your skin to heal speedily and successfully, thereby reducing scarring. Dilute essential oils in a carrier oil before application to the skin. Use up to 12 drops in 6 to 8 teaspoons of a carrier oil such as sweet almond or grapeseed oil. The exception is lavender oil, which can be applied undiluted. Here are some specific suggestions:

● **Recent wounds or burns** Try aloe vera gel, or lavender, helichrysum, sea buckthorn or carrot root essential oils. An infusion of lady's mantle or St John's wort (especially for burns) can be applied as a cool compress to the affected area. Calendula (marigold) ointment is renowned for its healing properties and can be used for a wide range of minor skin injuries.

● **Sunburn** Sooth inflamed skin by applying witch hazel as a liquid or gel, or calendula or aloe vera gels. Another option is to apply a cool compress soaked in an infusion of dried marigold flowers, or apply neat lavender essential oil or sea buckthorn essential oil diluted in a carrier oil. It's worth noting that, contrary to popular belief, the application of yoghurt is not an effective remedy for sunburn.

● **Scars** Rosehip seed oil is reputed to encourage healing of scars and stretch marks. Alternatively try diluted clary sage oil (not to be used during pregnancy) or neroli oil, or undiluted lavender oil.

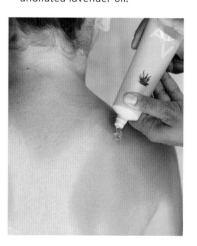

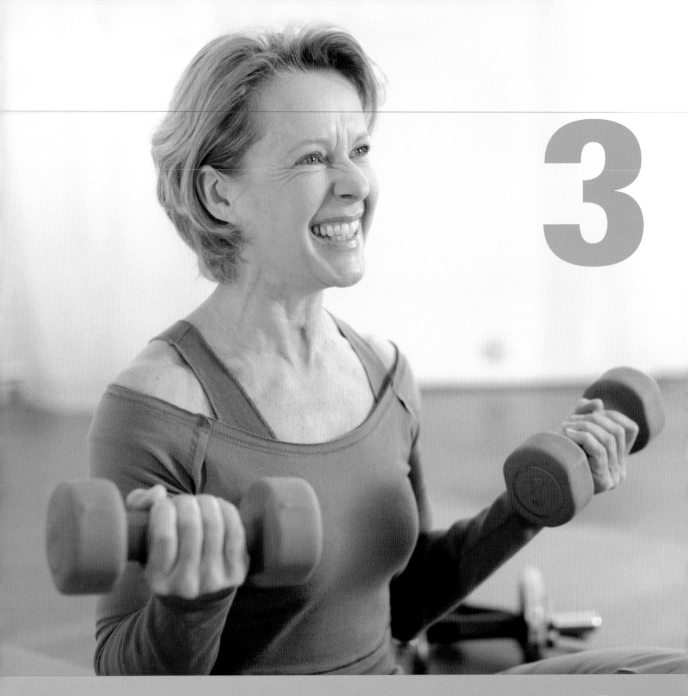

3

Get moving again

A condition that restricts your mobility is bound to reduce your enjoyment of life. It's reassuring to know that simple measures can soon get you back to living life to the full

Regaining your mobility

Accidents apart (see *Repairing damage*, pages 66–83), most mobility problems are caused by musculoskeletal conditions that affect the bones, muscles, joints, tendons, ligaments, cartilage and other connective tissue. These often cause pain and stiffness in areas such as the back, neck and limbs. Musculoskeletal problems are the second most common problems seen in general practice. Back pain accounted for one in five of these consultations, with knee problems prompting one visit in ten. More than 3 million Australians – 3 in 20 people – are affected by arthritis, and most people experience a musculoskeletal condition at some point in life, but there are now many effective medicines and therapies.

The following pages explain what you can do in conjunction with your doctor's advice to regain mobility, including advice on exercise and other aspects of lifestyle, work and medical treatments.

FIRST STEPS

If medical treatment is necessary, experts agree that certain factors – including pain control (see pages 214–239), having accurate information, believing that recovery is possible and getting on with life – all help the healing process. Here are some ideas:

Educate yourself Find out as much as you can about what may be causing your problems and how best to manage them. There are many patient education and self-management programs for specific disorders. For example, visit Arthritis Australia (www.arthritisaustralia.com.au), Chronic Pain Australia (www.chronicpainaustralia.org.au) or Pain Australia (www.painaustralia.org.au).

Seek advice quickly If the immobility and pain continue untreated, your body may experience changes that make recovery more difficult. Timely advice from a professional may help avert further damage.

Think positive A positive attitude will help you make progress and overcome difficulties. Focus on what you can do rather than what you can't.

Stay active With all musculoskeletal problems, it's important to keep moving. This may not be possible initially if your pain is severe, but don't put your feet up for too long. Resume everyday activities such as walking to the shops, going to work and light gardening as soon as possible. Range-of-movement exercises are especially important for musculoskeletal health. See those outlined on page 98.

Do what you can Don't give up. Try to exercise for at least 5 or 10 minutes each day, even if you feel tired. Movement is energising and you may find you can do more once you start.

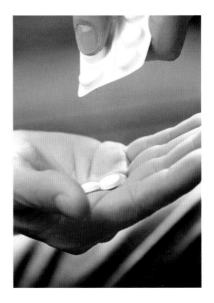

Effective pain relief will help to get you moving

Sleep well A number of musculoskeletal problems, especially fibromyalgia (see page 235), can disturb sleep. Disrupted sleep can, in turn, worsen inflammation (redness, swelling and/or pain), which is often a feature of these disorders, though not of fibromyalgia. If pain is keeping you awake, ask your doctor or physiotherapist for advice; it may be possible, for example, for you to time your medications to provide more relief at night. See also *Sleep*, pages 30–33.

Eat an anti-inflammatory diet Research shows that eating too many fatty and sugary foods worsens the pain, swelling and redness that characterise inflammation. Counter inflammation by eating plenty of fresh fruit and vegetables and a good intake of omega-3 fatty acids, found in fish and fish oils and foods such as walnuts, hempseed and linseed. Because inflammation fuels bone loss, such a diet may also help to slow osteoporosis, according to a study reported in the *Journal of Clinical Endocrinology & Metabolism* in 2008.

ACTIVITIES TO PROMOTE MOBILITY

Exercise helps to keep limbs and joints supple and maintain general fitness. The following forms of exercise are suitable for most people, but stop if any activity makes your pain worse. Your choice will depend on personal preference and the severity of any musculoskeletal condition you have (for specific advice on exercises for people with back problems, see page 89, and for arthritis, page 98):

Walking Helps build fitness and maintain bone density, is convenient and suitable for everyone.

Low-impact aerobics Involves large muscle groups used in continuous rhythmic activity, with at least one foot in contact with the floor at all times, which minimises impact. It improves general fitness, especially of the cardiovascular system, and is ideal for people who want to avoid high-intensity exercise.

Cycling An aerobic exercise (one that strengthens the cardiovascular system) that is non-weightbearing and therefore does not cause impact on the joints. Start gently, and stop if it exacerbates joint pain.

Powerplate Found in many gyms, this static vibrating 'plate' may help to strengthen muscles and bones.

Pilates Very good for flexibility, can be adapted to many fitness levels and needs, develops core strength (see page 75) and good posture.

Tai chi A gentle and complete system of exercise that puts joints through a full range of movement.

Weights Strength training with free or fixed weights can help strengthen muscles and stabilise joints, but go for light weights and build up repetitions.

Yoga Very good for flexibility of all joints. Choose gentle varieties, such as Hatha or Iyengar yoga, and work to your own ability level.

Water-based exercise Swimming and aqua-aerobics are ideal, maintaining general fitness and exercising the joints, which are supported by the water.

Dance This form of exercise improves balance and coordination. If you have musculoskeletal problems, try slow and low-impact types of dance, such as some ballroom and therapeutic dance, rather than higher-impact types, such as salsa and tap.

Back to health

Four out of five people experience low back pain at some time in their lives and it is a major cause of mobility problems. Learning how to protect and strengthen your back will help you recover and safeguard against future back pain.

Most back trouble has no obvious cause (termed 'non-specific'). It may be the result of misuse and strain from everyday activities, such as lifting and carrying, driving or sleeping in one awkward position or sitting or standing for too long in the same position. These kinds of strain can cause the muscles to go into spasm, causing pain and stiffness. Pregnancy, being overweight, stress, lack of fitness and poor posture can also put stress on the back. Back pain in itself does not pose a serious risk to health, but it can have a major impact on your quality of life.

The loss of mobility that often follows a back problem is not usually caused by mechanical damage to the joints or supporting tissue, but rather due to the understandable desire to avoid any movement that causes pain. Lack of use can cause the back muscles to weaken over time, often compounding the problem.

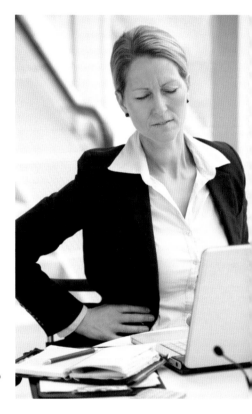

Everyday back care

It is important to rule out any serious underlying cause for your back pain, so be sure to consult your doctor before embarking on a self-help program. Your doctor will also be able to provide you with effective pain-relieving medication – a key component of your recovery. You can learn more about targeted pain relief in *Back pain* (pages 234–235). When you have a back problem it is essential to keep mobile. The sooner you put into place measures to protect your back (see *Back recovery in action*, pages 89–90), the faster you're likely to get better. Here are some other key pointers to help you get better:

Avoid prolonged bed rest Research shows that resting in bed for longer than three days can delay healing – while immobile, the unused back muscles become stiff and weak and other muscles take over, throwing the spine out of balance. People who stay active when suffering back problems tend to have better function and less pain.

Those with sedentary jobs are as likely to experience back pain as those who do physical work

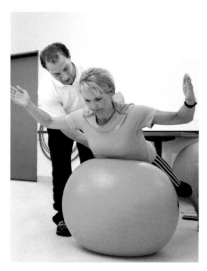

ON THE BALL

An exercise ball can be a useful aid to recovery. It forces you to engage the abdominal and back muscles to maintain proper posture and balance, which over time strengthens and stabilises the back. Ask a physiotherapist or fitness instructor for suitable exercises.

Pace yourself Too much activity can be as detrimental as too little to a bad back, so learn to pace yourself and don't do too much too soon, especially when the pain starts to subside.

Keep on working Research shows that people who continue to work during a bout of back pain recover more quickly.

Balance it According to research published in the journal *Pain* in 2009 both low and high extremes of physical activity are linked to an increased risk of chronic low back pain. Maintain a balance and don't overdo or underdo it.

Relax, relax Feeling tense may cause muscle spasms, which can exacerbate pain and stiffness; and undue worry about whether you're going to get better, for example, can add to the stress.

ACTIVITIES FOR BACK RECOVERY

Experts from different countries differ in their recommendations about the role of exercise in the treatment of chronic back pain. This is because this is a difficult area to do conclusive research in. Regardless of whether or not your therapist recommends formal activities, your goal should be to strengthen the muscles that support the back, improve flexibility and increase stamina. Ask your GP whether this type of program could help you. Even if you are not enrolled in a formal course, your goal should be to include a variety of physical activities in your life. Here are some ideas to consider:

Walking is a simple and effective low-impact aerobic activity that should cause minimal pain if your back is strained. Using a pedometer will help you record your progress and provides an incentive. Try to work up to 10,000 steps a day.

Swimming is a gentle way to exercise and strengthen the back muscles. Front crawl or backstroke is better for your back than breaststroke, which can strain the back muscles if you keep your head above water.

Yoga strengthens back muscles and improves flexibility and balance. US studies suggest that people with low back pain who do yoga have less disability, pain and depression. A UK pilot study published in the journal *Complementary Therapies in Clinical Practice* in 2010 found that people with chronic low back pain who practised yoga for 75 minutes a week over three months suffered significantly less discomfort.

Pilates classes are an effective way to strengthen the muscles of the abdomen and back that support the spinal column (see also *Improving core strength*, page 75).

BACK RELEASE

Physiotherapist Michele Harms recommends this simple at-home exercise to help prevent or relieve back problems. Repeat it 10 times:

1 Lie on your back on the floor or on a firm bed, with your knees bent and feet flat.

2 Flatten your spine against the surface by tightening your stomach muscles so that your navel moves towards your spine and your pelvis gently rocks backwards.

3 Hold for 5 seconds, remembering to breathe, then relax.

4 Then, in a controlled way, roll your knees slowly from side to side.

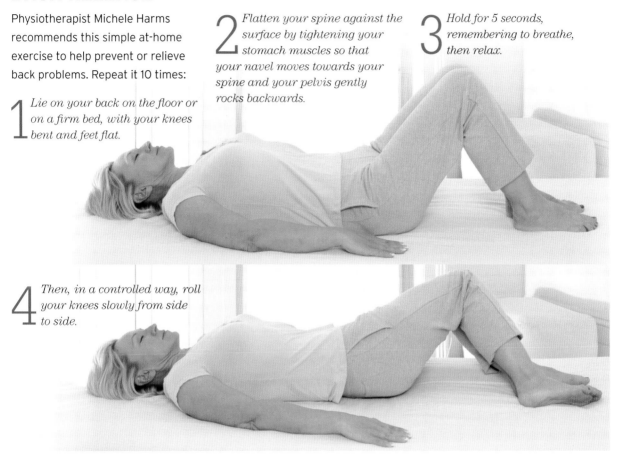

Back recovery in action

When recovering from an episode of back pain, you'll need to adjust the way you handle day-to-day activities in the home and at work. Yes, you need to keep moving, but you also must avoid any strain that could upset your recuperation. Here are some useful tips:

IN THE KITCHEN

- Make sure work surfaces and sinks are high enough to work at comfortably without the need to stoop.
- Use long-handled mops and brushes and an upright vacuum cleaner.
- Store saucepans at waist height and keep heavy appliances on the worktop to avoid bending and lifting.

IN THE GARDEN

- Check that your equipment is right for your size and build. Avoid using anything that's too heavy or awkward to lift.
- Look for specially designed spades, hoes, forks and rakes to relieve stress on your joints.
- Choose a small lightweight mower or whipper snipper.
- Dispose of grass clippings and other garden waste regularly to avoid the need to carry heavy loads.
- Take regular breaks between heavy tasks.
- Store tools tidily so you don't have to stretch awkwardly to reach for what you want.
- Rather than moving heavy bags of soil, mulch or fertiliser, divide them into smaller, more manageable loads and use a wheelbarrow to move them around.

At work

Here are six ways to modify your working environment when you return to work:

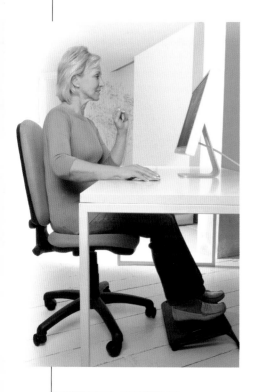

- **Change your hours** Shorter periods of desk work in front of a computer screen are more manageable than long hours. Try to take a 15-minute break every few hours or even arrange a shorter working day.

- **Adjust your tasks** A temporary change to your work can help to lessen the strain on your back. If your job includes lots of lifting and carrying, ask if you can switch to lighter tasks until you feel better. This will allow your back time to recover.

- **Check your desk** Place your monitor about an arm's length away from your eyes with the top of the screen at eye level. Keep other equipment within easy reach so you don't have to keep stretching or twisting to pick them up. Use a headset if your job involves regular long phone calls.

- **Be chair aware** Make sure your chair is at the right height and angle for your desk/workstation (see *Sit correctly*, below). Adjust your chair so that your forearms are resting comfortably on the desk and your elbows are roughly at right angles.

- **Sit correctly** When sitting, keep your shoulders back. Use a small cushion in the small of your back for lumbar support, if you have low back pain. When sitting, your hips should be slightly higher than your knees so that your upper legs are sloping down. If necessary, rest your feet on a footrest or a stack of books.

- **Break up the day** Get up and move around as often as you can. Make a drink, talk to colleagues in person rather than sending emails, do some photocopying or filing – anything that gets you moving.

FOCUS

Back to work

For many conditions affecting mobility, experts advise that it is best to carry on working or return to work as soon as you can. There will be good and bad days, but keeping yourself busy can help take your mind off the pain as well as ensuring that you remain active.

THE EARLY WEEKS

If back pain has forced you to take time off work, take the following steps to enable you and your employer to make any necessary adjustments. The same advice applies for a broad range of musculoskeletal problems. Within a week of your return to work:

- Explain to your employer or line manager how your problem is affecting your ability to work and discuss ways to make your working life easier.
- Consider consulting an occupational health professional (if available), a physiotherapist, chiropractor or osteopath. Your GP can advise whether this may be useful in your case.

Arrange a follow-up discussion with your boss for the following week. If back pain (or other problem) is still affecting you at work within two weeks of your return, further steps may be advisable. Consider making a plan with your doctor and employer to help you cope and recover. And you'll need to agree a timetable for checking that the plan is working. If it's not, you may have to make adjustments with the help of your GP and employer.

AFTER AN EXTENDED ABSENCE

If your symptoms are severe and intractable, you may not be able to return to work in the short term. If you find yourself in this situation, taking the following steps during your absence may make it easier when you do eventually resume work:

- Keep your employer up to date with any changes in your health.
- Work out a plan for returning to work or set up regular review dates.
- Explore any changes that could be made to ease your return (see *At work*, facing page).

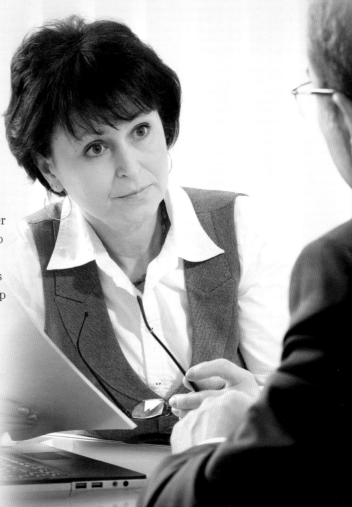

Action on arthritis

Arthritis is one of the leading causes of reduced mobility and can affect people of all ages. Medical understanding of this group of disorders is increasing year by year, and there is now a wealth of accessible treatments to help you maintain an active life.

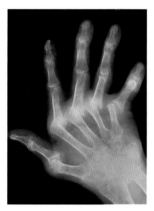 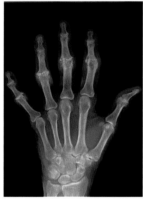

A JOINT PROBLEM

Both main types of arthritis can affect the hands. Above left is an X-ray that shows the distortion caused by RA and, above right, one showing the enlarged finger joints typical of OA.

True or False?

Osteoarthritis is a normal part of ageing

False Although OA becomes more common as people get older, it's far from inevitable. What's more, there are effective treatments and plenty you can do to ease the pain and symptoms and prevent it from getting worse.

Arthritis is an umbrella term that describes more than 200 different joint disorders, which have the following symptoms in common: pain, stiffness, restricted mobility, inflammation and swelling. The two main types of arthritis are osteoarthritis and rheumatoid arthritis.

Osteoarthritis (OA) is the most common form; it affects 1.6 million people in Australia – 7.8 per cent of the population. It is the result of changes in the cartilage (the protective covering of the bone ends). The main symptoms are pain, swelling and stiffness (after inactivity or on waking). These symptoms typically affect the finger and thumb joints, the neck, lower back, big toes, hips and knees.

Rheumatoid arthritis (RA) affects about 450,000 Australians. It most commonly first develops between the ages of 30 and 50, occurs when the immune system attacks and destroys the joint tissues, leading to inflammation. Other parts of the body such as the lungs and blood vessels may become inflamed too, and RA can also cause bone loss, which may lead to osteoporosis. The disease often proceeds in fits and starts, with periodic flare-ups. As well as arthritic symptoms, sufferers may experience fatigue, fever, malaise (a general feeling of being unwell), depression and irritability.

WHAT TO EXPECT FROM YOUR DOCTOR

For both types of arthritis your GP should discuss the following areas with you:

- exercise
- weight loss
- footwear
- hot and cold packs
- pain-relief strategies.

Your GP may recommend regular medication to relieve your pain (many helpful medicines are available over the counter), and may suggest joint replacement if you're in severe pain from OA of the hip or knee. For RA, a specialist can prescribe disease-modifying antirheumatic drugs (DMARDs) to minimise joint damage, reduce pain and help you to live as normal a life as possible. For information and advice on pain relief, see Chapter 9 (pages 214–239).

You should have regular check-ups to assess how your condition is being controlled and how it's progressing. You may be offered physiotherapy to increase joint flexibility and build up your muscle strength and an appointment to see an occupational therapist if RA affects your ability to use your hands or interferes with everyday life. Surgery may be advised if you have severe RA or your symptoms get worse despite treatment.

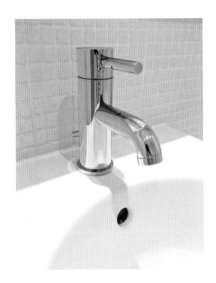

Living positively

The development of new and effective treatments, including painkillers and DMARDs, physiotherapy and surgery, has revolutionised the treatment of arthritis. But there are also ways in which you can help yourself to live as full and active a life as possible. Here are some ideas:

Protect your joints Canes to aid walking, splints to support the wrist or hand and devices to help with everyday tasks can all ease pressure on the joints. You also need to find ways to alleviate joint strain when doing everyday tasks. For example, when pouring water from the kettle, use two hands: one to hold the handle and the other to support the side of the kettle (use a folded tea towel or oven gloves to avoid getting burnt). The booklet *Looking After Your Joints When You Have Arthritis*, available online at www.cks.nhs.uk/patient_information_leaflet/arthritis, contains plenty of ideas. Arthritis Australia has good advice on its website (www.arthritisaustralia.com.au).

Manage stress Dutch researchers writing in the journal *Arthritis Research & Therapy* in May 2010 suggested that stress may exacerbate rheumatic diseases – especially those involving severe inflammation, such as RA – by altering the way the immune, nervous and hormonal systems work. Moderate your lifestyle to minimise stress and use techniques such as breathing exercises and relaxation to help you deal with it.

Simple adaptations to fittings in the home, such as lever controls for taps, can make all the difference

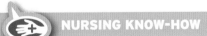

NURSING KNOW-HOW

Balance activity and rest

Professionals with experience in caring for people with arthritis suggest they do better if they have several short spells of rest throughout the day. Spending long periods in bed can weaken the muscles, reduce fitness levels and make symptoms worse.

Joint-replacement surgery

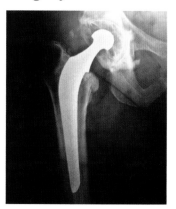

Surgery such as a hip-joint replacement (shown in the X-ray above) can help alleviate pain and improve movement – depending on the severity of your arthritis and the strength of the surrounding muscles. Ask your doctor what degree of improvement you can expect from the operation. You may want to consider surgery if:

Arthritis stops you sleeping at night.

Lack of mobility makes everyday activities difficult – for example, going up stairs, going to the toilet or working.

Your symptoms mean that you put off doing activities you enjoy such as visiting friends or taking a holiday.

Your medication is ineffective.

For more information visit: www.arthritisaustralia. com.au/images/stories/ documents/info_sheets/2013/ SurgeryforArthritis.pdf.

Take control Numerous studies indicate that feeling helpless makes any pain and disability worse. Research shows that people with self-management skills are more able to cope both physically and mentally, have a better quality of life, experience less pain, make fewer visits to the doctor and have a greater sense of confidence in their ability to cope. To find a course, contact your local Arthritis Australia office by calling 1800 011 041.

Enlist support Having a strong support system that includes friends and family can help you to maintain a positive attitude, as well as providing practical help when you need it.

Managing everyday life

Having arthritis shouldn't mean a future of disability and dependency. With a little forethought and planning, you should be able to adjust your surroundings and everyday life so you can cope with household tasks and maintain mobility and independence. Here are some suggestions:

AT HOME

Distribute tasks Spread household tasks over several days rather than trying to do them all at once. Don't do all the housework yourself – ask the rest of your family to help if you can.

Make it easy on yourself Keep utensils and cleaning materials within easy reach; have a stool handy to sit on while you prepare food, do the ironing, etc.; move objects from room to room on a trolley; fill the kettle with just the amount of water you need so that it's easier to carry and pour; wear thick gloves to reduce joint strain when holding tools and heavy objects.

Adapt it Fix handrails to walls, get lever taps fitted, use a long stick with a rubber end to operate push-button appliances, use a long-handled brush or sponge for washing-up or cleaning.

Take a shower If getting in and out of the bath is difficult, install a walk-in shower instead. You can have a seat attached to the wall so that you can sit down while you wash.

Let stronger parts take the strain Ease strain on smaller, weaker joints by using larger parts of your body to carry heavy items. For example, carry shopping bags using your forearms or the palms of your hands, rather than your fingers.

Select the right shoes For everyday wear choose well-cushioned lace-up or bar shoes with good arch support. If your feet are uncomfortable,

Case Study

A JOINT REPLACEMENT STORY

How one man's determination kept him mobile despite multiple operations

Terry Lawrence, 65, from Melbourne, is a retired public health worker. He describes his joint-replacement surgery below.

Ten years ago I never imagined that I would be so active and pain-free. I started getting a lot of pain in one of my knees when I was in my mid-50s, and the GP diagnosed osteoarthritis. The pain got so bad that in the end I had to have my knee replaced. I was devastated: I thought that was something that happened to people in their eighties. But within six weeks I was back taking my two dogs on their 2-km walks. Since then I've had to have both my shoulders replaced and I will probably have a hip replacement too, so it looks like I will soon be fully bionic.

I don't want to make it sound as if joint replacement is a perfect cure: you have a plastic or metal joint put in and you are always aware of that. But the recovery is very quick and I had no pain after it was done. OA is a chronic condition. I can't run around with my grandchildren as I could have done if I didn't have it and if I get down on the floor to play with them it's hard to get up again. But I don't let it defeat me. I've learned to pace myself, but as a former single parent, I'm used to being on the go all the time. I have to make myself take a break and put my feet up. I was worried I might not be able to cycle any more after my hip replacement, but my friend showed me an electrically assisted bicycle and I plan to get one of those so I can still join my friends for bike rides. 99

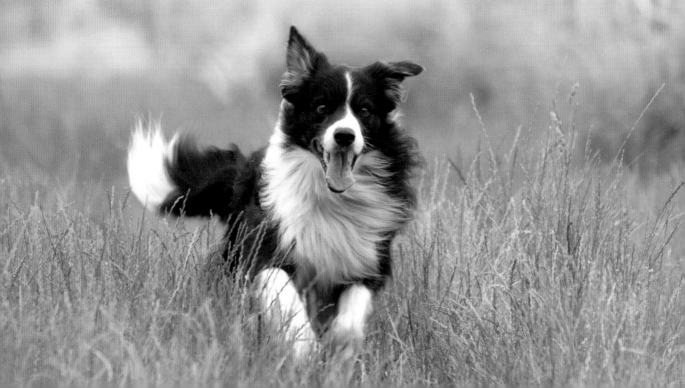

it may help to have an orthotic – a special insole – fitted. Avoid raised heels, but if you like to wear them occasionally, choose heels no higher than 2.5 cm.

AT WORK

Pace yourself Intersperse more demanding activities with less demanding ones. Change activity, stretch or rest at the first hint of discomfort. Don't wait until you're in pain.

Learn to prioritise Do activities in order of importance and think about what you could eliminate, postpone, delegate or get help with.

Assess how you work Do you spend a long time doing the same or similar repetitive tasks? Is your posture contributing to any pain or discomfort? Could a change of activity or posture help?

Seek solutions Would it be possible to work fewer hours or go part-time, job share, work flexitime, change your job, work from home from time to time or retrain for lighter work? If you've had time off, speak to your employer about a phased return. See *Back to work*, page 91.

IN THE BEDROOM

When it comes to sex, the traditional 'missionary' position can be uncomfortable if arthritis affects your hip, knee, leg or arm. Experiment with different ways to give and receive pleasure – for example, using your hands or a vibrator, or practising oral sex, and try positions that put less strain on the joints, for example:

- The 'spoons' position (side by side with the man behind – good if the woman has hip problems).
- The woman lying on her back with her knees together and a pillow under her hips and thighs (good if the woman has hip or knee problems or cannot move her legs apart). The man lies over her with his legs either side of hers.
- Side position facing each other (good if the man has back problems).
- The man on his back with pillows for support (good if the man has hip or knee problems).

Eat to beat arthritis

There is little scientific evidence to support many of the 'fad' diets that claim to beat arthritis, but there is an increasing acceptance that certain dietary measures can play a role in countering inflammation and therefore help to ease many of the symptoms of arthritis, as well

---

True or False?

Losing weight can help to slow the development of arthritis

True Even a small weight loss can make a big difference to your symptoms. According to research, each half kilo of weight lost will result in a four-fold reduction in the load exerted on the knee per step taken. But that's not all. Several studies show that loss of fat rather than loss of weight is what's important. That's because fat that accumulates around the organs produces inflammatory chemicals, and inflammation is a feature of many types of arthritis.

as protecting you against heart disease and metabolic syndrome (page 101), which are risks for people with RA. According to a review published in *Best Practice & Research Clinical Rheumatology* in 2008, the following food choices may help:

Eat a balanced diet with plenty of fresh fruit and vegetables: these are rich in antioxidant vitamins and minerals, such as vitamin C, vitamin E and selenium, which can help reduce the inflammation of many types of arthritis.

Take a vitamin E supplement This may help ease pain for some people with RA. Ask your doctor before taking any supplement.

Get enough vitamin C (found in most vegetables and fruit). It may slow the progression of OA.

Include copper (found in calf's liver, sesame seeds and raw cashew nuts) and zinc (from milk, shellfish, meat and dairy products) in your diet. This mineral may help maintain the health of connective tissue according to some studies.

Have healthy fats Replace spreads and oils made from 'vegetable' or sunflower oils with canola and olive-oil based products: these contain fatty acids with anti-inflammatory properties.

Eat fish Researchers advise eating two portions a week of oil-rich fish, such as salmon, mackerel, sardine or fresh tuna, and taking high-strength fish oil capsules (look for one supplying around 190 mg EPA and 120 mg DHA – both of which are essential fatty acids – a day) for at least three months. Fish may not suit some people with RA who have a particular genetic profile, however, so if there's no benefit or if your symptoms worsen, stop taking the supplement.

Check for food intolerance This may be a factor for some people with RA. Common culprits are corn, wheat, pork, oranges, milk, oats, rye, eggs, beef and coffee. Keep a diet diary to help you identify trigger foods.

Enjoy a Mediterranean diet (one that is high in fresh fruit and vegetables, and fish, with only moderate amounts of red meat and dairy products). This balance of foods may help ease pain and early-morning stiffness.

Gout guidance

Gout, which causes similar symptoms to some types of arthritis, occurs when the body is unable to manage the breakdown and excretion of chemicals called purines, found in many protein-based foods. When this happens, the body produces higher-than-normal levels of uric acid. The acid builds up and forms crystals, which accumulate in a joint (often the big toe) causing pain and inflammation.

Attacks of gout often come on suddenly. Anti-inflammatory drugs, and sometimes stronger painkillers, are prescribed; the inflamed joint may also be immobilised with a splint and ice applied.

To prevent further gout attacks:

Avoid alcohol.

Lose weight if you need to.

Ask your doctor if any medications you are taking cause elevated blood levels of uric acid (for example, thiazide diuretics) and if you can avoid taking them.

Cut down on purine-rich foods. These include anchovies, asparagus, consommé, herring, meat gravies and broths, mushrooms, mussels, offal and sardines.

Add cherries to the diet, as these reduce the number of acute attacks of gout.

Include oily fish in your diet for optimum joint health

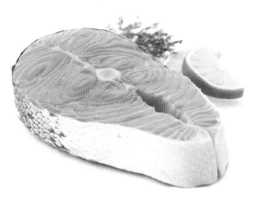

Moving on

According to the US Arthritis Foundation, exercise is the most effective non-drug treatment for reducing pain and improving movement in people with OA, and it can also help reduce pain and stiffness in those with RA. It can strengthen the muscles that support the joints, improve joint stability and help to maintain flexibility. It can also reduce bone loss, aid sleep, lessen pain, improve mood and help control weight.

YOUR EXERCISE PLAN

Aim to include endurance, strength and stretching exercises in your exercise regimen as well as building more physical activity into your everyday life. Take it slowly and bear in mind that it can take up to three months to start feeling benefits. Never force a painful joint. However you choose to exercise, you need to plan a program that

RANGE-OF-MOVEMENT EXERCISES

Daily activities, such as housework, going up and down stairs, dressing, bathing, cooking, lifting and bending, don't put your joints through their full range of movement. It's a good idea, therefore, to do daily range-of-movement exercises, as advised by your physiotherapist, to improve your joint flexibility. Ask your GP to refer you to a physiotherapist, who will be able to offer advice specific to your condition. Physiotherapist Michele Harms suggests the exercises (right) for key joints typically affected by arthritis:

KNEES

1 *Sit on the bed with your legs straight out in front of you, or lie down if it's more comfortable.*

2 *Working one leg at a time, pull the toes towards you, tighten the thigh muscles and press the back of the knee down onto the bed.*

3 *Slowly relax then gently bring your knee as close to your chest as the pain allows. Repeat for the other leg.*

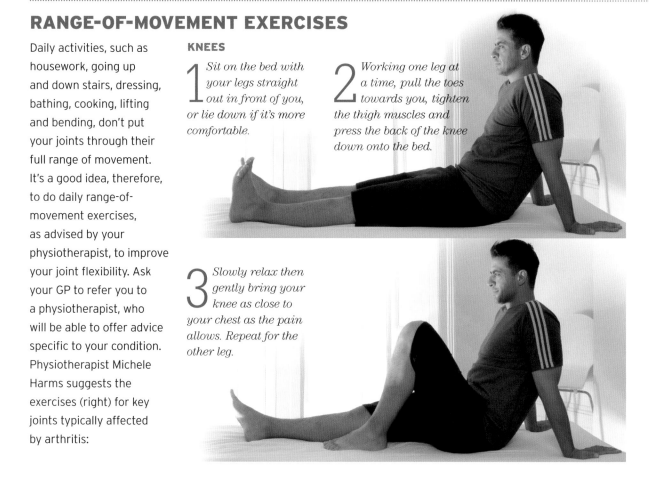

meets your changing needs over time. You should also avoid high-impact exercise, such as jogging, and wear supportive, shock-absorbing footwear when you exercise.

CHOOSE YOUR ACTIVITY

If you need to improve your general fitness, walking is perhaps your best option. It is low impact and reduces the risk of osteoporosis. Use your walking aid if you normally have one (make sure it is the right height). Swimming is also an excellent choice for strengthening muscles without putting strain on your joints. It also benefits your heart.

Some gyms have instructors trained to help people with health problems. You may be eligible for an 'exercise prescription' from your GP, which entitles you to regular gym sessions. Remember, you are likely to ache and be stiff when you start any new exercise, but if you feel unusual pain during or after exercise, consult your doctor.

WRISTS

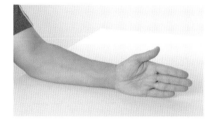

1 Sit with your forearm resting on a table and your thumb uppermost.

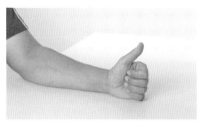

2 Gently curl your fingers inwards into the palm.

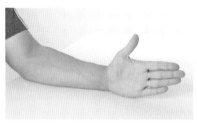

3 Slowly stretch them backwards, opening your hand and straightening the fingers. Repeat with the other hand.

HIPS

1 If you're able, lie on your side with your lower knee bent and your other leg straight.

2 Lift the straight top leg towards the ceiling.

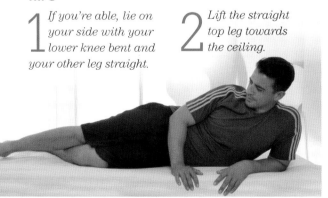

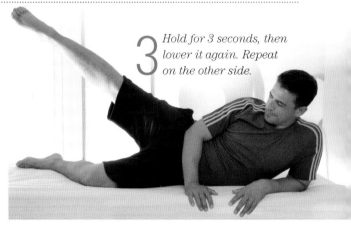

3 Hold for 3 seconds, then lower it again. Repeat on the other side.

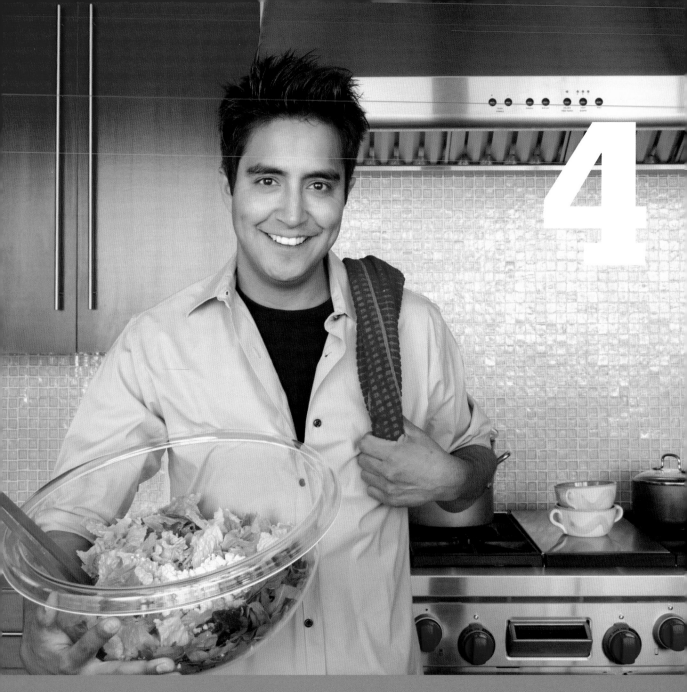

Dealing with diabetes

A diagnosis of diabetes can be a wake-up call that
sets you on the path to a healthier, fuller life

You've been diagnosed – what next?

Some 180 million people have diabetes worldwide and, if trends continue, this could double by 2030. If you're one of those affected, you may fear that a constant round of medications, injections and clinic appointments is all that lies ahead. But by making some lifestyle changes and possibly taking medication, you can lead a full life and may even feel healthier and fitter than you did before.

Diabetes results in high levels of glucose (sugar) in the blood. It occurs when the pancreas – an elongated oval gland about the size of your hand that sits behind the stomach – stops making the hormone insulin, or does not make enough insulin, or the insulin it produces does not work as well as it should (insulin resistance). Insulin is a chemical messenger in the blood that enables blood glucose to enter body cells to be used as fuel. If the amount or action of the insulin is inadequate, glucose levels in the blood become too high.

KNOW YOUR TYPE

There are three main types of diabetes, outlined below (rarer types exist, usually either inherited or linked to damage to the pancreas).
Type 1 The commonest type in childhood, type 1 occurs when the body's immune system destroys the insulin-producing cells in the pancreas. It's treated with insulin.
Type 2 This is the most common type, and it tends to appear after the age of 40, although children and teenagers can develop it too, and it's often linked to being overweight. It occurs when the pancreatic cells don't produce enough insulin or the body develops insulin resistance (see above). Treatments include weight loss for those who are overweight, a healthy diet, regular activity and medication and/or insulin.

Testing times

To diagnose diabetes, your doctor may do a fasting blood glucose test in the morning, before you've eaten anything, and/or an oral glucose tolerance test (OGTT), in which your blood glucose is tested before and 2 hours after you have a glucose drink. The test involves taking a sample of your blood.

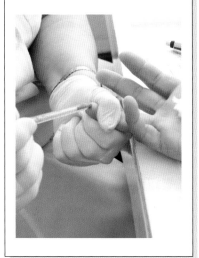

I've heard about metabolic syndrome. What is it?

The condition metabolic syndrome is actually a cluster of risk factors - high blood pressure, excess fat around the middle, high cholesterol and insulin resistance. Left untreated, the condition makes people more vulnerable to heart disease and stroke, and insulin resistance often leads to type 2 diabetes. There may be no obvious symptoms. If you are concerned, consult your doctor who can conduct tests and possibly prescribe medication. Lifestyle changes, such as losing weight and taking exercise, may also delay - or prevent - the onset of diabetes at this stage.

Gestational diabetes During the second half of pregnancy, a woman's placenta makes hormones that block the action of insulin to ensure that her baby gets enough glucose. To compensate, the pancreas makes more insulin, but about 1 in 20 pregnant women can't make enough, which results in a rise in blood glucose levels. This condition, called gestational diabetes, usually disappears after the baby is born, but if you've had it, you have a 50 per cent risk of developing type 2 diabetes within ten years. The risk factors include smoking, being overweight, having a family history of type 2 diabetes and being over the age of 35.

SYMPTOM WATCH

Insatiable hunger (in type 1), raging thirst and a constant need to urinate, especially at night, are the classic symptoms of diabetes. Others include blurred eyesight, frequent infections, itchy skin, unexplained weight loss (in type 1), tiredness and cuts and bruises that take a long time to heal.

Type 1 symptoms are usually obvious and appear quickly, within days or weeks. Type 2 develops slowly, often without specific symptoms, and may be detected only by chance at a routine check-up. See your GP if you have symptoms or risk factors (see *Are you at risk?*, left).

First steps

Discovering you have diabetes can come as a shock, and it's natural to worry about how it will affect your life. But it can be reassuring to know that you won't be tackling it alone. Once diagnosed, you'll have regular medical check-ups and the chance to discuss how your condition will

The support of your diabetes health-care team will be vital in the months and years following your diagnosis

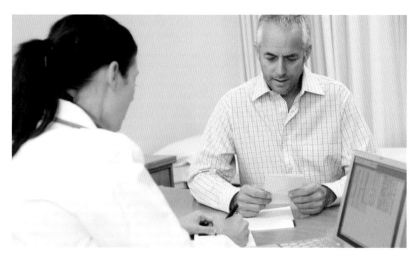

KNOW YOUR DIABETES HEALTH-CARE TEAM

Listed below are some of the key doctors, nurses and other specialists who may be involved in your care. For a list of the regular checks you will need, see page 118.

Endocrinologist This doctor specialises in diabetes and will oversee your care, usually in their rooms or at a hospital clinic.

Credentialled diabetes educator A diabetes educator is a nurse with advanced skills, who will play a vital role in giving you the skills and support to manage your condition, particularly in the first year after diagnosis.

General practitioner (GP) You GP will coordinate the whole health-care team. Care may be shared between the GP and endocrinologist or the GP may be the main carer, with occasional specialist consultations.

Practice nurse The nurse at your general practice may be responsible for a lot of routine care, such as reviewing blood glucose level logs.

Dietitian Your dietitian will assess your eating habits and help you make the best lifestyle and food choices so you can manage your diabetes effectively.

Podiatrist A footcare specialist will check the health of your feet regularly if you develop problems.

Eye-care specialists An ophthalmologist or optometrist will perform regular eye examinations and tests to check the health of the front and back of your eye.

Psychologist A specialist in counselling can help those with diabetes who may be having difficulties making the psychological adjustment to living with their condition.

Exercise physiologist/physiotherapist Exercise is an important part of managing diabetes, and this team member will work out the best exercise and activities for you.

Dentist People with diabetes need good dental care, so you should see your dentist for regular check-ups.

Pharmacist It's best to always go to the same chemist, so that the pharmacist can keep an eye out for medication errors and give you personalised advice.

---

be managed with the support of your diabetes health-care team (see above). From now on, you will work with them to control your diabetes and minimise the risk of complications, such as heart disease, stroke, nerve damage and kidney or eye problems. Here are some tips on getting the most from your time with the team:

- Make a list of questions to ask. Don't be afraid to raise them for fear of seeming silly or anxious or taking up too much time.
- Work with the team to set realistic goals and decide how you can meet them. These are the basis of your care plan.
- See a specialist dietitian (usually part of your health-care team) to discuss your diet and any changes you may need to make.
- For further help, contact Diabetes Australia. Their website is full of useful information (www.diabetesaustralia.com.au) or talk to someone on their information line (1300 136 588).

Type 2 diabetes is only mild

False Sadly there's no such thing as 'mild' diabetes. But with lifestyle changes and medication, if necessary, you can live a healthy, active life.

True or False?

Adapting to treatment

Since the 1970s, new treatments and technology have revolutionised diabetes care. These include more effective oral and injectable medications, improved types of insulin, useful devices such as blood glucose meters, insulin pens and insulin pumps. Specialists also have a better understanding of how to reduce the risk of complications.

Questions to ask

Ask your doctor the questions below to help you get to grips with your medication regime as quickly as possible:

- *What is this medication and what is it for?*
- *How long will it take to work?*
- *How much should I take?*
- *How often and when should I take it?*
- *Do I need to take the medication before, with or after a meal?*
- *Are there specific foods or drinks that I should avoid?*
- *Are there any side effects?*
- *Is there any situation that would cause me to change the amount of medication I take?*
- *Can this medication cause low blood glucose (hypoglycaemia), and what should I do if this happens?*
- *How should I store this medication?*

Most people with diabetes have to take lifelong medication. Australians with diabetes can get subsidised diabetes-related products through the National Diabetes Services Scheme (www.ndss.com.au) and medications through the Pharmaceutical Benefits Scheme.

TEAM SUPPORT

It is natural to worry how you will manage your treatment – especially if you need injections. Talk to your health-care team. Finding the drug regime that is right for you may also involve a certain amount of trial and error. Your health-care team will support you until you feel confident with your treatment.

 NURSING KNOW-HOW

If you forget to take your tablet

Some oral medications for type 2 diabetes are taken at specific times in relation to meals. If you forget to take one of these, skip that dose and take the next one when due. NEVER double your dose. For medications on other schedules, take the missed dose when remembered, unless there is less than 2 hours until the next dose is due. Talk to your doctor if you often forget your medication. There are aids that can help make remembering easier.

MONITORING YOUR BLOOD GLUCOSE

To gauge how well your treatment is working, it is best to check your blood glucose at regular intervals – your health-care team will advise how often you should do this. Modern glucose meters ensure that the procedure is quite straightforward and a spring-loaded lancing device makes it simple and painless to take blood. Your health-care team can also help you choose a style of meter that suits you. Diabetes Australia provides useful background information. The latest innovation is glucose watches, which can be used without having to draw blood. But they are likely to be expensive and there is some debate about their accuracy.

Living with insulin

Insulin, the hormone that people with diabetes lack, is the keystone of treatment in type 1 diabetes, and involves daily insulin injections for life. If you have type 2 diabetes, you may also have to take insulin at some point. The fact that the hormone has to be injected, as well as the lifelong duration of the treatment, can be difficult for some people to come to terms with. However, your health-care team will teach you how to manage your injections. The vast majority of people adjust to insulin self-administration quickly. The introduction of insulin pens, which have an integral insulin reservoir and a simple dosage control, to replace standard syringes has made injection even easier for many people.

PUMP IT UP

An alternative to injections is the insulin pump, which uses continuous subcutaneous insulin infusion (CSII). This small device delivers a continuous dose of insulin through a thin tube, usually in the abdomen. This method of administration may be a good choice for those whose type 1 diabetes has not been adequately controlled by multiple insulin injections or for whom multiple injections may not be practical (notably children). A pump is not an easy option and requires the user to adhere to a regular glucose testing routine for successful use. If you're interested, your health-care team will discuss the pros and cons with you.

CREATE A ROUTINE THAT WORKS FOR YOU

To control your diabetes effectively, you need to establish a routine for taking medication when your body needs it; this is determined by your intake of food and how much energy you expend. Initially you will have to monitor your blood glucose levels several times a day, at least, and discuss

TESTING YOUR BLOOD GLUCOSE

The typical stages involved in self-testing are shown below, but be sure to follow the instructions for the kit you are using. Your doctor will tell you the blood glucose level range you should be aiming for (see page 114).

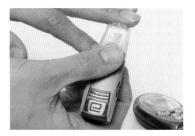

1 *Put a new test strip in the meter. Use the lancing device to draw a drop of blood from the side of a finger.*

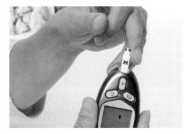

2 *Touch the drop of blood against the test strip in the meter.*

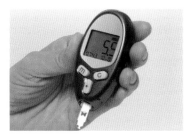

3 *Wait for the result to appear on the meter screen. Discard the used test strip.*

the results with the appropriate members of your health-care team, as instructed by your doctor. The team will create a workable schedule with you, taking into account your lifestyle and daily routine. For most people with diabetes, injecting insulin quickly becomes a normal part of daily life. A strong incentive to stick to your routine is knowing that it will help you to avoid diabetes complications, such as foot ulcers, sight problems and even kidney failure (see *Staying on track*, pages 117–119).

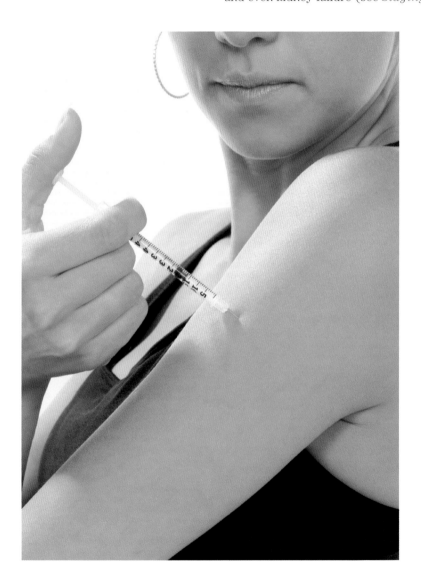

Change insulin injection sites every week or so for the best results

CHOOSING WHERE TO INJECT

The four main injection sites for insulin are the stomach, buttocks, thighs and upper arms. Of these, insulin is most rapidly absorbed from the abdomen. Administer each injection about 4 cm away from the previous one, and change sites every week or so. Repeatedly injecting into the same place may cause a fatty lump to develop, which can interfere with insulin absorption and affect your ability to control your blood glucose.

BE 'HYPO-AWARE'

Hypoglycaemia – a 'hypo' – occurs if your blood glucose level drops to less than 4 mmol/l (see *Glucose guidelines*, page 114). Hypos can happen if you are on insulin or tablets for diabetes. They may result from taking too much insulin or other diabetes medication, missing or delaying a meal, not eating enough carbohydrates, taking more exercise than usual, hot weather, having too much alcohol or drinking alcohol without food. Over time, there is a risk that you may become 'hypo-unaware' (see *Restoring 'hypo awareness'*, page 118).

Managing hypos

You should be aware of the key signs of a hypo, and make sure your friends, family and colleagues are also aware. Immediate action - by you or someone else - is needed, and treatment depends on the severity. Advice is given here for mild, moderate and severe hypos, and key symptoms are listed below. If possible, test your glucose level before treating a hypo.

MILD HYPOGLYCAEMIA

In a mild hypo you are aware of the symptoms and able to act on them yourself.

1 Stop and take a rapidly absorbed carbohydrate. Examples of readily available and effective sources of carbohydrate include:

● a sugary drink (not diet drinks) or fruit juice
● glucose, in the form of tablets or gel
● a couple of teaspoons of sugar, honey or jam.

Repeat if there is no improvement in 5–10 minutes.

2 Follow this up by eating a more slow-release or starchy carbohydrate snack such as a sandwich, piece of fruit, bowl of cereal, biscuit and milk, or a meal if you're due one.

MODERATE HYPOGLYCAEMIA

In a moderately severe hypo you may be confused and unable to take the necessary action yourself.

1 Others may need to take the initial action needed to restore your blood glucose levels. They should squirt or rub a glucose gel or something sweet, but not solid, such as syrup, jam or honey, into the inside of your cheeks. The outside of your cheeks should be gently massaged to aid absorption.

2 Once you're able to, have a sugary drink, followed by a starchy snack.

SEVERE HYPOGLYCAEMIA

Severe hypos result in loss of consciousness and possibly seizures. In this situation you need urgent medical help. If someone whom you know to have

SYMPTOMS OF HYPOGLYCAEMIA	
You may notice	**Other people may notice**
● hunger	
● trembling or shakiness	● pallor
● sweating	● glazed eyes
● anxiety or irritability	● slurred words/ inability to speak
● fatigue	● lack of coordination
● palpitations	● mood changes
● tingling lips	● confusion
● headache	● irrational behaviour
● blurred vision	

diabetes or who is wearing a diabetes identification tag (see page 115) loses consciousness, take the following steps:

1 Do not give him or her anything by mouth, but if you can do so, give a glucagon injection. Glucagon is a hormone that triggers the liver to release stored glucose. It takes around 15 minutes to restore consciousness in someone having a hypo.

2 If this is not possible or the person fails to regain consciousness, call an ambulance without delay.

3 Once the person has regained full consciousness following a glucagon injection and can swallow again, offer a sugary drink and a starchy snack as described under mild hypoglycaemia, step 2.

Lifestyle tweaks to boost your health

It's true that your life will change - possibly for ever. But it's important to remember too that this is an opportunity to make some relatively simple lifestyle adjustments - to your diet, exercise habits and mental attitude - that will benefit your health for years to come.

True or False?

There is no cure for diabetes

Largely true Although in rare cases a pancreas transplant can offer a cure for type 1 diabetes, this is not widely available. Type 2 diabetes is also usually considered incurable. But several studies have found that in people who are very obese, a stomach bypass (bariatric surgery) can actually cure type 2 diabetes - often within days. The reason? It's not known, but some scientists think the accelerated transit of nutrients from the upper part of the stomach to the gut improves the body's ability to use glucose. Others speculate that an unknown chemical, in the bypassed part of the stomach, promotes insulin resistance and diabetes.

Eating your way better

A healthy diet can help keep your blood glucose, blood fats and blood pressure in check and lower the risk of complications whatever kind of diabetes you have. You'll probably find that eating healthily is much more enjoyable than you think.

These days, people with diabetes are advised to stick to a diet that's much the same as the healthy diet recommended for everyone (see pages 22–26), but with some provisos. Here's how to stay on track:

Be consistent Always eat three meals a day, and space them out over the day, just as everyone should do.

Include carbs Include starchy carbohydrate (carb) foods, such as bread, pasta, rice, noodles, cereals and potatoes, in every meal. This will help to stabilise blood glucose levels throughout the day. Starchy carbs that contain higher levels of fibre, such as wholegrain products, are digested more slowly, helping to keep your glucose levels steady.

Match meals with medication Too little food in relation to medication – especially insulin – can cause hypoglycaemia (see page 107), while too much can result in high blood glucose (hyperglycaemia). Your diabetes health-care team can help you strike a balance. It's best to match your insulin dose to food intake, not vice versa.

COUNTING CARBS

Carb counting, a method of matching your insulin dose to your intake of carbohydrates, can give you better blood glucose control and a more flexible lifestyle. It's a very good way to help manage your blood glucose if you have type 1 diabetes. It's less useful if you have type 2, as the insulin-to-carb ratio is likely to be different due to insulin resistance. Carb counting involves identifying carbohydrates in food and using this

Balance your food groups

Whether you have type 1 or type 2 diabetes, to keep healthy and maintain your current weight, your daily diet should include foods from the five main food groups in roughly the proportions shown on the plate, right.

Every meal doesn't have to contain precisely these proportions – and foods and drinks high in fat and sugar can be omitted – but it is important to get most of your kilojoules from fruit and vegetables, and from starchy carbohydrate foods such as bread, rice, potatoes and pasta. Maintaining the plate balance shown here will help to keep your blood glucose levels steady.

If you need to lose weight, you should try to increase the proportion of fruit and vegetables to around 50 per cent and cut down on milk and dairy products, and non-dairy sources of protein, without reducing the amount of starchy carbohydrates you eat. When you're on a weight-loss diet, high-fat and high-sugar foods should be kept to the minimum.

These are only general guidelines; your dietitian will give you advice tailored to your individual needs.

Fruit and vegetables (excluding potatoes)

Bread, rice, potatoes, pasta and other high-carbohydrate foods

Meat, fish, eggs, beans and other non-dairy sources of protein

Foods and drinks high in fat and/or sugar

Milk and dairy products

information to calculate the amount of insulin needed in relation to your energy needs. You can get books, leaflets and web-based tools showing the amount of carbohydrates in particular foods and most nutrition labels show grams of carbs per serving. To learn how to count carbs, ask your dietitian, or diabetes educator. More information is available at www.diabetesaustralia.com.au.

IF YOU NEED TO LOSE WEIGHT ...

If you're overweight, losing just 10 per cent of your body weight can improve your insulin sensitivity and glucose tolerance as well as reducing your blood pressure and cholesterol levels. If you have diabetes, it can sometimes be hard to slim down because certain treatments (in particular some medications used in the treatment of type 2 diabetes) may cause you to gain weight. Your dietitian or diabetes educator can help you find the best combination of medication, diet and activity.

The best way to shed kilograms is to make small, healthy changes to what you eat and increase your activity levels rather than going on a strict diet. Diabetes Australia advises filling half your plate with vegetables or salad, a third with starchy foods and most of the rest with low-fat protein such as lean meat, fish, chicken, lentils or beans.

The GI factor

Increasingly, experts think that levelling the rise in blood glucose after a meal is a vital tool for managing diabetes effectively. One popular way to do this is to select foods with a lower glycaemic index (GI). The GI scores carbohydrates by how quickly they are absorbed and how rapidly they push up blood glucose. Pure glucose is almost instantly absorbed and scores 100.

Before the GI diet came to prominence in the early 1980s, scientists thought so-called 'simple' carbs – found in sweets, pastries, cakes and so on – were absorbed and boosted blood glucose faster than 'complex' carbs – contained in foods such as baked potatoes, legumes and wholegrain cereals. The GI changed all that, as some complex carbs – baked potatoes, for instance – were found to raise blood glucose almost as fast as simple foods such as cornflakes. Both have a high GI.

GI OR GL?

What the GI doesn't take into account is portion size. Carrots have a high GI, for example, but you'd have to eat vast amounts to have a noticeable effect on your blood glucose, because, by weight, they contain few carbs. That's why today the glycaemic load (GL), which ranks foods according to the amount of carbs in a typical portion, is regarded as more reliable.

A growing number of studies show that low-GI/GL diets increase sensitivity to insulin, leading to better control of blood glucose and lower levels of fats in the blood. There's also evidence that they can help control weight partly by making you feel fuller for longer. The chart (above right) shows some food swaps you may want to make for better blood glucose control. The GI and GL of a wide variety of foods can be found at www.glycemicindex.com.

GL-FRIENDLY FOOD SWAPS

Instead of	Go for
Chips	Sweet potato wedges
White rice	Basmati rice, quinoa, bulghur wheat, pearl barley, pasta cooked al dente
White bread	Coarse wholegrain bread, sourdough bread, dense rye bread
Cornflakes/rice cereal	Porridge oats
Sweetcorn	Beans and lentils
Crisps and other salty snacks	Unsalted nuts
Sweet drinks/ fruit juices	Skimmed milk or vegetable juices

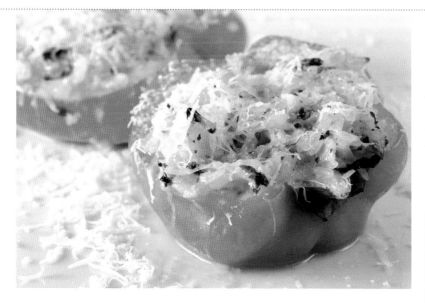

Go for meals that are full of vegetables for optimum control of your diabetes

Take it slowly and aim for a modest loss of 0.5–1 kg a week, aiming initially for no more than a 10 per cent weight loss. If, despite your efforts, you cannot reach a healthy weight (that is, your BMI remains 27+), weight-loss medication or even weight-loss (bariatric) surgery (see *True or False?*, page 108) may be recommended.

WATCH YOUR TRIGLYCERIDES

You probably know about cholesterol in your blood and why you should keep it in check (see page 128). But did you know that triglycerides – another type of blood fat – are also closely linked to metabolic syndrome, type 2 diabetes and cardiovascular disease? Cutting down on carbohydrate intake (especially high-GI carbs), reducing alcohol intake, taking regular exercise and losing weight all help lower triglyceride levels. Fish oils are especially effective – another good reason to include oily fish in your menu.

GO MEDITERRANEAN

A Mediterranean diet can help delay the need for blood glucose-lowering medication. So says a study of 215 overweight newly diagnosed people with type 2 diabetes published in the journal *Annals of Internal Medicine* in 2010. The study compared the standard low-fat, kilojoule-restricted diet usually recommended by the American Diabetic Association for people with type 2 diabetes with a Mediterranean diet containing a high proportion of vegetables, fruit, grains, legumes and nuts with some cheese or yoghurt, fish, poultry and eggs. The overall proportion of kilojoules derived from carbohydrates in such a diet is relatively low (less than 50 per cent) and its fats are mostly monounsaturated, mainly olive oil.

The carb debate

According to most diabetes specialists, a low-fat, high-carb diet is best for treating diabetes. But some experts argue that when it comes to maintaining a healthy weight and lowering blood pressure, a low-carb diet is as good or better – especially for those with non-insulin dependent type 2 diabetes. The low-carb proponents also point to the benefits of this approach in reducing the levels of damaging triglycerides and boosting levels of 'good' HDL fats in the blood – important in reducing your risk of heart disease and stroke.

There is no consensus among doctors, so the best approach is to discuss all dietary options with your health-care team before making any changes; sudden reductions in carbs could put you at risk of hypos, particularly if you are on insulin.

It's also important that you do not replace the carbs with unhealthy fatty foods. Eating more foods with a lower glycaemic load (see facing page), such as vegetables and fruit, is a better option.

After four years, just 44 per cent of people on the Mediterranean diet needed blood glucose-lowering medication compared with 70 per cent on the low-fat diet. Those eating the Mediterranean way also lost more weight and had lower levels of blood fats and blood pressure.

EASE UP ON ALCOHOL

Your liver normally releases glucose that has been stored as glycogen to offset falling blood glucose levels, but if it's processing alcohol it may not work as effectively. If you're on insulin and some oral medications, such as sulphonylurea drugs, even a small amount of alcohol can cause hypoglycaemia shortly after drinking and for up to 16 hours afterwards. A useful tip for those who continue to enjoy the occasional tipple is always to accompany it with a low-fat snack. And be aware that keeping your alcohol intake low will help keep your blood pressure low.

Get active

Being active is vital for your health, regardless of your circumstances, and especially if you have diabetes. Pick activities you enjoy and get moving – you'll feel much better for it. Becoming more active will help to improve your insulin sensitivity (which means that you'll need a lower dosage of insulin or other medication), lower your blood glucose, control your weight, lower your blood pressure and levels of harmful blood fats, and help shift any stubborn abdominal fat – and that's on top of other benefits such as increased stamina, strength and flexibility, and improved sleep.

If you haven't exercised for a while, have your cardiovascular risk factors, such as cholesterol and blood pressure, and other diabetes complications assessed. Ask your doctor or physiotherapist for advice on safe activities before starting.

EVIDENCE FOR THE BENEFITS

A 2005 Italian study of 179 people with type 2 diabetes, reported in *Diabetes Care*, found that previously inactive people who did the equivalent of a 5-km daily walk had lower blood pressure, lower unhealthy blood fats, lower blood glucose and a lower risk of heart disease risk after two years – even without weight loss. Those who were most active also saw a reduction in their weight, BMI and waist circumference. Better still, a quarter were able to stop taking insulin. For maximum benefit, the researchers recommend walking for an hour a day at 5 kph, or 45 minutes a day at 6.5 kph. And the findings of a study reported in the journal *Nature* in

Top Tips

Safe drinking with diabetes

It's generally safe to have a little alcohol as long as you stick to the following guidelines:

- Never drink if your blood glucose is low or your stomach is empty.

- Don't exceed 2 standard drinks on any given day (both men and women). See page 26.

- Check your blood glucose before drinking and before going to bed. Always eat a small, low-GI snack with an alcoholic drink.

- Always wear medical ID (see page 115). To those who don't know you have diabetes, the symptoms of a hypo can be similar to drunkenness.

- If you're watching your weight, choose lower-kilojoule drinks such as dry white wine. And don't forget to count alcohol in your daily carb or kilojoule allowance.

May 2010 suggest that exercise revs up the breakdown of stored glucose, blood fats and amino acids, as well as improving blood glucose control.

GET STARTED...

Choose light to moderate activities if your diabetes is not well controlled. Here are some tips for moderate exercise activities: brisk walking (outside or on a treadmill), swimming or aqua-aerobics, cycling (outside or on a stationary exercise bike), dancing, yoga, gardening, golf and racket sports such as badminton or tennis (doubles games tend to be less strenuous). Water-based exercises have the advantage of putting less strain on the joints.

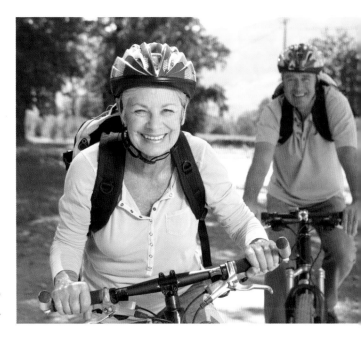

Exercise can be fun to share with a friend or partner

YOUR ACTIVITY PROGRAM

If you've been inactive or only moderately active in the past few months, the following outline exercise program will help you get into your stride and begin building exercise into your lifestyle. In this context, mild activity is defined as exercise that doesn't make you out of breath and moderate exercise is exercise that makes you slightly breathless but not totally worn out.

Weeks 1–4	
Previously inactive	5-10 minutes of mild activity daily building up to 20 minutes of mild to moderate by the end of week 4.
Previously moderately active	15-20 minutes of moderate activity daily building up to 30 minutes by the end of week 4.
Weeks 5–20	
Previously inactive	Increase the length, frequency and intensity every two to three weeks until you are exercising moderately for 30-60 minutes three to five times a week.
Previously moderately active	Increase the length and frequency of exercise until you are exercising more energetically for 60-90 minutes three to five times a week.
Weeks 21 and beyond	
All	Do 60-90 minutes most days of the week. Add in new activities and increase intensity to keep your body on track. To fit this much exercise into your life, try adopting the NEAT approach (see page 114).

Measuring blood glucose

In most countries blood glucose is measured in millimoles per litre (mmol/l), a measurement of the weight of glucose per litre of blood. In the US, mg/dl (milligrammes per decilitre) is the usual unit used, although many US medical journals use both systems.

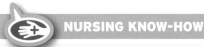

NURSING KNOW-HOW

Glucose guidelines

When exercising, you may need to take less medication or more food to balance your energy requirements. Check your blood glucose immediately before and after exercising and again a couple of hours later. Take advice from your diabetes health-care team and be prepared to adapt your insulin regime to meet your changing needs.

- Aim for a pre-exercise blood glucose level of 5.6 to 13 mmol/l. If it's above 13 mmol/l or below 5.6 mmol/l, postpone your workout until it's within the optimum range.

- Stop exercising if your blood glucose falls below 4 mmol/l or you experience signs of a hypo. Take the usual steps and only resume when it exceeds 4 mmol/l.

- If you exercise in the afternoon or evening, keep an eye on your blood glucose level before sleeping. If it's low, have a snack to avoid a hypo.

... AND KEEP GOING

Finding the motivation to keep on exercising after the initial novelty has worn off can be a problem. Here are some ways to boost your motivation in the first place and keep up your long-term momentum:

Get NEAT Being more active generally – what experts call non-exercise activity thermogenesis or NEAT – can burn an extra 1500 kJ a day, which is equivalent to about a sixth of a woman's recommended daily kilojoule intake and about a seventh of a man's. Adopting a NEAT lifestyle is straightforward – just take every opportunity you can to exercise when moving from one place to another. Take the stairs instead of the lift, walk to the shops instead of driving, walk or cycle to work instead of driving or taking the train. It doesn't matter what exercise you do – just do it.

Set goals Choose which activities you want to do and for how long, then work out how to achieve this. Start slowly – for example, three 5–10 minute walks a week – and build up gradually to 30 minutes most days. Keep a record of what you do, along with any changes in your blood glucose, blood pressure and weight, to keep you motivated.

Exercise in chunks Short of time? According to experts, 10-minute bouts are as good as exercising all in one go.

Ring the changes Avoid boredom by varying your activities. Pick something you enjoy – dancing may be more appealing than jogging. Or how about something you enjoyed at school, such as basketball, hockey, netball or skipping?

Find a friend It's more enjoyable to exercise with a friend and you're more likely to stay on course if you've made a commitment to someone else.

Stay on track Find a way to keep track of your achievements – keep a diary, wear a pedometer or use a recording device such as a Nike+iPod (a sensor you wear in your shoe that sends messages to your iPod).

Be prepared Always carry a starchy snack, such as an energy bar or banana, as well as a fast-acting carbohydrate source, such as glucose tablets or gel, in case you have a hypo while you are exercising. Make sure you drink plenty of fluids before, during and after exercise and never drink alcohol before exercising, as it increases the risk of hypoglycaemia.

Stay safe Always carry or wear some medical ID in case you run into difficulties. Make sure your exercise companion, trainer or fitness centre staff are aware that you have diabetes and know what to do if you have a hypo.

Be consistent Take particular care if planning to exercise while an insulin injection or insulin-stimulating medication is active in your body, adjusting your treatment and/or food intake according to the guidelines advised by your health-care team (see *Glucose guidelines*, facing page).

Mood matters

Diabetes can affect your mood – and not always for the better. In many studies, low glucose levels have been linked to depression and other 'cognitive' changes, such as poorer memory, attention and concentration. However, learning to manage your emotions can ease the blues and help you feel happier.

Watching what you eat and drink, taking medication or insulin and all the other lifestyle changes that are necessary when you have diabetes can make you feel as if you no longer have control over your life. Having diabetes may also impact on your relationships, your job and your leisure activities. These factors can all cause your self-esteem and confidence to plummet and may lead to depression and/or anxiety.

This will usually ease as you learn more about diabetes and gain confidence in dealing with it. But if you continue to feel anxious or depressed, your doctor can help. Psychological therapies such as cognitive behavioural therapy (CBT, see page 252) may be useful, and some health authorities run workshops designed to help with emotional difficulties.

WHAT DOES DIABETES HAVE TO DO WITH IT?

Don't fall into the trap of blaming yourself for feeling despondent about your condition. There is plenty of evidence that diabetes directly affects the parts of the brain and the chemical systems that control mood and behaviour. Glucose is the brain's main fuel and your brain is dependent on a continuous supply to work properly. It's not surprising, therefore, that fluctuations in blood glucose can leave you feeling low.

SEX AND DIABETES

Making love is important for your happiness and health, and diabetes needn't mean that you can no longer have a satisfying sex life. However, there are specific problems that you may need to overcome. Men with

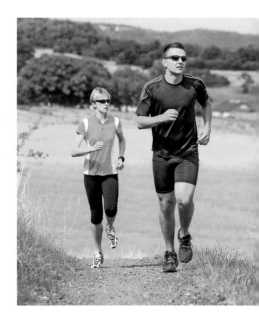

With the right support, people with diabetes can achieve high levels of fitness

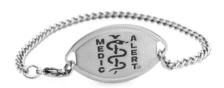

DIABETES ALERT
All people with diabetes should wear a tag (bracelet or necklace) that gives details of their condition. This is important if you need urgent medical attention and are unable to tell the doctors yourself. The MedicAlert Foundation is a charity that supplies tags (www.medicalert. org.au) at a cost (but if you're having financial difficulties you can discuss this with them on 1800 882 222).

diabetes may experience erectile dysfunction (ED), meaning they can't get or maintain an erection, whereas women may experience problems with libido and/or arousal. Why? Physical and chemical changes in the body caused by diabetes, some medications and depression are the main causes, and these may act in combination.

It's not always easy to talk about sex-related problems, but it's worth plucking up the courage to approach your GP or a member of your diabetes health-care team, as there are plenty of treatments available. Sexual difficulties are more common than you may think, and your team will be used to talking about these types of problems and will not be embarrassed. They will identify the underlying cause or causes and offer appropriate treatments as for other aspects of your diabetes care.

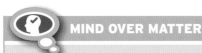

MIND OVER MATTER

Mind your mood...
dealing with your emotions

If you're feeling anxious or depressed about your condition, here are four great ways to stay on top of your emotions:

1 Control stress Techniques such as visualisation and relaxation can reduce levels of the stress hormones cortisol and adrenaline, which are linked to high levels of blood glucose and insulin resistance.

2 Think differently Research suggests that thinking of yourself as 'a diabetic' can cause you to feel bad about yourself because you're allowing the diabetes to define who you are. Conversely, thinking of yourself as 'someone who has diabetes' restores self-esteem.

3 Stay on course People who feel in control of their diabetes not only have better blood glucose levels but also better mental health and quality of life. Get educated and take an active role as the heart of your health-care team.

4 Cultivate mindfulness A study of 81 people with type 2 diabetes reported in the *Journal of Consulting and Clinical Psychology* in 2007 found that practising acceptance and a calm awareness of bodily sensations, feelings and consciousness - known as mindfulness - helped them cope and care for themselves better and led to lower blood glucose levels. Look on the internet to find a course near you.

SLEEP TIGHT

Sleep disturbance is linked to poor blood glucose control. Follow the sleep advice on pages 30–33 and try these tips for managing your night-time glucose levels:

- Check your blood glucose level before you go to bed – if it's too high or too low it can interfere with sleep.
- If you have experienced night-time hypoglycaemic episodes, set your alarm for 3 am over a week and check your blood glucose level. If it's below 4 mmol/l, have a snack.
- Keep a high-carb snack, such as a banana or cereal bar, by your bed to eat if you wake in the night – along with some water.
- If your blood glucose is often low in the early hours, you may need to adjust your insulin regimen or eating plan. See your doctor.
- Seek your doctor's advice if you think you may be suffering from sleep apnoea (see facing page).

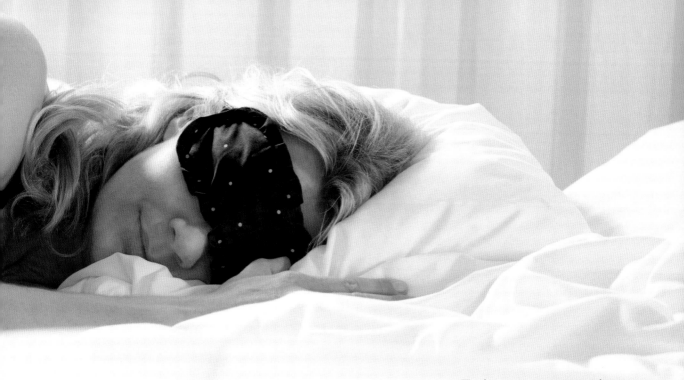

To improve your sleep,
keep your blood glucose
levels steady at night

Staying on track

Once you're used to living with diabetes, continue to stick to your care plan, follow a healthy lifestyle and go for regular check-ups to ensure your diabetes remains under control and complications are kept at bay. Uncontrolled diabetes can lead to many health problems, including narrowing and furring of the large arteries, which can cause heart attacks and strokes, as well as foot problems (due to poor blood circulation), kidney failure, eye problems and gum disease.

MONITOR YOURSELF

Some complications creep up with few or no symptoms. Taking time to make the daily checks below will help you spot changes early. In addition, check your weight weekly. Keep a diary – record your blood glucose levels, any problems you experience, plus the results of your medical checks (see page 118). Show this information to your health-care team.

Feet Check for cuts, blisters, sores, swelling, redness or soreness.

Teeth Clean and floss at least twice daily and use a mouthwash.

Blood glucose Most people on insulin treatment need to check their blood glucose level at least four times daily (or as advised by your health-care team). Those with non-insulin dependent type 2 diabetes should follow the advice of their health-care team.

Could you have sleep apnoea?

Sleep apnoea, a sleep-linked breathing disorder that causes snoring and daytime sleepiness, can alter the way your body deals with glucose. Avoiding alcohol in the evening, losing weight, lying on your side and aids such as nasal strips to improve breathing can help. In more severe cases, according to a study published in *Current Diabetes Reports* in February 2010, wearing a special mask to improve breathing (known as continuous positive airway pressure or CPAP) can improve your insulin sensitivity, blood pressure, levels of blood fats and abdominal fat, and the working of your heart.

Restoring 'hypo awareness'

Over time many people with diabetes become less 'hypo aware'. A clue can be if your blood glucose is regularly lower than your target level. If you are experiencing episodes of hypoglycaemia without apparent warning signs, seek medical help, as you may need to adjust your insulin regime. It is also very important that you do not drive. You may be able to restore your hypo awareness; ask your doctor about this. Research shows that going on a 'structured education course' such as DAFNE is one way to help restore hypo awareness.

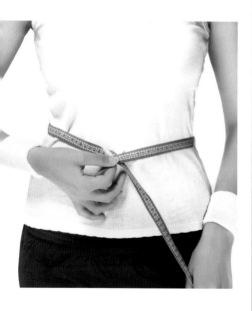

Measure your waist circumference every three months

CHECKS BY YOUR DIABETES HEALTH-CARE TEAM

To track your diabetes and its potential complications, you need to have regular check-ups that include the relevant tests outlined in the table below, unless otherwise recommended. A pregnant woman with gestational diabetes should follow the monitoring schedule advised by her health-care team.

WHAT IF I BECOME ILL?

Being sick takes an extra toll if you have diabetes because it can throw off your blood glucose and put you at risk for significant short-term complications. Blood glucose can rise dramatically when you're ill. The

DIABETES TESTS

How often?	What kind of test?
Every 3 months	● Do a SNAP check (smoking, nutrition, alcohol use, physical activity)
	● Measure weight and waist circumference
	● Check blood pressure
	● Check blood glucose logs
	● Examine your feet
	● Check your medications
Every 6 months	● Check your HbA1C
Every year	● Check that your immunisations are up to date
	● Do a full physical examination
	● Check your cholesterol
	● Check on your kidneys, with a blood and a urine (microalbuminuria) test
	● Organise a home medicines review
	● Decide whether you need a visit to the endocrinologist, diabetes educator, dietitian, exercise physiologist, podiatrist, dentist or psychologist
Every 2 years	● Refer you to an ophthalmologist or optometrist

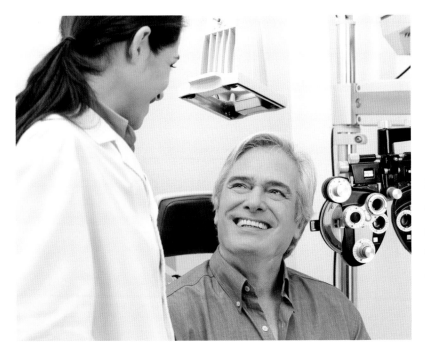

See your doctor or optometrist if you develop problems with your vision when you're ill

best way to deal with sickness is to know what to do in advance. Speak with your doctor, diabetes educator and dietitian to work out a strategy you can quickly put into action the next time a cold, the flu or some other ilness strikes.

During illnesses, such as colds, flu or stomach upsets, drink plenty of sugar-free fluids, check your glucose levels more frequently and adjust your medication as necessary. If you have type 1 diabetes you may need to test your urine or blood for ketones; test strips are available on prescription. Be sure to seek your doctor's advice if any of the following situations occurs:

- A blood pressure check shows that your blood pressure has risen above 130/80.
- You have blurred or double vision, see rings, flashing lights or spots, or have pain, pressure or problems seeing objects out of the corner of your eyes (see the doctor or optometrist).
- You develop blisters, ingrown toenails, or cracked skin on your feet, arms, hands or legs, or your feet feel numb, you feel shooting pains or develop a foot infection (see the doctor or podiatrist).

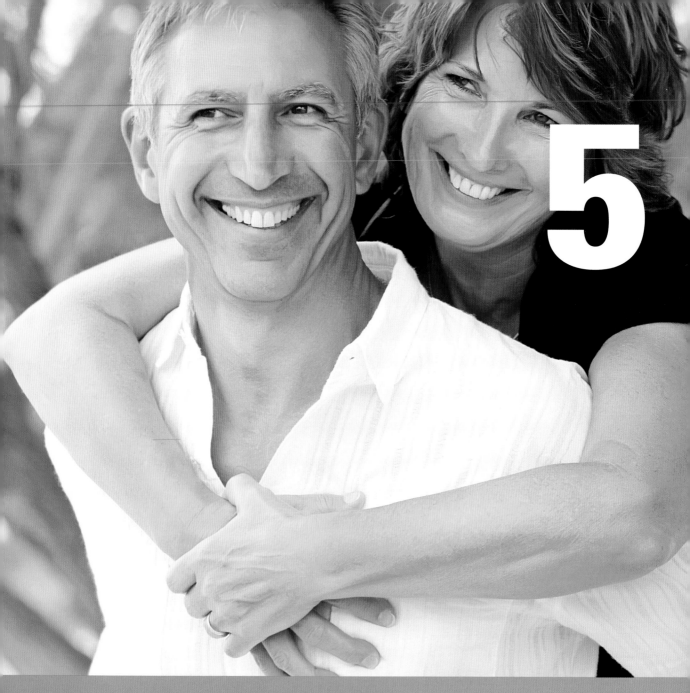

5

Mending your heart

Recovering from a major heart problem requires excellent medical care but you, too, have a key role to play

Overcoming heart disease

Medical science has transformed the treatment of heart disease in the past 50 years and now most people survive a major incident. But full recovery and a good future quality of life also depend on making important healthy lifestyle changes that help the heart to heal.

A FULL LIFE AHEAD

A diagnosis of heart disease no longer means slowing down or putting your life on hold for good. Improved surgical techniques and a wider range of medications allow many people to have as full a life as before their diagnosis – going on holiday, getting back to work, seeing friends and family and enjoying activities such as sport, gardening and dancing. For some people, medical treatment for heart disease can even bring about an improvement in their quality of life. The key to optimum recovery, however, involves more than taking pills – you will need to allow yourself enough time to recover from immediate problems and have the determination to make healthy lifestyle choices for the future.

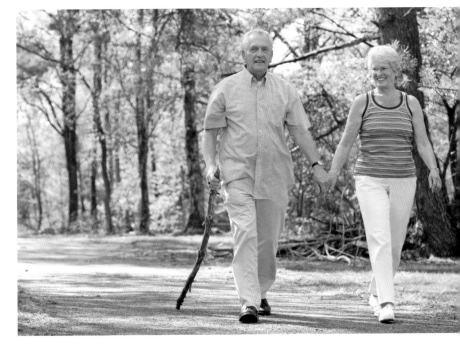

COMMON CONDITIONS

When your condition was diagnosed, your doctor may have explained that there are many different types of heart disease, stemming from a variety of causes and ranging in severity from mild to life threatening. Below are some of the more common conditions that affect the heart and circulation.

Coronary artery disease (also known as ischaemic heart disease) is characterised by narrowing of the coronary arteries – usually as a result of the build-up of fatty deposits, known as atheroma. The narrowing reduces the supply of blood and therefore oxygen to the heart muscle, and the main symptom is recurrent chest pain (angina), most commonly after exercise. A further danger is that narrowed coronary

You can look forward to a full and active life after a diagnosis of heart disease

Keep taking the pills

Medications are very likely to be part of your recovery program. Medications treat heart disease in different ways: they may target the heart directly, by affecting the way it works, or indirectly, by lowering blood pressure or cholesterol (see also *Get the most from your medicine*, pages 312–339).

Aspirin improves blood flow in narrowed coronary arteries by reducing the stickiness of blood cells called platelets, cutting the risk of clotting or a blocked artery.

Beta-blockers block the effects of stress hormones, which make your heart beat faster. They cut the risk of a heart attack by preventing angina attacks, reducing high blood pressure and improving heart function. They can make an abnormal heart rhythm regular. Medications in this group include atenolol, bisoprolol and metoprolol.

Calcium-channel blockers help to dilate constricted blood vessels improving angina, high blood pressure and heart function. Medications in this group include amlodipine, diltiazem, nifedipine and verapamil.

Diuretics (water tablets) remove excess water from the body and are used to treat high blood pressure and heart failure. Medications in this group include bendroflumethiazide, furosemide and indapamide.

Nitrates dilate the coronary arteries to improve blood flow to the heart muscle and are used to relieve angina. Glyceryl trinitrate (GTN) comes as tiny pills or a spray to put under the tongue during an attack. Isosorbide mononitrate (ISMN) is taken daily to prevent attacks.

Statins reduce the risk of having a heart attack by reducing the amount of cholesterol in the blood.

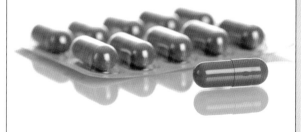

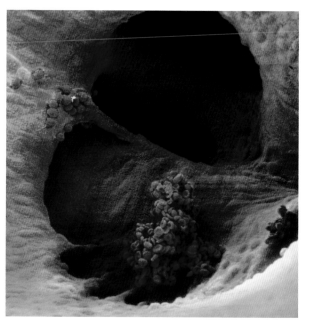

HEART ATTACK IN WAITING
This image of a thrombus (blood clot) in an artery supplying the heart shows a heart attack waiting to happen. Once detected, medical intervention – for example, with clot-busting medications – can disperse clots to minimise the risk of a blocked artery.

arteries are more susceptible to blockage by a blood clot – coronary thrombosis or heart attack – in which the blood supply to a part of the heart muscle is cut off completely. This is a life-threatening condition, which can also weaken the heart muscle as a result of oxygen deprivation.

High blood pressure (hypertension) is very common in older people. The condition increases the risk of the formation of abnormal blood clots and therefore adds to the likelihood of a heart attack or stroke (see *What happens during a stroke*, page 146).

High blood cholesterol – above normal levels of LDL (low-density lipoprotein) cholesterol – is a prime cause of artery narrowing, as it can build up and gradually thicken the walls, restricting blood flow. The fatty deposits, known as plaque, may also rupture, causing the formation of a blood clot, which could block vital blood flow to the heart muscle.

Abnormal heart rhythm A variety of problems are caused by dysfunction of the electrical system that controls the heartbeat, leading to irregular rhythms. These are described in more detail on page 124.

These and other heart conditions are all highly treatable by medical interventions in conjunction with measures within your control. A diagnosis of heart disease could be the spur that encourages you to adopt a much healthier lifestyle. From the outset you can begin to take charge of your recovery with the support and advice of your medical team.

RECOVERING FROM HEART DISEASE

The first steps involve being well informed about the nature and severity of your condition. Find out as much as you can, so that you are better able to make the changes needed to maximise your chances of a good recovery. Here are some ideas to help:

- Make a thorough list of questions to ask your doctor. You should never hold back from asking questions for fear of seeming stupid or taking up too much time.
- Get to know your medical team. Make sure you and your family know how to contact the different specialists who will be able to help you with different aspects of your recovery program, from your cardiology consultant, to specialist nurses, physiotherapists, dietitians and counsellors.
- Educate yourself about your condition by visiting the National Heart Foundation's website or calling their information line (www. heartfoundation.org.au and 1300 362 787).
- If you've had a heart attack, make sure your doctor refers you to a cardiac rehabilitation program. Most such schemes provide a supervised safe exercise program combined with relaxation, counselling and dietary advice. See also *Life after a heart attack*, pages 138–139.

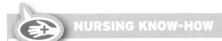

NURSING KNOW-HOW

Brush your teeth

Brushing and flossing are important for everyone but especially so for people with heart disease. Inflamed gums can release pro-inflammatory chemicals that increase the risk of a number of serious conditions, including heart attack. The Australian Dental Association recommends using a soft brush.

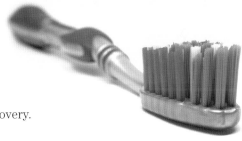

FOCUS

Recovering your rhythm

A heart arrhythmia is caused by a fault in the electrical circuit that keeps the heart beating regularly. The heartbeat may be erratic, or quicker or slower than normal, producing symptoms such as faintness or shortness of breath. Once it is diagnosed, treatment can quickly regulate the problem.

Over one million people in Australia have an arrhythmia. The most common are harmless 'extrasystoles', felt as a missed beat or extra beat. Other arrhythmias include:

Supraventricular tachycardia affects people of all ages. Symptoms include a fast heartbeat, which may occur after exercise, at times of stress, or without warning or obvious cause.

Atrial fibrillation (AF) affects mainly those over the age of 50, and is a leading cause of stroke.

Bradycardia causes a slow heartbeat that can reflect physical fitness, but could be a sign of heart disease or of degeneration of the electrical system.

Ventricular tachycardia (VT) is caused by a fault in the electrical system in the lower heart chambers causing the heart to beat so fast it cannot pump sufficient blood to the brain.

TREATMENT OF ARRHYTHMIAS

Your treatment will depend on the type of arrhythmia, your general health and age.

- Following advice on lifestyle, you will probably be prescribed anti-arrhythmic medications (see *Get the most from your medicine,* page 331).
- Some people may be treated by catheter ablation (the destruction of abnormal heart tissue by tiny electrical impulses).
- Many people have a pacemaker fitted. This small device is placed under the skin of the chest, and uses electrical pulses to prompt the heart to beat normally. A pacemaker is usually visible beneath your skin.

- If you have a ventricular arrhythmia, you may be fitted with an implantable cardioverter defibrillator (ICD), which delivers an electric shock to the heart if it senses a dangerous abnormality. The shock may be so small you're not aware of it, or you may feel a jolt. Having an ICD fitted can be unsettling but most people value the reassurance it provides.

 SELF-HELP

Beat the abnormal beat

Here are some tips to help yourself if you've been diagnosed with arrhythmias:

- ✔ Give up smoking.
- ✔ Cut down on, or give up, alcohol and caffeine.
- ✔ Find ways to reduce the stress in your life.
- ✔ Avoid using over-the-counter medications that contain stimulants such as pseudoephedrine, which is often found in cough and cold remedies.
- ✔ Do not take diet pills, many of which contain stimulants such as ephedrine.
- ✔ Avoid energy drinks, which contain stimulants.
- ✔ Limit exposure to chemical fumes.

Keep pace with a pacemaker

If you have a pacemaker, you need to know what may interfere with its operation and what is safe.

- Household equipment, such as televisions and microwaves, will not affect your pacemaker.

- Most types of hospital and dental equipment don't cause any problems, but inform your doctor or dentist that you have a pacemaker fitted.

- Magnetic resonance imaging (MRI) machines can disrupt pacemakers. Check with your doctor.

- Avoid treatment with electrical nerve stimulators, such as TENS machines.

- Shop and airport security machines. Walk through quickly and don't stand near to them for long. If you show airport security your pacemaker ID, you may be given a manual body search instead.

- Avoid carrying magnets, mobile phones or hi-fi equipment close to your pacemaker.

- Avoid falling asleep while using an iPad, since it can fall onto your chest and interfere with your pacemaker.

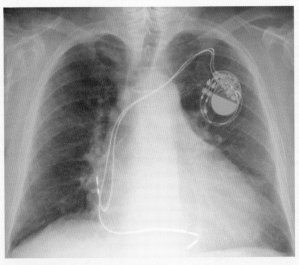

PACEMAKER IN PLACE
A pacemaker, seen in this X-ray, is fitted under the skin of the chest and has wires that transmit electrical signals to the heart muscle to trigger normal heart rhythm.

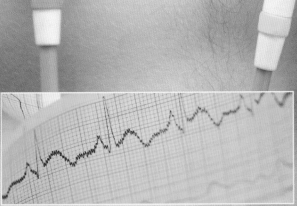

READING YOUR RHYTHM
An ECG (electrocardiogram), which picks up signals via electrodes on your chest, shows electrical activity in your heart and helps your doctors choose the right treatment.

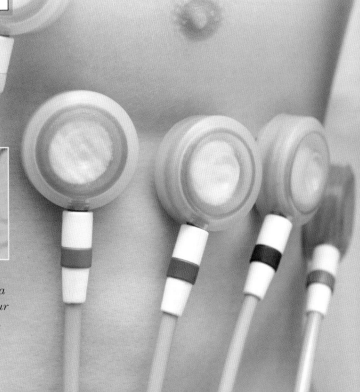

Helping yourself

A global study called INTERHEART has found that 90 per cent of first heart attacks can be attributed to nine risk factors unrelated to where you live, how old you are and your ethnic background – in other words, factors within your control.

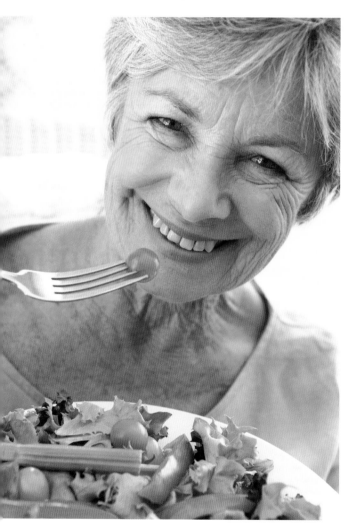

Healthy changes to your lifestyle can be enjoyable as well as good for your heart

Most heart disease is not inevitable. The Interheart study pinpointed the following controllable major risk factors: smoking, high blood cholesterol, high blood pressure, diabetes, obesity, stress, lack of daily fruit and vegetables, excess alcohol intake and lack of daily exercise. If any affect you, you must tackle them as part of your recovery. Keep diabetes, high blood pressure or high blood cholesterol under control by taking your medicines as prescribed and carefully follow your doctor's lifestyle recommendations.

ADJUST YOUR LIFESTYLE

Whatever your heart problem, stopping smoking is a priority (pages 136–137). Not only will this give your heart the best chance of recovery, your general health and fitness will improve dramatically. Other essentials are:

Healthy diet (pages 127–130) Stepping up your fruit and vegetable intake to at least seven a day has been proved to reduce heart problems.

Weight reduction (pages 130–131) Losing excess weight will be of benefit in many areas of your life.

Daily exercise (pages 134–136), which can be gently tailored to your age and ability. Do not be put off by thinking you have to go to a gym; simple measures such as walking to the next bus stop or walking up stairs instead of taking the lift count as daily exercise and are easy to incorporate into even the busiest life. If you are fit and active, you are less likely to develop type 2 diabetes or heart disease. Being overweight is a risk factor for both.

Control stress There is a link between stress and heart problems, and stress is something you can learn to control (pages 140–141).
Moderate your alcohol intake Drinking more than the weekly allowance (see page 26) can affect the health of your heart in the long term. However, many studies have shown that drinking a small amount, particularly red wine, can have a protective effect on your heart and circulation. People who drink a little tend to have better heart health than teetotallers.

Eating your way to a healthy heart

One of the most positive ways you can help yourself during your recuperation is to improve your diet. Major US studies have proved conclusively that an unhealthy diet is a leading cause of heart disease – and that eating the right food can be as effective as medication or any other medical intervention in recovering from heart disease.

The good news is that a heart-healthy diet is versatile enough to suit all dietary preferences. Build it around the advice given in the panel *The top 10 healthy heart foods* (page 128) and *What can I eat?* (page 129). Start by making a few easy adaptations and experiment a little more as you feel the benefits. Improving your diet can also help you to avoid becoming overweight, which could further affect your heart and increase the likelihood of developing type 2 diabetes.

GOOD AND BAD FATS

Although your heart-friendly diet should be generally a low-fat one, you need some fat in your diet for energy and to help absorb important nutrients. There are different types:

● Unsaturated fat – liquid at room temperature – is kinder to the arteries, protects against irregular heartbeats, helps to lower blood pressure and reduces the risk of heart attack. Unsaturated fat is divided into polyunsaturated fat, such as fish oil and sunflower oil and monounsaturated fat, including olive oil, canola oil and nut and avocado oils. Coconut and palm oils are, however, saturated fats.

● Saturated fat – mostly animal fats that are solid at room temperature – raises harmful blood cholesterol and increases the risk of heart disease. This is the type of fat you should cut down on. Examples include butter and lard.

True or False?

Statins are 'miracle' drugs that reduce your risk of having a second heart attack, whatever you eat

False Statins do not cancel out the problems of a poor, fatty diet. Changing to a healthy diet is the best way to help your recovery from heart problems and increase your chances of living a long and healthy life. Statins help but they are much more beneficial if taken with a healthy diet.

Choose unsaturated fats, such as olive oil, over animal fats

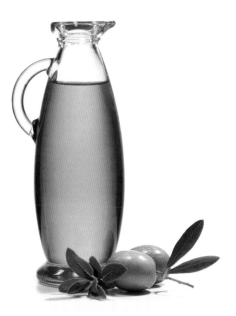

The top 10 healthy heart foods

The first eight foods in this list are the building blocks of your new healthy eating plan; the final two are 'treats' that should be taken in moderation. Variety is the key to success so this is your chance to be creative in the kitchen.

1 Oats contain a high proportion of soluble fibre, which reduces 'bad' LDL cholesterol.

2 Yogurts and spreads containing plant sterols (similar to good cholesterol) can reduce blood levels of LDL cholesterol by up to 10 per cent.

3 Olive oil is a potent mix of antioxidants that reduce LDL cholesterol while leaving your HDL cholesterol untouched.

4 Salmon and fresh tuna contain high levels of omega-3 fatty acids. Eat three portions a week if you've had a heart attack.

5 Tomatoes and tomato paste are packed with vitamins and the antioxidant lycopene, which has beneficial effects on the heart.

6 Walnuts and almonds are rich in essential fatty acids that help to keep your blood vessels healthy by lowering cholesterol levels.

7 Apples contain quercetin, an anti-inflammatory chemical that can help prevent blood clots.

8 Onions and garlic help reduce blood cholesterol, as well as improving circulation and discouraging blood clotting.

9 Red wine has been shown to clean up the walls of the arteries. But be careful not to exceed healthy guidelines.

10 Dark chocolate is rich in heart-friendly flavonoids that keep cholesterol from gathering in blood vessels. It also slightly lowers blood pressure. Eat no more than 45 g daily.

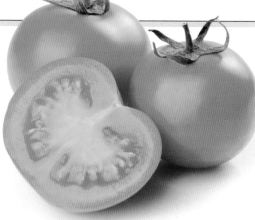

Tomatoes are packed with heart-friendly lycopene

Trans fats (or artificial trans-fatty acids) are considered even more dangerous than saturated fat for raising cholesterol levels. Many doctors believe that the chemically altered vegetable oils, often 'hidden' in processed foods such as biscuits and pastries, are such a serious threat to heart health that they should be banned. Check food labels for the words 'hydrogenated' or 'partially hydrogenated vegetable oils' and avoid products that contain them.

WHAT YOU NEED TO KNOW ABOUT CHOLESTEROL

Cholesterol is a fatty substance that is found naturally in the blood. It is vital for many functions, such as making cell walls and hormones. Cholesterol may be low density (LDL) or high density (HDL). LDL is considered 'bad' because too much causes atherosclerosis (fatty deposits in the arteries). HDL is 'good' because it gets rid of excess LDL. The more HDL in your blood, the lower your risk of developing heart problems and the better your chances of recovery from existing problems. One of the aims of a heart-healthy diet is to cut down on your saturated fat intake, which will reduce the amount of LDL in your blood. (Go to www.heartuk.org.uk for more information about cholesterol.)

CUT DOWN ON SALT

Common salt (sodium chloride) raises your blood pressure, which puts extra strain on your heart. To help you recover from heart disease,

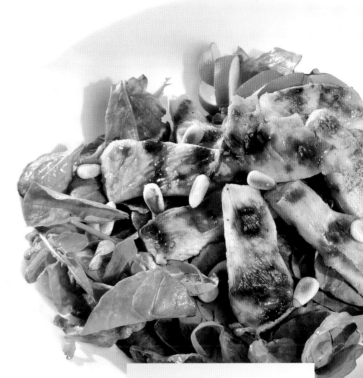

A low-fat diet, high in fresh vegetables, can be a delicious way to boost heart health

you must cut back on salt; you should eat no more than 6 g of salt (2.3 g of sodium) a day. Your taste buds quickly adjust to eating less. To help reduce your salt intake try the following suggestions:

- Sprinkle less or preferably none on your food. In cooking, use lemon juice, vinegar, spices and pepper as alternative flavourings.
- Buy low-sodium salt, which contains potassium. Sea salt, rock salt and natural salt are high in sodium.
- Avoid processed foods, tomato ketchup, stock cubes or other manufactured stock, sausages, bacon and other cured meats, all of which contain high levels of salt.
- Find low-salt alternatives of crisps, crackers, tinned soups and even breakfast cereals.

WHAT CAN I EAT?

A heart-healthy diet is a healthy, balanced eating regime but there are some foods that are especially good for your recovering heart (see panel, facing page). Aim to restrict your intake of saturated fat, replacing it with unsaturated fat. Eat two to three portions of fish a week, especially oily fish, such as salmon, mackerel and trout. You need to eat at least seven portions of fruit and vegetables every day, and select different colours for the healthiest choice. Keep your intake of milk, cheese, butter and red meat to a minimum and avoid foods such as pastry, biscuits and cakes. Use low-fat dairy products where possible. Include wholegrain bread, wholemeal pasta or brown rice with every meal along with a low-fat source of protein such as chicken breast.

Adopt low-fat cooking techniques, such as grilling or roasting, stir-frying, steaming and cooking without oil, such as in a griddle pan or in a parcel of greaseproof paper. Try partnering 'good' and 'less good' foods. For example, wholemeal crackers and cheese or grilled meat with a tomato and onion salad are healthy combinations.

Top Tips

Supplement dos and don'ts

DO take coenzyme Q10 if you're also taking statins. This naturally occurring enzyme has been shown to counteract in some people a common side effect of these medications: muscle cramps.

DON'T take St John's wort or ginkgo. Both these herbal remedies have been shown to interact with several heart disease medicines, according to the British Heart Foundation.

DON'T take vitamins as a substitute for your seven daily portions of fruit and vegetables. They are not as nutritious and cannot provide the variety of vitamins in fresh produce.

WHAT CAN I DRINK?

Moderate drinking, that is the equivalent of a small glass of wine a day, may protect against heart disease in men over 40 and postmenopausal women. Alcohol can help raise the levels of HDL cholesterol in the blood, which in turn reduces its stickiness, lowering the risk of heart attack. Red wine, which contains a polyphenol called resveratrol, is thought to be particularly beneficial. Regularly drinking more than a glass of wine a day increases the risk of high blood pressure. Binge drinking can cause abnormal heart rhythms and regular heavy drinking leads to enlargement of the heart, known as cardiomyopathy.

Reducing the strain

Being overweight is bad for health in general, and your heart in particular. If you are one of the many overweight people with heart disease, you probably know that losing weight will give a huge boost to your chances of a lasting recovery. Most people think that carrying around any extra weight puts strain on your heart, but the real problem is fat around your waist, known as visceral or 'active' fat, according to the British Heart Foundation (BHF). Active fat pumps out chemicals that inflame and narrow your blood vessels, raising blood pressure. It also changes the way in which the

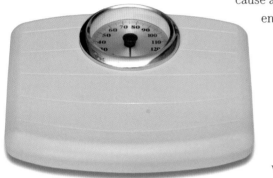

Losing weight from your waist keeps the fat from your arteries

---

Five top weight-loss myths

Half-truths and myths regarding losing weight are everywhere. Here some frequently quoted myths are debunked to give you the best chance of success:

1 Cutting out all snacks can help you lose weight Snacking itself isn't the problem; it's the type of snack. Many people need a snack between meals to maintain energy levels, especially if they're active. Choose fruit or vegetables instead of crisps or chocolate.

2 A radical exercise regime is the only way to lose weight Not true. Sensible slimming involves making small changes that you can stick to for a long time. To lose 450 g a week, most people need to use up 2,100 kJ more per day than they consume. Eat less, exercise more, or, for best effect, do both.

3 Slimming pills are effective for long-term weight loss They're not. Slimming pills alone will not help you keep the weight off in the long term. They should be used only when prescribed by a doctor to support a healthy eating plan.

4 Drinking water helps you lose weight Water won't cause weight loss but it does keep you hydrated, and might help you snack less; thirst can be mistaken for hunger. Water is certainly better for you than sugary drinks.

5 Skipping meals is a good way to lose weight Skipping meals is not a good idea. It will result in tiredness and poor nutrition – and may lead to snacking on unhealthy, high-fat, high-sugar foods.

body handles fat circulating in the body. 'Belly fat causes fatty tissue to grow inside the walls of your arteries, over time building up a bulge that restricts how much blood can get to your heart, and eventually causing a heart attack,' explains the BHF. The good news is that if you take steps to reduce weight, active fat starts to disappear long before you can see any change in body shape.

SLOWLY DOES IT

Crash diets are not a healthy option. Rapid weight loss almost inevitably involves losing essential water and muscle. What is more, your body tends to adjust by burning kilojoules more slowly. The best way to lose weight is by reducing your kilojoule intake to a realistic amount. Sticking to between 6,300 and 7,500 kJ a day helps most people (men need to eat more than women). Aim to lose about 0.5–1 kg a week. You are more likely to keep the weight off for good by this steady route.

BURN OFF THE KILOS

You can lose weight more quickly if you combine physical activity with your diet. It doesn't matter what sort of exercise you choose to do. Even low-intensity exercise – for example, walking, gardening and housework – burns kilojoules and helps you lose weight. The National Heart Foundation recommends 30 minutes of moderate activity on at least five days a week. The secret is to find an activity that you enjoy and can easily be incorporated into your life.

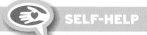

SELF-HELP

Am I overweight?...
an easy way to find out

Weighing yourself or looking in the mirror tells you only half the story. Try one of the following methods to find out whether your weight is hampering your recovery chances:

- **BMI (body mass index)** Work out your height in metres and multiply the figure by itself (your height squared). Weigh yourself in kilograms. Divide your weight by your height squared. Various websites will do the calculation for you, using metric or imperial units. Go to www.mydr.com.au/tools/bodymass. If your BMI is 25 or above, whether you're a man or a woman, you need to lose weight.

- **Your waist size** To measure your waist, breathe out and put a tape measure around the narrowest point between your lower ribs and your hips (usually just above the navel). If the measurement is greater than 80 cm for a woman or 94 cm for a man, you're at increased risk of heart disease.

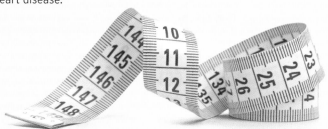

- **Your body shape** People who store most of their body fat around their waist ('apples') are more prone to heart disease than who have more fat around the thighs and buttocks ('pears'). To work out whether you are an apple or a pear shape, measure your hips and waist. If the ratio between the two is higher than 0.8 if you're a woman or 0.95 if you're a man, you need to take action. (Go to www.mydr.com.au/tools/waist-to-hip-calculator for if you'd rather not do the maths.)

Bypassing problems

Since it became a standard treatment for clogged coronary arteries in the 1970s, bypass surgery has given thousands of heart disease patients the chance to live a normal life. This operation rapidly restores the blood supply to the heart muscle, preventing recurrent angina and significantly reducing the risk of a subsequent heart attack.

When angioplasty, in which a balloon is inserted into an artery or arteries that have become clogged by a build-up of fat or cholesterol, is either unsuccessful or inappropriate, bypass surgery is usually recommended. The artery or arteries to be bypassed are narrowed, slowing or even stopping blood reaching the heart and thereby causing angina (chest pain) or a heart attack. Coronary artery bypass surgery involves re-routing or bypassing the affected artery. In the operation, a segment of healthy blood vessel is taken from another part of the body and used to make a detour around the blockage. The result is improved blood flow to the heart muscle. This operation has a high rate of success, but the speed of recovery can depend on how you prepare yourself beforehand and the actions you take afterwards.

AFTER THE OPERATION

Knowing what lies ahead can help you recuperate. There will be hurdles to overcome on the road to recovery but being prepared can help. Once you leave hospital, you'll need to convalesce for several weeks and it's best to have someone at home with you at this time. Try to arrange a network of family and friends to be available to help you. See also *Before and after surgery*, pages 196–213.

1 **Pain** Once the anaesthesia drugs have worn off, you'll be given oxygen and pain relief. It is important for your pain to be well controlled in order to move on through the stages back to health.

2 **Getting moving** Once you're breathing on your own, you'll be encouraged to start moving by sitting on the edge of the bed and walking a few steps to a chair. Rehabilitation can be a long process but it's helpful to know that moving will become much easier the more you try.

3 **Weakness and fatigue** Your body has had a severe shock and extreme fatigue is normal for a few days or weeks. If you find activity exhausting,

---

SELF-HELP

Countdown to surgery

How you prepare yourself for heart surgery can make a big difference to the success of the treatment. Make every effort to quit smoking and, if you need to lose weight, start a healthy eating plan before your operation. It is important to get your teeth checked before any heart surgery to be sure you are free of gum and other mouth infections, because bacteria in the mouth can enter the bloodstream and infect the heart valves. You should also prepare yourself emotionally. There is evidence that those who are psychologically prepared have fewer complications, less discomfort and a quicker recovery. Take the time to learn some relaxation techniques. Try yoga, meditation, hypnosis or simply listening to a relaxation tape or calming music.

always have a rest. It is best to build up gradually to avoid being discouraged. Accept that progress might be slow and be guided by your body.

4 **Emotional upheaval** Once you're on the road to physical recovery, you might become aware of emotional and psychological problems. Depression is common in the weeks following a major operation so be kind to yourself (see also *Regaining your emotional health*, page 212). Try to avoid any stressful situations. Be honest and open about your feelings.

The support of loved ones can speed your recovery

MILESTONES TO FULL RECOVERY

Recuperating from major heart surgery can take many weeks so you need to be patient, have a lot of help and listen to your body. This should give you an idea of what you can expect to be able to do:

24 hours	You will spend the first 24 hours after your operation in an intensive care or cardiac recovery unit.
One week	Expect to spend another six or seven days in a high-dependency unit or on a cardiac surgical ward. The physiotherapists will give you breathing exercises and you will be encouraged to walk in the ward for a few minutes three or four times daily. You will not be discharged until you are able to walk up and down stairs.
2 weeks	You're on the road to recovery. Walk 7 to 10 minutes two to three times a day and get dressed every day even if you don't go out.
4 weeks	You may be able to go back to light work provided you feel well enough and up to the demands of your job. Check with your doctor. Start driving a car but stop every 1 to 2 hours to stretch your legs; go swimming but don't pull yourself up by the steps; walk 15 to 20 minutes once or twice each day.
6 weeks	You can resume your sex life. Don't expect too much at first. Medication can cause lack of interest in sex. You're bound to feel anxious after major surgery. Men who have had bypass surgery can take Viagra safely, under medical supervision.
3 months	You can play tennis, dig the garden and mow the lawn without worrying.

Exercise your heart

Exercise is vital for your heart and is one of the cornerstones of your recovery program. There is very strong evidence for the heart-strengthening benefits of aerobic exercise. It involves working your large muscles hard so they require more than the usual amount of oxygen. This will force the heart muscle to work harder, helping it to become stronger.

If you have heart disease, take your time building up aerobic strength, starting gradually and initially working out only under the supervision of a physiotherapist or other qualified practitioner. Provided you exercise regularly, you will soon regain confidence in your capacity for vigorous activity.

HOW KEEPING ACTIVE HELPS YOUR HEART

Understanding precisely how exercise can help your heart is a powerful incentive to get you moving. Among its many benefits, exercise can:

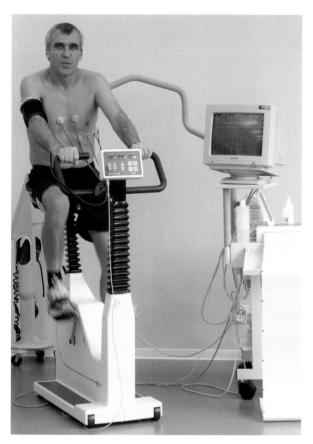

An ECG to test your fitness for exercise is a wise precaution

- Lower blood pressure, reducing the strain on the heart and increasing 'good' HDL cholesterol that transports fat away from the arteries and back to the liver for processing.
- Improve circulation, which prevents the formation of blood clots that can lead to a heart attack.
- Help you control your weight; thereby reducing the extra load of fat you are carrying and the workload that your heart has to undertake.
- Strengthen and enlarge heart muscle so it can pump more blood around the body and sustain its maximum level with less strain. The resting heart rate of those who exercise is slower because less effort is needed to pump blood.

How long should I exercise?

Exercising to strengthen your heart muscle involves speeding up your heart rate and keeping it elevated for a period of time. You should aim to build up to exercising for 30 minutes at least five days a week.

SAFETY FIRST

Before you start exercising, check with your GP or cardiologist. Your doctor may organise a stress test, which involves having an ECG test while on a running machine or exercise bike to find out how much activity is safe for you.

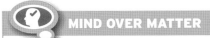

MIND OVER MATTER

Feeling good helps your heart

Exercise can lift your mood by promoting the release of endorphins – feel-good hormones. Not only do you feel better, but these hormones help to alleviate stress and anxiety that can slow down your recovery from heart disease.

Discuss what your target heart rate should be. A healthy person's target heart rate is 60–85 per cent of their maximum heart rate (220 minus their age). If you are taking medications that slow your heart rate, such as beta-blockers or calcium-channel blockers, you may not reach your target despite intense exercise.

Be kind to your heart by starting exercise slowly with a warm-up and slow down gradually ('warm down') before the end of the session. The ideal level of exercise is where you get warm and slightly out of breath but are still able to talk. Avoid exercising after a heavy meal, in cold weather or if you have a viral illness such as a cold. If you have high blood pressure, especially if it's not well controlled, avoid intense exercise such as heavy weightlifting. If you have angina, don't do regular exercise that causes chest pains or makes you too out of breath.

Invest in a pedometer and aim for 10,000 steps a day

TOP FITNESS CHOICES FOR HEART HEALTH

It is important to find a type of exercise that fits into your lifestyle and doesn't become a chore. If you find it hard going, you're less likely to keep it up and it's essential that exercise becomes part of your life. Here are some ideas to start you on the right road:

Go for a brisk walk Start slowly, and only increase the distance and speed when you feel able to. Wear good shoes and loose clothing. To make it more interesting, go with a friend or borrow a dog.

Add extra walking into your day Walk to the next bus stop or train station, walk up the stairs or escalator instead of taking the lift, think twice about taking the car to the local shops.

Swim If you have mobility problems or osteoporosis, swimming is a gentle but effective form of exercise.

Cycle You can cycle for pleasure or take your bike to work and avoid the daily commute.

Dance Whatever your style you're sure to find a class or club that caters for you. Dancing on your own at home is just as effective.

Jog Whether you go solo or with a friend or group, set your own pace and build up gently.

Keep-fit class Being in a group provides many people with much needed motivation.

Garden The heavy work, such as digging, is good exercise but be careful not to cause sprains and strains in other parts of your body.

Energetic housework This can count towards your daily exercise.

Clearing the smoke

Stopping smoking is the kindest present that you can give your heart. Compared with non-smokers, smokers have double the risk of having a heart attack and increase their risk of dying from heart disease by 60 per cent (85 per cent in heavy smokers). Smoking causes one in five deaths from heart disease. The benefits of stopping smoking are as valuable for those who already have heart disease as for those who have not yet developed heart problems.

WHY SMOKING IS BAD FOR YOUR HEART

Each breath of cigarette smoke triggers several dangerous responses in your heart and blood vessels:

- Fatty deposits form on artery walls, narrowing them, which can lead to angina, heart attack or heart failure.
- Carbon monoxide flows into your bloodstream and reduces the amount of oxygen available to your heart.
- Nicotine enters your bloodstream, stimulating the production of adrenaline, making your heart beat faster and raising blood pressure. Nicotine also increases the production of fibrinogen, the protein that causes your blood to clot, and this increases the likelihood of abnormal blood clots (thrombosis).
- Smoke introduces toxic chemicals that increase the stickiness of blood, causing it to thicken or clot, increasing the risk of a heart attack.

HOW TO GIVE UP SMOKING

In Australia, former smokers outnumber current smokers, and about a quarter of all Australians have managed to give up – this should be encouraging if you're finding it tough. There are many ways to try to stop smoking. A lot will depend on your personality and motivation

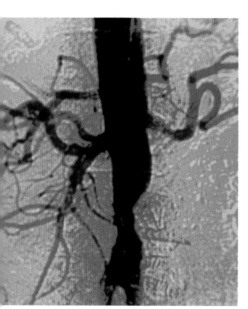

DANGEROUSLY NARROWED
This view shows an abdominal aorta narrowed by the build-up of atheroma (fatty deposits). Smoking is one of the prime causes of atheroma and therefore of heart disease of many kinds.

so what has worked for a friend or relative may not work for you. Joining a group or seeing a therapist means you have support and you are more likely to succeed. It is important not to treat a relapse as an excuse to start smoking again. Cutting down does not always lead to quitting, but for some people giving up smoking gradually makes the process more bearable. Here are some tips for giving up:

Go 'cold turkey' Choose a day on which you'll have your last cigarette. You'll give yourself the best chance if you avoid highly social or stressful days such as Christmas or a time of demanding commitments. If you're a woman, don't stop just before a period.

Hypnotherapy There's much anecdotal evidence that a few sessions with a hypnotherapist can change the way you think about smoking and make it easier to break the habit.

Nicotine replacement therapy Whether you use gum, patch, inhaler, lozenge or pill, it's well documented that taking nicotine without the tar and carbon monoxide in tobacco is a successful way of breaking the smoking habit – especially if you are also using another method of quitting.

Ask your doctor to prescribe a quit-smoking medication, such as varenicline or bupropion. These medications help to suppress the desire to smoke.

Go online Go to the Australian Government's QuitNow site (www.quitnow.gov.au) for top tips and information, and to access the Quit Coach.

Call for help Call the Australian Government's Quitline (13 78 48), a telephone information and counselling serving, for support. You can also order a free Quit Pack.

WHAT HAPPENS WHEN YOU STOP SMOKING

Your body responds to being smoke-free after only 20 minutes. Look out for these changes to encourage you to quit:

After 20 minutes	Blood pressure and heart rate begin to drop.
After 8 hours	Carbon monoxide level in the blood decreases. You can cope better with physical exertion and may manage with less medication.
After 24 hours	Carbon monoxide is eliminated from the body. The heart's supply of oxygen increases substantially, reducing the chances of chest pain following exertion.
After 14 days	Blood circulates more efficiently.
After 1 month	Skin appearance improves.
After 3 months	Lung function begins to improve.
After 1 year	The risk of having a heart attack reduces by up to 50 per cent. If you've had a heart attack, quitting smoking reduces your risk of a subsequent fatal heart attack by 25 per cent.

 SELF-HELP

Quit the habit

However determined you are, there may be times when you struggle. Remember, you will get there in the end, even if it takes more than one attempt. To stay on track, try to:

✔ Keep busy.

✔ Drink plenty of fluids.

✔ Take exercise.

✔ Buy yourself a special treat with the money you're saving.

✔ Avoid other smokers.

✔ Find a quitting partner.

✔ Avoid triggers.

✔ Think positively.

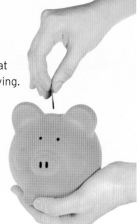

FOCUS

Life after a heart attack

Recovering from a heart attack isn't just about beating physical symptoms. It's also about minimising the risks of it happening again and laying the foundations for good health in the future. As part of getting well, you and your family may need to make significant lifestyle changes.

According to recent research, modifying certain key aspects of everyday life can dramatically reduce the risk of suffering a second heart attack. Changes discussed elsewhere in this chapter include stopping smoking, reducing cholesterol levels, exercising and avoiding stress. Your recovery program will involve a wide variety of lifestyle and relationship adjustments. These hints and tips may help you feel more in control of the factors that will speed your recovery:

1 Dress every day as if you're going out – it reminds you and your family that you're on the road to recovery and the next phase of your life.

2 Take up any available offer of cardiac rehabilitation (provided free by public hospitals). Evidence shows that starting gentle exercise with the support of physiotherapists and nurses is the best possible way of fast-tracking recovery from a heart attack or cardiac surgery.

3 Talk to your family about the importance of exercise in your recovery, and explain that it's safe to sweat or pant a little. Help them to understand that by exerting yourself, you're actually making your heart stronger. Having your family worry unnecessarily can trigger anger, frustration and a feeling of powerlessness.

4 Never stop taking your medications without medical advice, even if you're having side effects – you might be putting your life at risk. Discuss any problems with your GP or cardiologist.

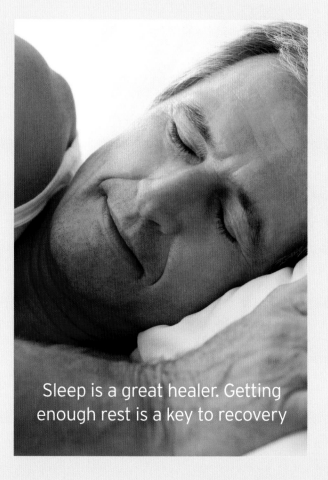

Sleep is a great healer. Getting enough rest is a key to recovery

FAMILY MATTERS

A heart attack is a life-changing event and it unsettles everyone in the family, particularly the patient's partner, but family ties can become stronger as a result of going through adversity. The lifestyle changes that are needed to lay the foundations for recovery require a tough, consistent approach. Family members of heart attack victims should consider these points:

- Coming home can be daunting after being in hospital, where help is always at hand; recovery can gather pace in the familiar surroundings, but be prepared for a period of adjustment.
- Patience and commitment to change are key and your relative will be counting on you for encouragement and support.
- Avoid being overprotective and try to remember the patient as the independent person from before the heart attack.
- Be understanding if your relative has a lapse from the recovery program, and don't allow him or her to be disheartened or give up.
- Be alert for signs of excessive anxiety or depression because they're easier to treat in the early stages before taking hold.
- Take one day at a time: focus on what your relative can do at that moment without worrying too much about what may or may not happen in the future.
- Try to carry on as normal as far as possible. Avoid changing your routine or cancelling important events to accommodate your relative.
- Ensure that you look after yourself – eat well, have enough rest and exercise and allow yourself some time away from the responsibilities of caring.

There can be a special joy in sharing the path to full recovery

Q&A

Is it safe to have sex after a heart attack?

Yes. As long as you've been given the all clear to have moderate exercise, you can have sex – usually two to three weeks after having a heart attack.

HELP FROM OUTSIDE THE FAMILY

Not everyone is lucky enough to have family support. But there is plenty of other help available through cardiac rehabilitation programs, which can give heart attack patients a 26 per cent greater chance of survival after five years. The efforts of nurses, dietitians, physiotherapists, psychologists and occupational therapists can improve quality of life, minimise anxiety and reduce the likelihood of return hospital admissions.

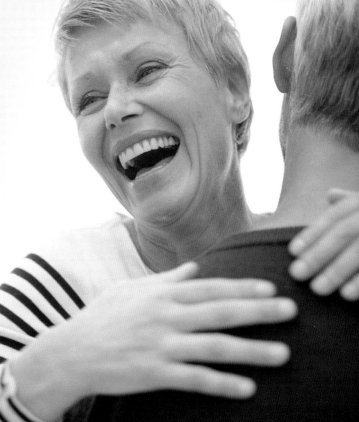

Stress and heart health

Anxiety and stress are normal and sometimes useful human emotions. Stress prompts the body to release a rush of adrenaline and other hormones, causing the heart to beat faster and raising blood pressure. If you are healthy, this response provides energy so that you can solve problems or react quickly to a threat to personal safety.

Feeling under pressure can all too easily become a fixed state of mind so that the body is permanently flooded with stress hormones. Because the stress is never dissipated, chronic physical symptoms, including raised blood pressure and psychological symptoms, such as feelings of hopelessness, despair and depression, start to affect health.

Are you stressed?

If you answer 'yes' to more than half of these questions drawn up by the Royal College of Psychiatrists, in the UK, you should talk to your GP about ways of combating unhelpful stress and make it a priority to find ways to relax and enjoy your life.

- Do you feel worried almost all of the time?

- Do you feel tired or lacking in energy all of the time?

- Are you unable to concentrate on a task for as long as you used to be able to?

- Do you have episodes of panic?

- Do you feel unusually irritable with tasks or people, or get angry quickly?

- Are you finding it difficult to get to sleep or are you waking earlier than usual?

- Do you ever experience a strong or rapid heartbeat (or 'palpitations')?

- Do you find yourself sweating a lot when you are not exercising?

- Do you have regular or constant pain or tension in your muscles?

- Do you find yourself breathing quickly or more heavily at times of anxiety?

- Are you experiencing indigestion or diarrhoea?

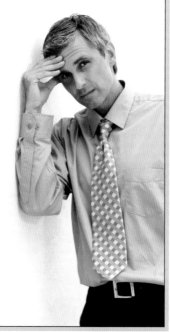

EFFECTS OF STRESS ON YOUR HEART

Stress contributes to heart problems rather than directly causing them. Much depends on how you cope when under stress – turning to cigarettes, alcohol or food in times of stress may have a knock-on effect on your heart. If you suffer from heart disease, any anxiety or stress in your life can bring on angina (chest pain). Finding ways to reduce stress and practising stress-mitigating measures will put you back on the road to heart health.

REDUCING STRESS THROUGH MEDITATION

Guided meditation is an easy way to learn to relax. Thanks to the MP3 player or iPod, you can lose yourself in centuries-old wisdom while travelling on a jam-packed train on the way home from work. Choose from hundreds of guided meditations that can be downloaded from the internet –

many of them specifically designed for people with heart disease. Make it part of your routine to unwind with your favourite meditation – no matter how busy you think you are.

LAUGH AWAY YOUR TROUBLES

Believe it or not, watching your favourite comedian or enjoying a funny cartoon is one of the best ways to combat heart disease. Research has shown that laughing out loud – whether it's helpless giggles or a full-blown guffaw – expands the inner walls of your blood vessels, boosting blood flow by 25 per cent. That's equivalent to the physiological impact of a stroll in the park or even being on a course of cholesterol-lowering medications. It's so good for you that heart experts recommend you aim for 15 minutes of laughter every day.

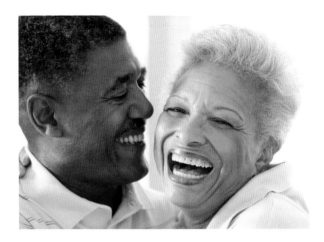

A stress-busting laugh is much more than light-hearted relief, it's a health-giving tonic

Top Tips

Ten top tips for reducing stress in your life

There's a lot you can do to reduce your stress levels without resorting to prescription medications. Take up as many of the suggestions as you can from the following list:

1 **Take care of yourself** Make sure you get plenty of sleep, eat a healthy diet, stop smoking and don't drink too much.

2 **Talk about it** Share your feelings on a regular basis with friends or family members. And then listen to *their* problems.

3 **Take aerobic exercise regularly** It's easiest to do if you find an exercise you thoroughly enjoy. Gentle exercise, such as yoga or Pilates, has been demonstrated to reduce stress.

4 **Try to enjoy your work** If you wake up dreading it, seriously consider searching for an alternative source of income.

5 **Know when to say 'no'** Living entirely for others is a major cause of chronic stress.

6 **Cultivate optimism** See the best in others and expect good things to happen.

7 **Set limits** Find a way to prevent other people's hurtful behaviour from upsetting your peace of mind.

8 **Organise your life** Getting rid of clutter will leave you with more energy and contentment.

9 **Have 'me-time'** We all need to be able to stare out of the window, read a book or enjoy a lazy, luxurious bath sometimes.

10 **Focus on deep breathing** It's a simple but highly successful stress-buster. You can teach yourself (see panel, page 250) or learn how to do this from a yoga teacher or in a special relaxation or meditation class.

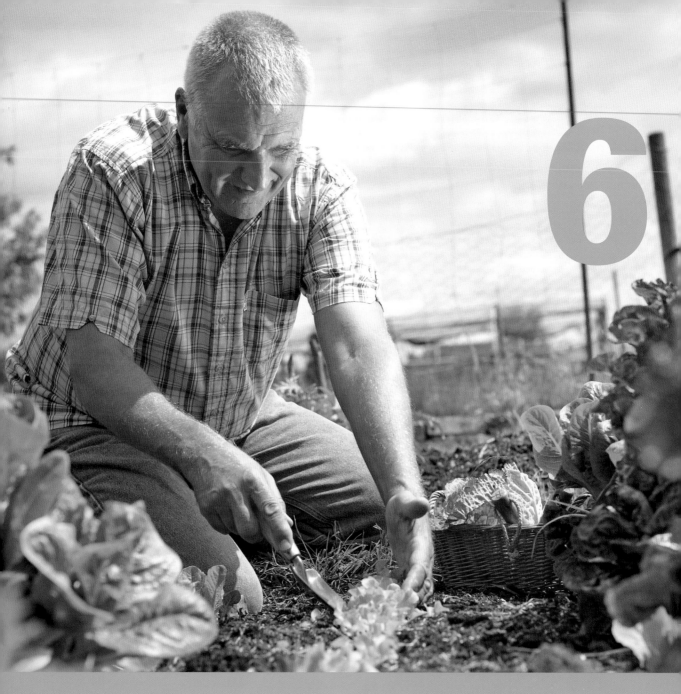

6

Recovering from a stroke

It can take time and determination but these days a high proportion of people get better and enjoy a full, active life

You've had a stroke. What now?

Although a stroke is widely viewed as one of the most frightening medical crises, there's increasingly good news about the potential for recovery. A stroke, also called a cerebrovascular accident (CVA), can strike at almost any age, but it is most likely from middle age onwards, with seven out of ten strokes occurring in people over 65. The severity of symptoms varies, but the degree to which a person is affected is not necessarily age-related. Being older doesn't mean a stroke will definitely be worse. Although strokes sometimes lead to devastating and permanent disability, many people suffer only temporary symptoms and make an excellent recovery. Some of the most common physical effects of a stroke are listed in the panel on page 144. The following symptoms may also occur but usually subside within a few weeks: shoulder pain, swollen hands and feet, incontinence, difficulty with swallowing and extreme tiredness.

PROMPT ACTION BRINGS SIGNIFICANT BENEFITS

Once diagnosed, stroke patients are more likely than ever to be treated by a highly specialist multi-disciplinary stroke team – possibly with drug treatment that dramatically reduces the risk of disability. Patients fare best when this treatment is followed seamlessly by well-organised practical, emotional and social support when they return home.

Recognising symptoms early (see *Take action FAST*, right) and getting treatment as quickly as possible are crucial. Changes to the connections between brain cells begin within 3 minutes of a stroke occurring. Accurate diagnosis and effective treatment in the hours after a stroke can make a big difference to your rate and extent of recovery.

DIAGNOSTIC TESTS ... WITHIN 24 HOURS

There are some essential tests that most hospitals will carry out. **Brain imaging** to assess your stroke symptoms. The test can be done using a CT (computerised tomography) scanner or by cross-sectional MRI (magnetic resonance imaging). The results ensure that the appropriate treatment is started as soon as possible. While a stroke expert may be able to assess the type of stroke simply from observing your symptoms, a brain scan should be carried out as quickly as possible to determine what type of stroke the patient has suffered. This is essential because different types of stroke can require radically

! ALERT

Take action FAST

With prompt treatment, much damage caused by a stroke can be kept to a minimum. If the condition is recognised quickly (whether by the medical profession, friends, family or colleagues), the outlook for recovery is much better.

You can use the FAST test to spot a stroke:

Facial weakness - can the person smile?

Arm weakness - can the person raise both arms?

Speech problems - can the person speak clearly and understand what you say?

If the answer to one or more of these is NO, it's:

Time to call 000 (in Australia).

Make sure the emergency operator and paramedics know that the person may be having a stroke.

The most common stroke symptoms

If you've had a stroke, you may experience some or all of the following in the immediate aftermath or weeks and months after the stroke. These symptoms can often be reversed or greatly alleviated with therapy:

Numbness or weakness (hemiparesis) or paralysis (hemiplegia), especially on one side of the body.

Stiffness of muscles and joints (spasticity) on one side.

Problems with walking due to dizziness, loss of balance or coordination.

Drooping facial muscles.

Confusion or difficulties with speaking or understanding speech and with reading and writing (aphasia – also known as dysphasia).

Vision problems affecting one or both eyes.

Severe pain, often developing weeks or months afterwards.

Problems of perception, for example in judging distance, rate of movement or recognising familiar objects.

Changes in mental processes such as learning, concentrating, remembering, making decisions, reasoning and planning.

Depression as well as anxiety, low self-esteem and loss of confidence.

different types of treatment. See *What happens during a stroke* (pages 146–147) for explanations of the types of stroke.

In fact, strokes caused by blood clots blocking blood flow to the brain are by far the most common. And one of the biggest recent changes in treatment has been 'thrombolytic therapy', whereby 'clot-busting' medications are delivered directly into the bloodstream. It must be delivered within 4½ hours of the onset of the stroke – the sooner the better. A scan should also be performed before aspirin or other blood-thinning (anticoagulant) medications are prescribed.

Swallowing test If you've had a stroke, your ability to swallow will usually be tested by a qualified health-care professional to ensure against the risk of choking. You will be given one or more teaspoons of water to drink. If you can manage this, you will then be asked to drink half a glass of water. More than one in three people who have strokes are unable to swallow properly for the first few days, which is dangerous because food and drink could enter the windpipe and then the lungs. If this is a potential problem, it should be identified as early as possible so that, if necessary, artificial feeding can be arranged. Later a speech and language therapist may be able to help you.

... WITHIN A WEEK

Some or all of the following tests and procedures will be carried out in the first week following a stroke.

Blood pressure and cholesterol checks These are needed so that appropriate medication can be prescribed.

Diabetes assessment People with diabetes whose blood glucose levels are not well controlled are at greater risk of having a stroke, so their diabetes treatment may need to be adjusted.

An ECG (electrocardiogram) to check for abnormal heart rhythm (atrial fibrillation) – this is present in around one in four sufferers.

An assessment by a specialist team Since suffering one stroke is a major risk factor for having another, a specialist team draws up a strategy to prevent this happening. For example, appropriate lifestyle changes, therapy and medication can reduce the risk significantly.

Surgery Anyone who suffers a 'carotid artery territory' stroke (related to the blood flow in the carotid artery in the neck) may be considered for urgent surgery in a specialist unit. This will involve opening up the artery in order to reduce the risk of another stroke.

A relative or friend may need to act as your advocate in the early days following a stroke

Keeping track

Understanding the treatment is important for all stroke victims. In some cases the person will be well enough to participate in decision making from an early stage, but in other cases a relative or friend may need to act as an advocate and intermediary. The following advice is valid for the stroke victim or someone acting on behalf of a loved one.

- *Ask questions – jot them down to help remember them, so that you can raise important concerns at the right moment.*
- *Make sure the clinical team is aware of any other health problems you may have. A friend or relative should provide this information if the patient can't.*
- *Talk to the nurse to ensure that health-care staff are taking every precaution to prevent MRSA and other infections during treatment.*
- *Make sure you know who is in charge of the case so that you can discuss any problems. If you are acting for the patient, ensure that the care team know your role, and put any request for a meeting with them in writing.*

FOCUS
What happens during a stroke?

Knowing how and why your stroke occurred can help you to understand your symptoms and begin to plan your path to recovery.

A CLOT (AN ISCHAEMIC STROKE)

Four out of five strokes are ischaemic; this means they occur when a blood clot blocks blood flow to the brain. There are two types of blood clot that can cause a stroke:

Cerebral thrombosis A blood clot that develops in an artery that supplies the brain.

Cerebral embolism A blood clot that travels from elsewhere in the body to an artery in the brain. People who experience blood clots may have chronic health problems that affect the normal flow of blood such as:

- Hardening of the arteries (atherosclerosis) as a result of high blood pressure, diabetes, high cholesterol or smoking.
- Atrial fibrillation or other irregular heart rhythms.
- Heart disease (coronary artery disease, heart failure, heart valve problems).

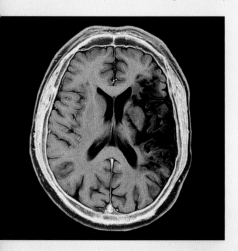

HAEMORRHAGIC STROKE
In this CT scan the blue area indicates the area of the brain affected by a haemorrhagic stroke several weeks previously.

A BLEED (A HAEMORRHAGIC STROKE)

This occurs as a result of bleeding into or around the brain. It can be caused by:

- An intracerebral haemorrhage: this is where a blood vessel inside the brain bursts.
- A subarachnoid haemorrhage: this occurs when a blood vessel on the surface of the brain bleeds into the area between the brain and the skull.

Strokes of this type are usually caused by long-standing high blood pressure or a ruptured aneurysm (a blood-filled balloon-like bulge in the wall of a blood vessel). They are often more severe than an ischaemic stroke and, although the symptoms are similar, early treatment is very different.

WHY DO THE EFFECTS VARY?

A stroke may cause only temporary symptoms such as facial palsy or a weakness in your arm that disappears within hours. This is known as a TIA (transient ischaemic attack, or 'mini-stroke'). In more severe cases, it could take months of therapy before you stand unaided, move your arms easily or recover your powers of speech.

This variation depends on the part of your brain that has been injured. The right half controls the left side of the body and vice versa. Common symptoms such as weakness or paralysis usually happen on the opposite side of the body to the side of the brain damaged by the stroke. If it is the left half of the brain that is affected, you're more likely to have problems with language (talking, understanding, reading and writing). If the right half is affected, you may have difficulties with perceptual skills (making sense of what you see, hear and touch) and spatial skills (judging size, speed, distance or position in space).

The severity of symptoms depends on the extent of the damage and whether it is caused by a clot or bleeding. Symptoms are also likely to be worse in those whose health is already poor.

Mini but not minor

A TIA (transitory ischaemic attack) is often called a 'mini-stroke'. It is a stroke with symptoms that last for less than 24 hours and which can be diagnosed by observation.

Having a TIA increases the risk of having a further stroke within five years – although it could occur within days or weeks of the first attack. If a doctor believes, or the FAST test (see page 143) shows, that you've been experiencing stroke symptoms for even a few minutes, it's essential to see your GP or an emergency department as soon as possible, ideally that day. The assessment will help doctors decide on the best medication for you and whether you need surgery.

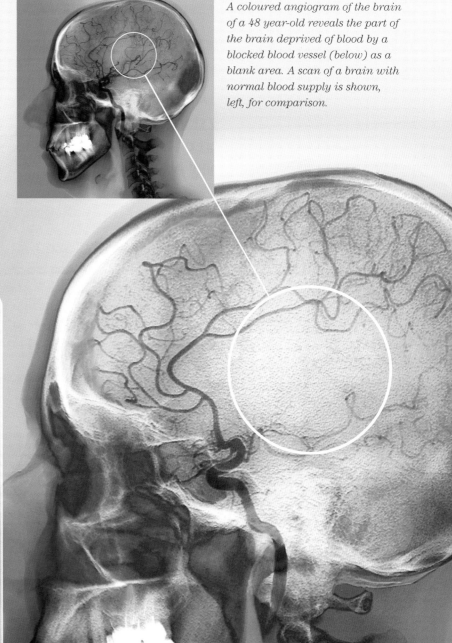

ISCHAEMIC STROKE
A coloured angiogram of the brain of a 48 year-old reveals the part of the brain deprived of blood by a blocked blood vessel (below) as a blank area. A scan of a brain with normal blood supply is shown, left, for comparison.

First steps on your road to recovery

The days following a stroke can be frightening and uncertain, but your recovery starts now. Your specialist team provides expert help, but the support of family and friends and your own determination and commitment also play a key role.

Doctors can try to predict your future health based on your physical condition before the stroke, your symptoms and your improvement so far – but only to a degree. There is no single rule book for recovery. Your own commitment to rehabilitation and maintaining good health is at least as important as the work of the medical team. And the contribution lifestyle changes can make towards reducing the likelihood of a second stroke is immense (see page 156). One thing is certain: the journey towards recovery will involve setbacks as well as achievements. It can be emotionally and psychologically challenging for the family as well as the stroke patient. If you accept this from the outset, your expectations about the rate of your recovery will be more realistic.

WAYS TO KICK-START YOUR RECOVERY

Remind yourself that – however unwell you feel now – your body has a huge capacity for healing: this can help you to feel more positive about your prospects for recovery. Trust your health-care team and focus on all the tasks they teach you, practising them between sessions, if you have the strength, but don't become overtired. It's your willingness to persevere that really counts.

Here are five of the best things that you and your family can do to help you on your way:

Get moving A pattern of taking control and doing as much for yourself as early as possible will pay huge dividends later on. The stroke may have affected your mobility, but the sooner you get out of bed and start walking around the ward (under supervision), the better your chances of making a good recovery. While you are still in hospital and have begun to walk, try to move on to taking regular gentle aerobic exercise under the guidance of a physiotherapist as soon as possible.

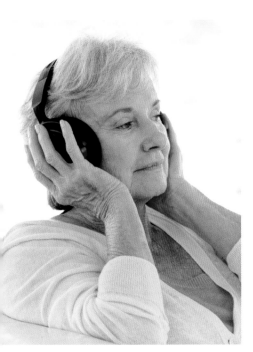

Listening to music can boost the recovery process

Focus on your muscles More than one in three stroke patients will suffer spasticity, meaning they have tight or stiff muscles. Moving your arms and legs can be difficult as well as painful, and simple daily activities become time-consuming for both you and your carers. Yet there are effective treatments for spasticity including medications and both physiotherapy and occupational therapy. Evidence shows that early treatment for this problem can make a significant difference to how severely you will be affected in the long term. Talk to your health-care team about the most effective rehabilitation program for improving your quality of life.

Listen to your favourite music Before you're ready to take control of your own recovery, your family can give you a vital head start by simply putting your favourite CD on an MP3 player, according to Finnish researchers. The study, reported in the journal *Brain*, showed that stroke patients who listened to their favourite music in the early days of recovery were better at remembering language later on than those who did nothing or just listened to audio books. They had better cognitive recovery and were less likely to develop depression.

Get the family involved While you're still in hospital, surround yourself with pictures of family and friends and ask them to bring

Who is on your team?
As you recover, the following key professionals are likely to be involved in your care and rehabilitation.

Consultant physician specialising in stroke heads the team of people involved in your recovery, although you may not see him or her very often. Once you are back at home, your GP is usually in overall charge of your medical care.

Nurses on the ward provide day-to-day care. When you return home, a community or district nurse will make regular home visits to monitor your medication, blood pressure and overall health.

Physiotherapist helps you with any balance problems, paralysis or muscle weakness and provides exercises to improve your movement and prevent your limbs becoming stiff and painful if they are weak. Eventually, this vital team member can advise you on returning to normal activity.

Speech and language therapist assesses any difficulties with swallowing initially. Once you return home, he or she can advise you on managing and overcoming communication problems, including speaking, reading and writing, often drawing on the support of family and friends.

Dietitian develops a nutritious diet that is safe and easy for you to eat if you're having swallowing problems, have lost your appetite, are underweight or have diabetes.

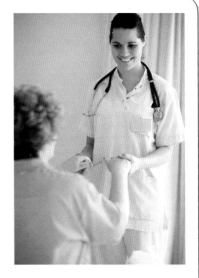

Occupational therapist (OT) helps with everyday activities at home including dressing, using the toilet and washing. Once you've returned home, the OT can also help you obtain useful equipment such as a wheelchair.

Depending on how the stroke has affected you, you may also be referred to one of the following:

Ophthalmologist vision can deteriorate following a stroke.

Clinical psychologist to help with emotional problems such as tiredness, mood swings, stress, anxiety and depression.

Chiropodist to help with foot care, especially if you have problems caused by paralysis and lack of movement.

Orthotist makes special bracing devices that can support and control your limbs, if this could help your mobility.

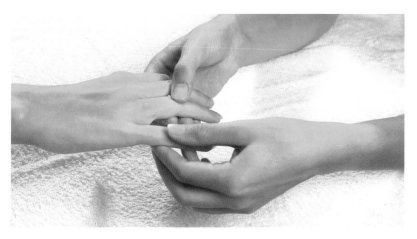

Your physiotherapist will help you to gently mobilise joints and limbs affected by your stroke

in much-loved objects, such as souvenirs and keepsakes. This reminds you why it's worth striving to return to normality. If your family stay by your side as much as possible, it will allow them to meet the rehabilitation team. Physiotherapists and speech therapists are often keen to work with the patient's family and advise on an ongoing rehabilitation program when the person returns home.

Get support The return home can be daunting since stroke patients are almost certain to be discharged from hospital while still experiencing some movement difficulties. However, community support services exist to assist you and your family through any problems. Continuing physiotherapy and occupational therapy, which includes planning the aids and equipment

EXERCISING YOUR FACIAL MUSCLES

If your facial muscles have been affected by a stroke, practising the following simple exercises will help strengthen them.

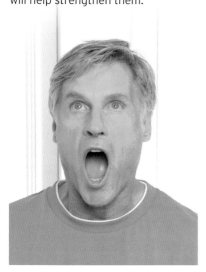

1 *Open your eyes and mouth as wide as possible, then squeeze them tight.*

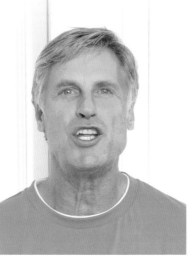

2 *Recite your vowels to work the muscles around your mouth.*

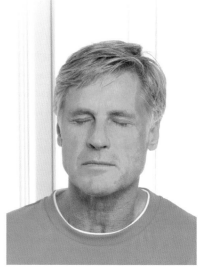

3 *Raise and lower your eyebrows.*

you will need to use around your home, should be organised before your discharge. Your GP can also advise you on getting support from local health and social services, including physiotherapy and advice from an occupational therapist. You might also find it helpful to contact the National Stroke Foundation for advice and support. Go online at www. strokefoundation.com.au, or call the StrokeLine on 1800 787 653.

Once you're home

The rehabilitation process continues in the weeks and months after you return from hospital. Your goal is to regain as much independence as you can as soon as possible. Coming home can be an uncertain time, and you may wonder how you'll manage with any disability that remains. The challenges you face will be individual to you, depending on the impact of the stroke and the extent of your recovery.

COMMITMENT TO REHABILITATION

Re-educating your body after a stroke is a vital part of a recovery and an ongoing commitment. By practising exercises suggested by your physiotherapist and other members of your care team, you can relearn any basic skills you may have lost, such as talking, eating, dressing and walking, as well as improving your strength, flexibility and endurance.

Once home, carry on with the approaches and exercises that you learned in hospital, developing ways to sit up in bed, get up and move around. Your physiotherapist will continue to focus on functional, task-specific movements around the home, with the aim of getting you mobile and able to perform practical day-to-day activities that will enable you to regain your independence as soon as you can manage.

SEEK STIMULATION

Mental and physical stimulation are vital for rediscovering yourself after your stay in hospital. One stroke patient recalls her experience: 'Anything stimulating can help. My week in hospital was completely unstimulating and I was left sitting around. As soon as I got home, I was able to watch TV and use the computer again … and here I am beginning to return to work within three months.'

Try to arrange regular challenges for your body and mind – for example, by setting goals for your physical exercise program or mental workouts such as puzzles. Just be careful not to be overambitious or to be disappointed if you don't reach your targets.

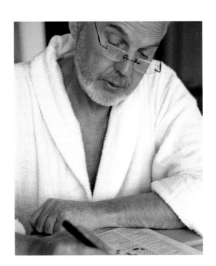

Doing puzzles isn't just a way of passing the time, it can be a key element of your recovery program

GET LOOSE, GET STRONG

Here are four daily exercises, devised by a physiotherapist with a special interest in stroke, to help you regain mobility. It's essential to take extra care with any joints that have been affected by the stroke. Talk to your physiotherapist before you start this or any other exercise regimen.

MOBILISE YOUR NECK AND HEAD

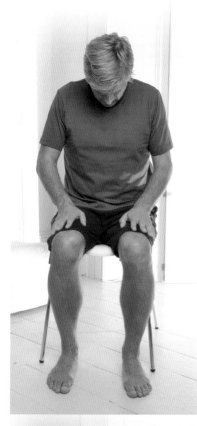

1 *In a sitting position, with both your feet flat on the floor, bend your head downwards towards your chest.*

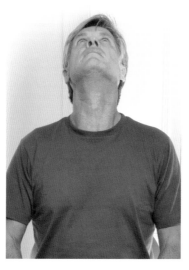

2 *Slowly raise your head to face upwards towards the ceiling, then move it down, so that you look straight ahead.*

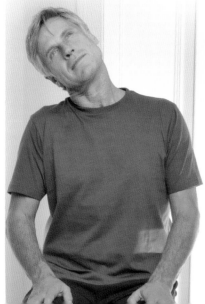

3 *Next, angle your head to bring your right ear down towards your right shoulder. Then straighten your head and repeat the movement on your left side.*

LOOSEN YOUR SHOULDERS

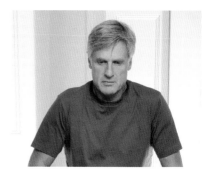

1 *Mobilise your shoulders by rolling them forwards several times.*

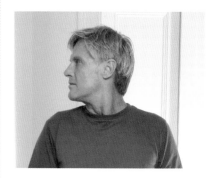

2 *Then, turn your head towards your right shoulder, as far as you can. Repeat the step looking over your left shoulder.*

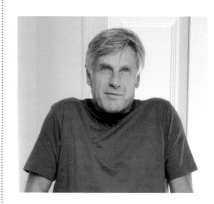

3 *Move both shoulders up and down, as if shrugging. Do this several times.*

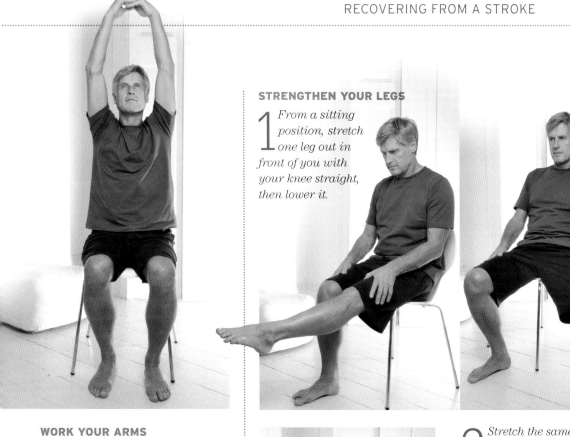

STRENGTHEN YOUR LEGS

1 *From a sitting position, stretch one leg out in front of you with your knee straight, then lower it.*

WORK YOUR ARMS

1 *Clasp your hands together on your lap, then slowly raise your clasped hands up over your head. Get advice from your physiotherapist if this is painful.*

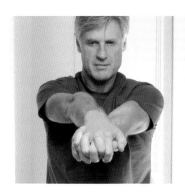

2 *Bring your clasped hands down to shoulder level. With a twisting motion of your arms, rotate your hands so that the top hand is at the bottom. Repeat a few times. Seek your physiotherapist's advice if this is painful or you have shoulder problems.*

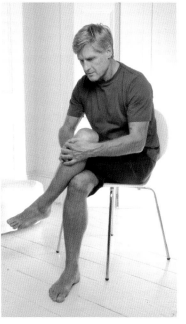

3 *Now cross the same leg over the other and lean forwards slightly in your chair, then back, before uncrossing the leg. Repeat all three steps on the opposite side.*

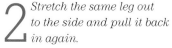

2 *Stretch the same leg out to the side and pull it back in again.*

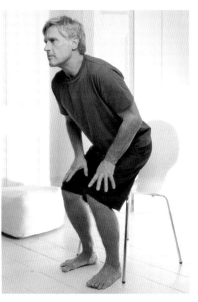

4 *Now put both feet on the ground and practise rising from the chair and sitting down again. Repeat a few times.*

MUSICAL SOLUTIONS

Curious as it may seem, singing is sometimes easier than talking. About one in five people lose the ability to speak after a stroke – yet many of them can communicate their words by singing them, researchers reported to the American Association for the Advancement of Science in 2010. The technique, officially known as Melodic Intonation Therapy, involves teaching people to sing words and phrases, including asking for the bathroom or stating that they are hungry or thirsty. Scientists believe the melody can help the brain rewire itself so that it can bypass the damaged regions of the brain. 'Music is a good medium to get parts of the brain responding that are not responding,' said Dr Gottfried Schlaug, a neuroscientist at Harvard Medical School.

Getting your friends and family involved

However good your medical and therapy team are, it's friends and family that can make the real difference to you. Here are ten ways they can support your recovery:

1 By accepting you as you are. They should help you to express your needs and fears and be supportive and full of praise for what you achieve.

2 By finding out how to help with particular problems – by asking the physio or speech therapist, or doing research on reputable websites such as www.strokefoundation.com.au.

3 By involving you in stimulating and challenging activities you can do together, such as card games, puzzles or board games – or virtual reality games on a computer or computer console. There's evidence that playing them can help improve mobility after a stroke.

4 By engaging you in conversations and avoiding questions that call for yes or no responses. They should ask open questions requiring you to speak in sentences - however long it takes, they should wait for the answer.

5 By bearing in mind if you're having trouble remembering words that you're more likely to recall the words to songs - so it may be worth singing together.

6 By avoiding doing everyday tasks for you that you can manage on your own, even though it may take longer. The more you're left to get on with things, the more confident you'll become.

7 By researching local rehabilitation classes and attending them together with you wherever possible.

8 By helping to maintain contact with your wider social circle so that your world does not 'shrink'.

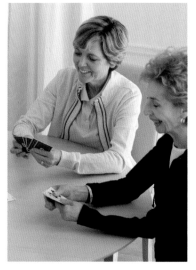

9 By recognising that depression is common following a stroke. It can have a negative effect on your recovery - but once you're aware of it, depression is relatively straightforward to treat.

10 By understanding that recovery can be exhausting and being aware of the healing power of sleep.

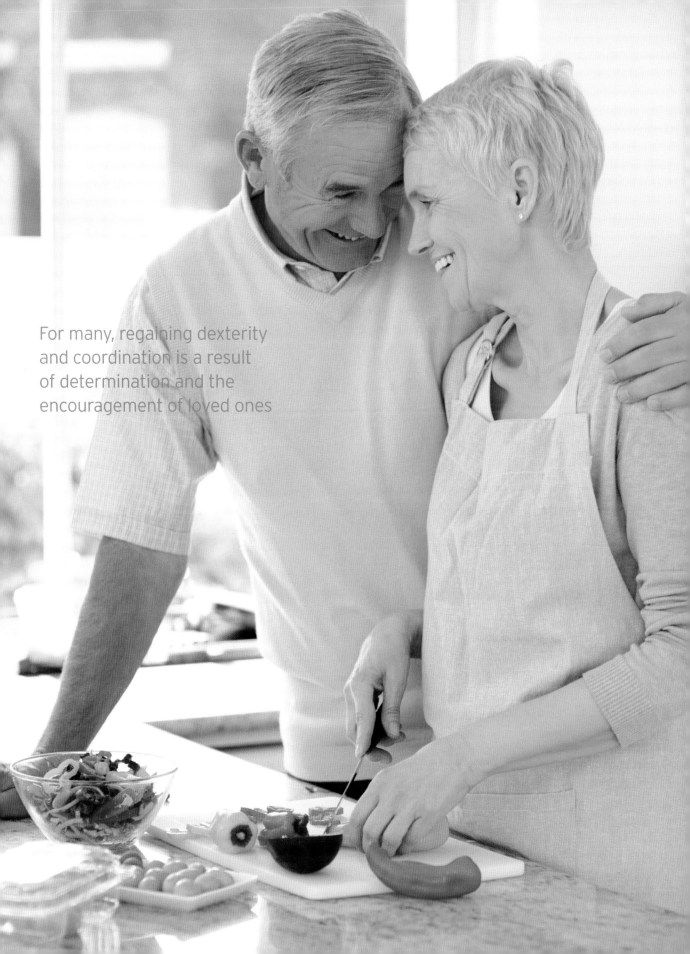

For many, regaining dexterity
and coordination is a result
of determination and the
encouragement of loved ones

Safeguarding health for the years ahead

Make it a priority to tackle the factors that contributed to your stroke. While having had a stroke is the main risk factor for having another, you can vastly improve your chances of a lasting recovery and reduce the risk of it happening again by addressing risk factors in your lifestyle.

While there are some factors you can't control – the risk is greater for older people, for men, and for those of Indian or African descent – the good news is that many strokes can be prevented. Indeed, scientists in the United States estimate that making lifestyle changes can halve the risk of having a stroke – with eight out of ten strokes being entirely preventable by simple measures.

Here are five important ways to cut your risk of a second stroke:

- Stop smoking – the habit doubles the risk of a stroke. For advice on quitting smoking, see *Clearing the smoke*, page 136.
- Keep your alcohol intake low. Excess consumption raises blood pressure, increasing your chances of having a second stroke.
- Eat a healthy diet to boost your energy and reduce excess weight. Being overweight, especially carrying excess fat around your abdomen, is strongly linked to raised blood pressure and therefore to risk of stroke. Salt intake also raises blood pressure, so avoid eating processed foods that contain high levels of salt and minimise the amount you add to food (see panel below, and *Cut down on salt*, page 128).

I've recently suffered a stroke. Now that I'm home, should I be following a special diet?

A 'stroke-healthy' diet is no different from normal healthy-eating guidelines described on pages 24-25. Make sure your diet is nutritious and balanced as well as being low in saturated (animal) fat, sugar and salt. Try to eat as much fruit and vegetables as you can manage and add wholegrain bread and pasta and brown rice to your diet. Eating oily fish regularly will also help to reduce your risk of stroke. And be sure to moderate your alcohol intake.

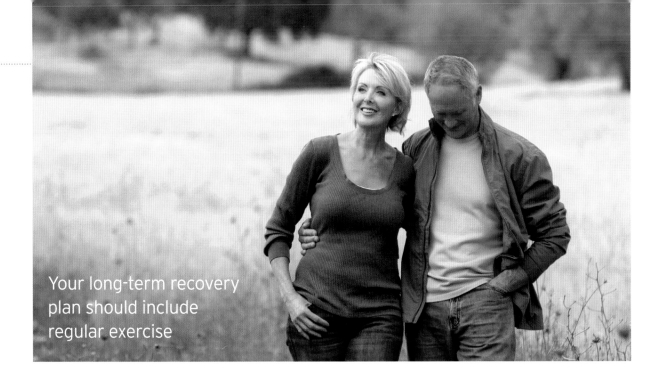

Your long-term recovery plan should include regular exercise

- Increase your level of exercise. Physical inactivity significantly increases your risk of a second stroke. Aim for 30 minutes of moderate exercise that raises your heart rate at least five times a week. Research shows that moderately active people have a 20 per cent lower risk of stroke than people with a sedentary lifestyle, while highly active people have a 30 per cent reduced risk of stroke.
- Reconsider your use of hormone-containing drugs (in contraceptive pills and hormone replacement therapy). They may raise your risk of a second stroke. It's wise to discuss alternatives with your doctor.

CONTROLLING CHRONIC HEALTH PROBLEMS

Once you've had a stroke, there are several key long-term conditions that you need to make an even greater effort to control, to reduce your risk of having a second stroke:

High blood pressure This is perhaps the most important. If your doctor prescribes medication for high blood pressure, make sure you take it and go for regular blood pressure checks.

High cholesterol levels Ask your doctor if you should be prescribed a statin to reduce levels of 'bad' cholesterol (see *Managing your medication*, page 158). There's evidence that almost everyone who's had a stroke will benefit from lifelong statin treatment; the exceptions are those with low cholesterol levels and those under the age of 40.

Abnormal blood glucose levels Keep your blood glucose levels as normal as possible. Follow the advice for type 2 diabetes (see pages 108–112).

Blood-thinning meds Depending on what type of stroke you have had, your doctor may put you on a blood-thinning medication, most commonly aspirin.

B vitamins aid recovery from stroke

Unproven A major Japanese study published in the journal *Stroke* in June 2010 suggests that taking folic acid and B6 supplements can prevent the worst consequences of stroke, significantly reducing the risk of death. As a result of this and other studies, there's a growing feeling that folic acid may be a useful treatment for anyone who has had a stroke or is at risk of having one in the future. But many doctors are not convinced. Even if you do decide to take B vitamins, it's still essential to follow the key steps for improving your lifestyle (see facing page).

True or False?

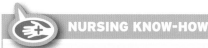

Managing your medication

Nurses in the community (or community nurses) report that people who are well organised and who fully understand their medication are more likely to keep to their regimen and do better in the long term. Here are some suggestions:

- Get a pill-sorting box with containers for your medication for each day of the week. Most pharmacies stock them.

- Make sure you understand why each type of medication is important. If you don't know, ask your GP or stroke specialist to explain.

- Find out from your doctor what your optimum blood pressure and blood cholesterol levels are. Keep on top of your levels yourself. Being interested and aware of your body will improve your motivation to keep these critical factors under control.

- Enlist the help of your partner or a family member to remind you when to take your pills. If necessary, put a note on your fridge.

Living with your medication regimen

Medication is vital in the immediate aftermath of a stroke. Most people are discharged from hospital with a prescription for several types of medications. It is crucial for your long-term recovery that you stick to the treatment plan prescribed by your doctor.

Research from the USA found that while the vast majority of stroke patients are still taking their medications after three months, that figure dwindles to one in three just a year later – with many thousands of patients regularly skipping doses. Researchers who followed 6,000 stroke patients after they had left hospital reported that failing to take medication as directed was one of the key factors that caused a second stroke.

MEDICATIONS YOU MAY NEED

The three most common types of medication prescribed for stroke patients are:

Statins to reduce cholesterol These medications work by controlling the level of cholesterol in the blood, which is a major risk factor in the build-up of plaque in the blood vessels and thus a clot. By taking a statin, in combination with other medication, you are also likely to suffer less extensive brain damage if you do have a stroke. There is convincing evidence that statins dramatically reduce the risk of a second stroke as well as the risk of a heart attack in people who have had an acute ischaemic stroke or a TIA (transient ischaemic attack).

Blood pressure medication Lowering your blood pressure will help to prevent further strokes no matter what sort of stroke you've had. Several different types of blood pressure medication are prescribed – including diuretics, ACE inhibitors and angiotensin receptor blockers (ARBs) – depending on your symptoms and how well you tolerate them. They are most effective if you also make lifestyle changes such as reducing your alcohol consumption, increasing your activity and exercise levels and eating a healthier diet. Your GP will monitor your blood pressure and adjust your medication over time.

Blood-thinning medications Depending on what type of stroke you have had, you may be put on the blood-thinning medications, typically aspirin for ischaemic strokes and warfarin for strokes caused by atrial fibrillation. All blood-thinning medications carry a risk of causing bleeding, but overall they do much more good than harm.

An active recovery

More than half of all people who have a stroke are left with long-term mobility problems or difficulties in balance and coordination. Exercising the affected parts of your body is key, but how much and what sort of exercises you're able to undertake depends on how much movement you've lost as a result of your stroke and on how active you were before. Here are four suggestions for increasing your strength and fitness, recommended by a physiotherapist with a special interest in stroke.

The support of an expert physiotherapist can be a key to progress

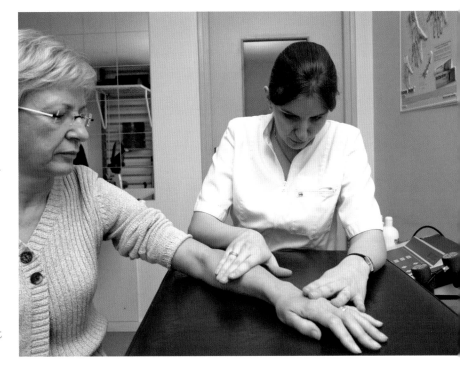

1 Challenge yourself to do a little bit more each day. Stand for longer, walk a bit farther, climb the stairs more than once a day.

2 Try not to do everything with your stronger side. Even if it takes a bit longer – for example, attempt activities that require you to move or put weight on your weaker leg.

3 Keep your muscles flexible by stretching and moving regularly. Extend and wiggle your fingers, make sure your foot is fully flat on the floor, stretch your back (arching and turning) and sit up straight.

4 Think of ways to incorporate exercise into your day or have a set time that you allocate for completing your exercises. Set yourself targets, such as increasing the number of exercises you attempt, or have a specific goal such as walking out in the garden again.

THE BENEFITS OF EACH EXERCISE TYPE

You're still finding your feet. But whether you're exercising at home, in the gym or during hospital visits, the following large-muscle exercises will do wonders to increase the speed at which you walk and your sense of independence when you undertake everyday activities. At the same time, these forms of exercise will improve your physical endurance and reduce your risk of cardiovascular disease.

Walking This is good for your leg muscles, balance, coordination, fitness and for strengthening your cardiovascular system.

Treadmill walking As well as providing all the benefits of regular walking, you have handrails to provide extra stability. Most treadmills also offer the facility to alter the speed and slope of your walk and to time your exercise.

Static bike or cycle ergometer (which measures the amount of exercise you do in a single session). This allows you to exercise from a seated position. It's good for leg muscle work, coordinated movement, seated balance and cardiovascular fitness.

Arm ergometer This is not a gym staple but it is usually available in hospital rehabilitation departments. It works like a bicycle for the arms and is good for the arm muscles and upper trunk, cardiovascular fitness and upper limb coordination and function.

Everyday activity Standing up from a chair or toilet, climbing the stairs to fetch your glasses or picking up something that you've dropped on the floor are all forms of exercise, too. Unless you really can't manage, don't ask for help – do it yourself.

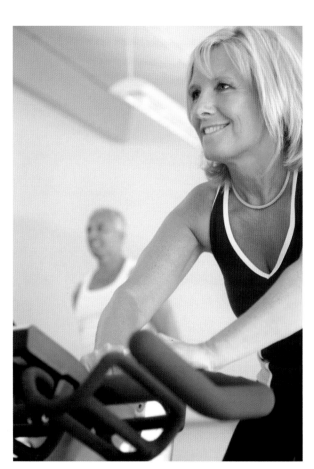

A gym can provide safe facilities for post-stroke workouts

AIDS THAT CAN REALLY HELP

After a stroke, you may find daily tasks such as getting around, cooking and bathing much harder than before, but you don't have to manage on your own. A number of aids designed to help those recovering from stroke to undertake everyday tasks are available through social services or your local occupational therapy department. Your GP can help you identify local suppliers of stroke-related aids and equipment.

Here's a list of basic aids that can help you live an independent life while you're recovering. Your occupational therapist will be able to advise you where to get practical and financial help for household adaptations:

Daily mobility If you are confined to a wheelchair, you may need to make adaptations to your home, including installing ramps and a stairlift. A wheelchair-friendly, low-level toilet and easy-access bath are other aids you may consider.

Independent living Household adaptations include fitting handrails on the stairs or in the shower and placing a non-slip mat in the bath.

Eating Try specialist equipment such as easy-grip cutlery and crockery that doesn't slip on the table.

Cooking Gadgets are available to help you open jars, pour a kettle or peel potatoes.

Washing Helpful implements include long-handled sponges and suction brushes.

Dressing Look for gadgets that help you do up buttons and make it easier to put on shoes and socks if you find it hard to reach your feet.

Taking control

Poor control of urination is a common problem after a stroke. There are usually a number of causes, such as nerve damage from the stroke or loss of muscle control as a result of a change of diet or being bedbound. The problem is often made worse by the fact that many stroke patients can't get to the toilet without someone helping them – and may have difficulty communicating their need.

The vast majority of people regain control quickly. If you need extra help, ask for a referral to a continence adviser. This specialist nurse will develop a rehabilitation plan including bladder retraining and pelvic-floor exercises to strengthen muscles, as well as the use of continence aids such as pads and bed covers while you're recovering. You could also ask your occupational therapist whether your home or toilet could be adapted for easier access.

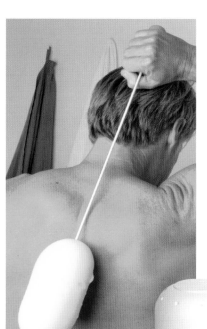

INCREASE YOUR REACH
A sponge on a handle can help you wash parts of your body that are hard to reach as a result of your stroke.

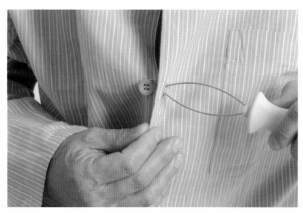

BUTTON UP
If a stroke has affected fine motor control of your hands and fingers, this handy aid can help you to fasten buttons on your clothing.

ON TAP
The twisting action required to turn on a tap can be difficult when you've had a stroke. These fittings, which convert conventional taps to lever-style control, are ideal.

LEARNING THE LANGUAGE

These are some of the phrases that medical professionals may use when describing different sorts of aphasia.

Receptive aphasia the term used when a person finds it hard to understand what is being said to them. Dysphasia is an alternative term.

Expressive aphasia when a person can understand what's being said but can't find the right words to express what he or she wants to say. Dysphasia is an alternative term.

Dysarthria when someone has problems forming words and speech sounds due to weak muscles in the mouth.

Dyspraxia occurs when the brain cannot properly coordinate the muscles used for speech.

Overcoming speech difficulties

Being able to communicate is something we take for granted, yet one in three people who survive a stroke are left with language and communication difficulties. Known as aphasia, or sometimes dysphasia, this condition occurs when the stroke damages the brain's ability to process language, which can lead to problems with speech, writing, reading and the ability to interpret what is heard. Yet whatever their communication problems, the common link in people with aphasia is that their intelligence and understanding remain unaffected.

As with all stroke symptoms, the impact of aphasia varies from person to person. The problem can last from just a few weeks to months but sometimes much longer, and signs of improvement happen slowly but surely. For those few affected with severe aphasia, it can mean years of being unable to speak (or having a very limited vocabulary) as well as the disabling loss of the ability to read, write or use numbers.

Carers need to be aware that people with aphasia, as well as having difficulties with speech, may have problems with reading, following what's happening on the television or radio, writing a letter or filling in a form, using the telephone, counting, numbers and money, and repeating their own name or the names of their family. Without sympathetic help, aphasia can be very distressing and may lead to social exclusion, loneliness, boredom, loss of confidence and the breakdown of relationships. However, with the knowledgeable support of friends, family and carers, as well as expert speech therapy, many of these communication problems can be overcome.

THE NATURE OF APHASIA

Unlike other neurodegenerative diseases that affect communication, such as dementia, aphasia damages the brain's language system but leaves the memory system intact. People with aphasia can access their memory system by sight, smell or sound, but they can't say simple phrases, for example, 'that's a telephone', according to Professor Richard Wise, consultant neurologist at Imperial College, London.

It is often too easy to assume that someone with aphasia has lost the ability to think and remember, rather than simply the ability to communicate. As a result, friends and family may find it hard to slow down or resist finishing the person's sentences. But by making small adaptations, they could help the person to develop new ways of participating in conversations (see panel, below).

'Most people are still unaware of ways they could change their communication practices to make sure people with aphasia can join in on an equal footing and thereby help them feel involved and valued,' says Carole Pound of Connect, the aphasia charity that publishes a helpful book called *Better Conversations* (available from www.ukconnect.org/publications.aspx).

ACCESSING HELP

It is important for someone who has suffered a stroke to be helped and encouraged. A speech and language therapist will first make a detailed assessment, either in hospital or after discharge. They may then recommend that you practise the following (carers, friends and family may be able to help with this and provide patient encouragement):

- Exercises to improve facial muscle strength (see page 150).
- Repeating simple words.
- The use of gestures.

Top Tips

Stroke victims are adults

Remember that someone with aphasia has not become less intelligent. Treat him or her as an adult. You may need to remind less tactful friends and relatives of this.

How to help someone with aphasia

Encourage a person with aphasia to join in with normal conversations. Here are some tips to make communication easier:

- Have a pen and paper to hand.

- Take plenty of time.

- Be clear and tackle one idea at a time.

- Don't pretend to understand. If you're having difficulty understanding someone, be honest and tell him or her, 'I'm sorry, I don't understand – let's try again.'

- Write down key words as you go through the conversation.

- Encourage the person with aphasia to use drawings – and use them yourself.

- Remember that communication is not about using perfect grammar and forming proper sentences, so don't feel that you must correct every mistake. This could be discouraging.

- Be positive and encouraging and always remind the person of any progress that he or she has made.

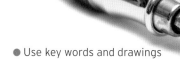

- Use key words and drawings to check back and summarise.

- Make use of expressive gestures to reinforce your meaning.

- Always check that you and the person with aphasia have both understood what each is saying to the other.

- Word and picture charts.
- Drawing or using a computer (the website www.aphasianow.org carries reviews by therapists of existing software packages designed for people with aphasia).

If a stroke has affected your speech, you or your family should ensure that you are fully informed about the help available. Ideally you should be offered several weeks of intensive language therapy, involving repetition and hard work.

Speech and language therapists play a crucial role in supporting people with aphasia. In a survey carried out by the Royal College of Speech and Language Therapists (RCSLT), in the UK, most people with aphasia said that therapy helped them remain independent, able to communicate, make choices and feel less isolated.

SHARING THE PROBLEM

If you have aphasia, there's evidence that spending time with people with similar language problems will boost your confidence and put meaning back into your life.

Here are some organisations that can put you in touch with fellow aphasia sufferers:

Australian Aphasia Association A support and advocacy association for people with aphasia, their families and the professionals who help them. It provides online resources and contact information for social aphasia groups across the country (www.aphasia.org.au).

National Stroke Foundation The National Stroke Foundation has lots of online resources, runs the StrokeLine (1800 787 653) and coordinates local stroke support groups (www.strokefoundation.com.au).

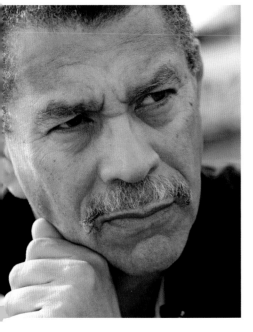

The loss of speech can often lead to feelings of isolation

Staying positive

Life doesn't stop when you've had a stroke – even if it sometimes feels that way. Instead of dwelling on what's been lost, it's worth focusing on what you're achieving and how your family and friends, physiotherapy and other support systems are helping you to get back to an independent life.

POST-STROKE MENTAL AND PHYSICAL FITNESS

Quite apart from worries about work and money, it's easy to be overwhelmed by feelings of anger, resentment, grief and a sense of 'why me?' following a stroke. People can feel that they're no longer the same person or that they don't belong to the outside world when they leave hospital. Such feelings are entirely normal. However justified they may be, it's important to recognise that too much negativity gets in the way of recovery. If you are struggling emotionally, ask your GP if a psychologist should be part of your chronic care team.

FOCUSING ON RECOVERY

Getting to the gym regularly and eating a healthy diet are relatively simple and enjoyable activity when life's going well. After a stroke, everything becomes more of an effort. But it is doubly important to exercise and eat well, as both will help to boost your spirits and counter any stress and depression you may experience.

Evidence from Cambridge University, published in the journal *Stroke*, shows that people who take 'a well-rounded approach' to their problems, including maintaining high levels of exercise and avoiding smoking and drinking too much throughout a difficult period, have a significantly lower risk of suffering a stroke or of having a second stroke if they've already had one. There's also evidence that strokes caused by a blood clot developing inside the brain (ischaemic strokes) are most common in people who've been suffering from a significant amount of stress over an extended period of time.

WAYS TO STAY POSITIVE DURING YOUR RECOVERY

After a stroke it's important to accept that you'll have bad as well as good days, that sometimes you'll go backwards as well as forwards, and not ask too much of yourself. Remember that recovery can often be gradual and even when progress is slow, it is still worth persevering. It's a good idea to practise the tasks therapists have taught you between therapy sessions. This will help keep you motivated. Look after your general health. Take any medication as directed. Plenty of sleep, a good diet (one that is high in fibre and lean protein, and low in salt, fat and processed foods) and regular exercise are essential to recovery.

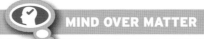

MIND OVER MATTER

How to melt your stress away

Being unable to do the things you could before your stroke is frustrating and stressful and you will need strategies to help deal with your emotions. But you can combat even the most severe stress by retreating to an inner sanctuary, say a sun-drenched beach. Using guided visualisation techniques, you can go there in your mind whenever you need to. You can also undertake gentle relaxation techniques while listening to soothing music. The internet is the best place to search for guided relaxation CDs or downloads to an MP3 player.

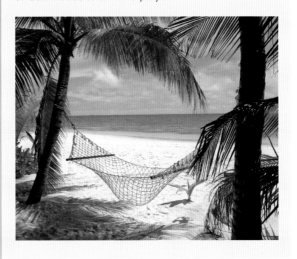

Here are some additional tips to help you on your journey to recovery:

- Don't overdo it. Becoming exhausted will set you back rather than push you forward.
- When you're discharged from hospital, you will probably be prescribed medication to take for the foreseeable future to protect against further attacks. It is important follow your doctors' instructions and take all medications exactly as prescribed.
- Try not to push people away. Even if you have difficulty communicating, spending time with your family and wider social circle is healthy.
- Don't despair. If you can't do everything you used to be able to do, there will be many things you can still enjoy and new possibilities to explore. Remember that recovery can often be a slow process, so you may need to be patient. While the most significant improvements occur in the first few weeks after a stroke, recovery can continue for months, evens years, particularly if care and rehabilitation begin early.
- If you are feeling sad, consider treatment, whether this involves seeing a therapist or clinical psychologist, or taking a course of antidepressant medication. You can discuss this with your GP.
- Join a self-help group for people who have had a stroke (see *Sharing the problem*, page 164). Participating in a self-help group could help you learn more about stroke, and give you the inspiration to move forward.
- Remember that acceptance, including acknowledging at some point that you may not make significant further progress, can bring peace of mind.

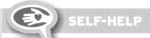

SELF-HELP

Finding the keys
managing memory loss

Simple tricks can help you get on with life while you try to overcome any memory problems.

- Have a notebook on the table all the time – use it to make lists and update them regularly.
- Aim to establish a routine – do certain tasks at regular times each day.
- Try not to tackle too many things at once and break down each task into smaller steps.
- If something needs to be done, make a note of it or do it right away.
- Use email to communicate with friends and family so that you don't have to rely on your memory while talking. Give yourself plenty of time to make a telephone call.
- Get into the routine of always putting things such as keys and other important items in the same place where they can be easily seen or found.

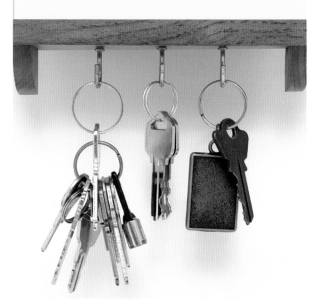

OVERCOMING THE HURDLES

How, by tackling small, everyday tasks, one stroke survivor fought his way back to a full, active life

Martin Stephen, High Master of St Paul's School, UK, and the author of the Henry Gresham crime thrillers, had a stroke in October 2005 when he was 56. His book *Diary of a Stroke* charts his recovery.

" Medicine isn't an exact science, my father always used to say. He also said that you always know those stroke victims who're going to get better. They fight it, they don't let it win. This memory comes at me with the force of the snowball that you didn't know was coming crashing on your cheek. "

Day 3 after the stroke

" My face is covered in stubble. I stink. I can't walk and I'm far from sure I can even manage a Zimmer frame. Yet I must, must get to the shower room, clean myself up and rinse away some of the horror that has happened to me … If I sit up with my legs over the edge of the bed, clench my fists and stick them ramrod straight down the side of my body so they jam hard into the mattress, I can keep myself upright. I inch my bottom forward on the mattress and feel my feet on the floor … My destination is six massive double steps away.

From somewhere I gather new strength … and make it through the door of the bathroom. It's far from a perfect shave. My face looks like a harvest field through which a drunkard has driven a combine harvester but it's the best shave of my life. "

By week 2

" I'm at home in comfortable surroundings and frightened that I will slip into lethargy. I divide up into two-hour stints. First there are the tennis balls – the idea is to bounce the tennis ball off a wall and catch it. The target is to catch the ball 2,000 times a day. It's an extraordinary high number when one comes down to actually trying to do it. 2,000 balls takes a long time.

Next is the handwriting. My signature is laughable, unrecognisable. I'm not depressed though. The rock fall of the stroke has buried the skill but it's been a part of me for so long that I'm sure it's still there. It just needs a massive slog of digging to unearth it.

I return to full-time work in January. When I come back from the Easter holiday, it is almost as if the stroke had never happened. Energy levels are good. The handwriting is indistinguishable from what it was before – only I know it takes that little bit of extra effort to get it right. "

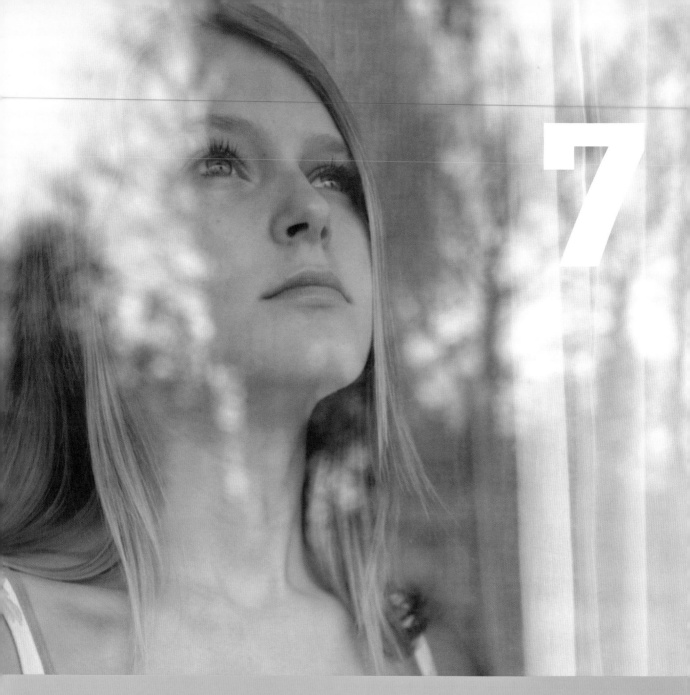

7

Confronting cancer

Although cancer can be one of the hardest diagnoses to receive, people living with cancer today have much more reason than those of previous generations to feel optimistic

Millions survive the 'Big C'

One person in three will develop cancer during their lifetime, but a higher proportion than ever before are overcoming the disease, with survival rates doubling in the last 30 years. Half of those diagnosed with cancer today will still be alive in five years' time and more than 40 per cent in ten years' time.

Earlier detection – partly thanks to screening programs – improved treatments and better after care are the main factors behind these figures. But it is also clear that patients themselves can do much more to increase their chances of coming through cancer – and the sooner after diagnosis they start, the better. 'Emerging evidence shows that lifestyle factors including physical activity and diet can influence the rate of cancer progression, improve quality of life, reduce side effects during treatment, reduce the incidence of relapse and improve overall survival,' says the British-based National Cancer Survivorship Initiative (NCSI). Research also suggests that being actively involved in the management of your illness may improve your chances of recovery.

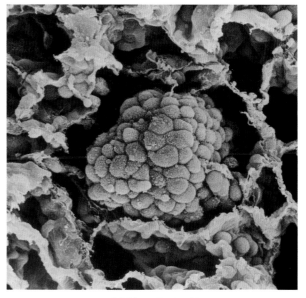

CATCH IT EARLY
This scanning electron micrograph (SEM) shows a small cluster of cancer cells in the air pockets (alveoli) of the lungs. Ever-improving techniques for early diagnosis of cancer offer the best chance of effective treatment and a lasting recovery.

WHAT IS CANCER?

Cancer occurs when the normal process of cell division gets out of control and the dividing cells have the potential to spread around the body, destroying healthy tissue. About 85 per cent of cancers are carcinomas, which start in the epithelial cells that line and cover the body and its organs. Much rarer are leukaemias and lymphomas – which occur where white blood cells are formed – and sarcomas – which grow in the connective structures of the body such as muscle and bone.

THE TREATMENT ARMOURY

Today, there is a vast armoury of different treatments available to fight cancer, including surgery, radiotherapy, chemotherapy, immunotherapy, biological therapy, hormone therapy and bone marrow transplants. Your treatment will depend mainly on where in the body your cancer is, how far it has spread and how aggressive it is. New research is revealing another factor that may influence treatment choices – the tumour's genetic characteristics (see *Cancer is more than one disease*, page 172).

Getting the diagnosis

Even if you were expecting bad news, immediately after diagnosis you may feel too shocked to absorb much of the information that your specialist gives you. If you are receiving the results of tests that could bring a cancer diagnosis, take a relative or close friend with you to your medical consultation. They can ask the difficult questions or write down the answers to your queries if you are too distraught to think clearly.

In most cases your oncologist (cancer specialist) will initially have discovered what type of cancer it is from a biopsy (in which cells are taken and inspected under a microscope). Further information about the rate of spread is gleaned from scans and blood tests. Once this is available, your treatment options will be discussed with you.

Questions to ask

To remember all the important questions, it may be easier to take along a previously prepared list when you meet your oncologist. These are the core questions, but feel free to add any more that are relevant to you:

- *What is the full medical name for my cancer?*
- *Where did the cancer start?*
- *Has the cancer spread and where to?*
- *Is it slow-growing or aggressive?*
- *What treatment will I need?*
- *Are there different treatment options and – if so – how will I choose between them?*
- *How successful is the treatment likely to be?*
- *What are the side effects of treatment?*
- *How ill will I feel and for how long?*
- *How long will I be off work?*
- *What support is there at the hospital where I'll be treated?*
- *What other support is available?*
- *What are the chances of recurrence?*

SOURCES OF SUPPORT

Ideally, your GP will be the lynchpin of a team of professionals working with you to treat your cancer. There is also a lot of support available to cancer patients, ranging from helplines to online forums (see *Getting the right support*, page 172). A good starting point is the Cancer Council, through its website (www.cancer.org.au) or helpline (13 11 20). When you're looking for information online, avoid any websites claiming to offer a cure (chances are they don't do anything of the sort!) and don't be afraid to ask your GP whether a particular site is reputable.

UNDERSTANDING SURVIVAL STATISTICS

If you ask about the long-term outlook for you, you will be given statistics on survival rates. Statistics tell you about the percentage of people with different types and stages of cancer who are alive and disease-free after five or ten years following different types of treatment. They cannot predict how well you as an individual will do. Your prognosis will depend on the stage and grade of the cancer, how early it has been detected and your age and general health. If you want to see survival statistics for a particular type of cancer, many are available on Cancer Australia's website, www.canceraustralia.gov.au/affected-cancer/cancer-statistics.

A positive approach

Positive thinking will not make your cancer disappear, but it can help you take control of your situation. The better you feel physically and psychologically, the better you'll be able to deal with the bumpy road ahead and develop ways of coping that are right for you.

DEALING WITH THE DIAGNOSIS

There is no 'right' way to deal with a cancer diagnosis, and everybody's experience of cancer is unique, explains Celene Doherty, Cancer Information Nurse Specialist with Macmillan Cancer Support, UK. 'It is devastating news that produces a wide range of emotions: everybody copes with it in their own way.' There's no one *right* person to talk to about having cancer, she says, but getting support really helps.

To begin building a positive attitude, accept both your negative feelings and the help you'll need to cope with them. At first you may feel shock and panic, then fear, anger, uncertainty and sadness. 'These feelings may stay or come and go. Allow yourself time to develop coping strategies that work for you.'

In her work, Celine has noticed that while some people gain comfort from telling lots of people about their diagnosis, others react differently and tend to withdraw from everyone other than their nearest and dearest. And those closest to you will want to be involved, she says. 'If you do not share your feelings with them, they may feel excluded from your illness and unable to support you as they – and perhaps you – would like.'

If you find it difficult to discuss, focus on telling one person: 'If you can find the courage to talk to just one person about how you feel, it can be the first step towards dealing with your emotions.'

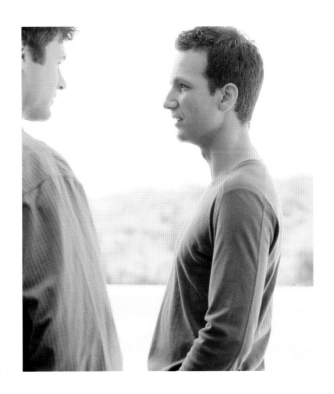

Sharing your feelings with someone sympathetic can help you cope

CAN YOUR MENTAL ATTITUDE AFFECT YOUR CANCER?

There has been much debate about whether staying positive improves cancer survival rates. A large 2007 study in the journal *Cancer* found that emotional wellbeing had no effect on survival, and another study reviewing past papers concluded that: 'There is little consistent

Should I get a second opinion?

Q&A

'Try to have a full and open discussion about your prognosis with your health-care team – rather than seeking a second opinion – as they know you and have all your test results,' advises Professor Karol Sikora, Medical Director of CancerPartnersUK, a private cancer treatment network. 'The most senior member of the team may not be the most informative. A young doctor or nurse can sometimes be more approachable.'

Cancer is more than one disease

Until now, cancer has been defined by where in the body it starts. But scientists are discovering that what really matters are the specific genetic mutations that make tumour cells multiply. They are reaching the conclusion that cancer is not a single disease.

They have found that two patients can have cancers in different parts of the body that are triggered by the same genetic defect and may respond to the same treatment. Conversely, two patients with cancer of the same body part may benefit from completely different treatments.

At Massachusetts General Hospital in Boston, the treatment of some patients is matched to the molecular profile of their tumour. This approach could transform the treatment of cancer. As we discover more about the DNA of different cancers, 'smart' treatments targeted at specific mutations can be developed.

evidence that psychological coping styles play an important part in survival from or recurrence of cancer.' So do not feel guilty if you cannot feel positive. Current thinking is that people should cope in the best way they can in order to feel physically or emotionally better, rather than to improve survival or prevent recurrence. Your mindset will colour your daily life but may not affect the course of your disease.

GETTING THE RIGHT SUPPORT

If you prefer not to talk to friends and relatives about your illness because you are afraid of distressing them or feel that you cannot be as honest as you want to, there are plenty of other places to turn to. Here are some ideas:

Counselling In one trial, women with breast cancer who received counselling felt more relaxed than those who did not. Blood tests showed that their immune systems were also boosted. You can find a counsellor specialising in cancer through your hospital or your GP.

Religion Some people find that they gain support from spiritual advisers when they are ill.

Helplines The Cancer Council runs a free, confidential telephone information and support service (13 11 20) that is available to anyone: cancer patients, people living with cancer, their families, carers and friends.

Online forums Online message boards or real-time chat rooms allow you to exchange experiences with others at any time of the day or night. Close friendships can sometimes be formed this way. Most cancer charities run online forums. Cancer Connections is a free, professionally moderated online support community where people affected by cancer can find support by participating in groups, discussions, blogs and webinars (www.cancer.org.au/about-cancer/patient-support/cancer-connections.html).

MIND OVER MATTER

You can cope ...
strategies to get you through

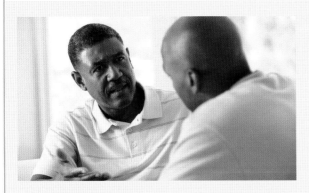

You may feel that life will never be 'normal' while you have cancer. But you will develop your own ways of dealing with the illness. There are no hard and fast rules – what works for one person may not help another – but you will soon discover what feels right for you. Here are some tips:

Previous coping mechanisms According to the Mayo Clinic in the USA, whatever has comforted you through rough times before is likely to help after a diagnosis of cancer - it may be the presence of a close friend, the inspiration of a religious leader or the pursuit of a favourite activity. You should turn to these sources of comfort again, but also be open to new strategies.

Work You may want to carry on working during treatment, but you may choose not to or you may be too ill. You do not have to tell your employer that you have cancer, but most people do. If you need time off or are not able to do your job effectively, it's helpful to have the support of your boss. You may also want to discuss your situation with your human resources department and trade union. Colleagues can be a great support, but you may wish to keep your work life separate from your illness.

Let others help Accepting help can be hard, especially if you are used to supporting others. But it is important to recognise the limitations imposed by your illness and its treatment and not to overstretch yourself when you are feeling unwell. You should also encourage your family to accept help from others; at some point they may need a break. If you don't have a wide network of friends and extended family, find out about support groups in your area from your GP or from the national cancer charities (see *Helpful organisations*, page 340).

Keep a journal People with cancer who write about their emotions can benefit physically and emotionally, perhaps because it prompts them to think more about their feelings.

Support groups If you prefer to share experiences face to face, ask your doctor whether there is a local cancer support scheme in your area. Some cancer charities and cancer support centres run 'living with cancer' courses or buddying programs, in which you are allocated a specific person to support you through your illness.

It's fine if you don't want to talk about your condition, but if you withdraw completely, it could be a sign that you are depressed. In this case you should see your doctor.

A STORY OF CARING SUPPORT

How other people helped a breast-cancer patient get through her illness and its treatment

Karin Mankour was 33 when she was diagnosed with breast cancer. Over two years she had a lumpectomy, radiotherapy, chemotherapy, hormone therapy, a bilateral mastectomy and breast reconstruction.

A fiercely independent human resources executive, Karin found her life turned upside down by cancer. From day one, she made use of a range of different support mechanisms and believes this network has played a vital part in her recovery.

The day I was diagnosed, I was given a breast-care nurse and she supported me right the way through, looking after my emotional wellbeing, fighting my corner to get certain treatments she felt I needed and helping me to make difficult decisions, for example about breast reconstruction.

Your family has a hard time too when you have cancer. Sometimes the low days sneak up on you and you don't want to share your dark thoughts with them. Once I found cancer support specialists, I called them all the time for emotional support and information.

Reading the online forums gave me a lot of reassurance. During cancer treatment, you get all sorts of strange symptoms and you want to know if they are normal. For

example, I developed painful sores in my nose. The specialist said they were nothing to do with Herceptin, but everybody on the forum was talking about them. It is so easy to panic and worry until you realise lots of other people have the same symptoms.

Karin also picked up useful tips from other patients going through chemotherapy and made friends with women of her own age.

We still meet every six weeks or so in our own little support group and it is very important to all of us – a safe space where we can say anything without worrying that it sounds as if we are whining.

A counsellor guided Karin through the trauma of mastectomy.

My counsellor helped me prepare for every aspect of the operation, including how it would be to wake up and look down at myself, the sense of loss and mourning. She was a wonderful woman who helped my life move forwards.

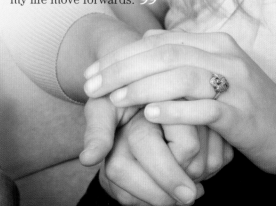

Look at your lifestyle

It may be hard to believe, but some people with cancer describe the illness as a wake-up call that gives them an opportunity to rethink their priorities. Faced with a life-threatening condition, they find themselves reassessing every aspect of their lives – work, relationships, diet, leisure. If you choose to – and have the strength – cancer can give you a chance to make a fresh start.

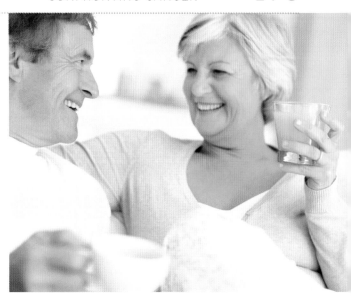

Choose fresh juices and herb teas over alcoholic drinks at this time

DITCH TOBACCO AND ALCOHOL

If you make just one resolution after a cancer diagnosis, it should be to give up smoking. Smoking is not just a cause of cancer; studies also suggest that patients are more likely to survive if they do not smoke. Smoking may also make some treatments less effective. 'Continuing to smoke exposes the body to high levels of carcinogens, which can cause further DNA damage to existing cancers, encourage the cancer to mutate into a more aggressive type or develop mechanisms to hide from the body's immunological defences,' says Professor Robert Thomas, editor of the Cancernet information website.

The Million Women Study has established that there is a link between alcohol consumption and some cancers, including breast, liver and bowel. A recent study of 365 women who had had breast cancer showed that those who consumed more than six alcoholic drinks a week had a 90 per cent greater risk of developing a second breast tumour.

EAT TO BEAT CANCER

If you already eat healthily, you will be starting your cancer journey in good shape. If not, now is the time to change your diet for the better. According to Cancer Research UK, a good diet can help your body to:
- cope with treatment side effects
- handle the most beneficial dose of certain treatments
- recover and heal faster
- fight off infections
- feel stronger, healthier and more energetic.

But cancer can do strange things to your appetite and eating habits. Anxiety, the illness itself and its treatments can all put you off food. Up to four people in ten have unintended weight loss or have problems with eating when their cancer is diagnosed.

Top Tips

Top Tips

Ease your eating problems

Try these tips to help you get over eating problems related to your cancer:

- **Poor appetite** Eat little and often – five or six times a day – and eat what you fancy. If you are losing weight, ask your doctor or nurse about food supplements to drink or sprinkle on your food.

- **Sore mouth or trouble swallowing** Choose soft foods such as soups, eggs and mashed potatoes. Avoid spicy or acidic foods and anything with a rough texture, such as toast.

- **Nausea** Cooking smells can make it worse. Choose cold foods such as sandwiches and salads or stay out of the way when hot food is being cooked. A drink of hot water poured over slices of ginger root may reduce nausea.

- **Diarrhoea** Go for low-fibre foods such as white bread, pasta and rice and peeled fruit. Drink plenty of fluids to replace what you are losing, but avoid citrus juices.

- **Constipation** Drink plenty of liquids and eat high-fibre foods such as wholemeal bread and pasta, brown rice and fruit.

Nutritionist Fiona Hunter advises: 'If you have no problems with your appetite, eat as healthily as possible. But if you have no appetite or it is difficult for you to eat, work around that and get as many kilojoules as you can into your body. You need to be well-nourished to fight disease: otherwise your immune system will not work as well as it should.'

IN THE LONG TERM

Most experts agree that what you eat can influence whether you develop cancer. But it is less clear whether diet plays a role in cancer progression or its recurrence. In its 2007 report on lifestyle and cancer prevention, the World Cancer Research Fund (WCRF) concluded cancer sufferers should follow the guidelines for cancer prevention. These include:

Eat more fruit, berries and vegetables Especially green, leafy vegetables; healthy oils such as unsaturated fats and omega-3 found in oily fish; nuts and seeds; unprocessed grains and legumes.

Eat less fast food Avoid these and other 'energy dense' highly processed foods and sugary drinks; cut down on red meat (no more than 500 g a week), smoked or cured meat including ham, bacon and sausages, and salt.

Avoid faddy diets Be wary of extreme diets such as the Gerson Regime, which involves eating large quantities of juiced vegetables and having coffee enemas. There's no scientific proof that it helps and it can cause unpleasant side effects.

SUPPLEMENT SENSE

There is also no good evidence that vitamin or mineral supplements make any difference to cancer patients. In fact, a WCRF report concluded that 'high dose supplements may be harmful'. In the view

Delicious fresh fruit
can be a regular
part of your diet

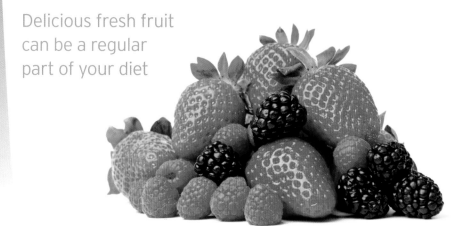

of oncologist Robert Thomas, supplements 'should not be required if individuals are able to eat a varied balanced diet' and should be avoided during chemotherapy as they may interfere with drug treatment.

GET OUT MORE

Exercise may be the last thing you feel like doing during cancer treatment. But research shows that it can help with the side effects of treatment, such as fatigue, pain and nausea, and can also improve your mood. What you can do will depend on the type of cancer, your treatment, stamina, strength and fitness. The UK National Association of Cancer Exercise Rehabilitation (www.nacer.org.uk/) suggests some gentle exercises and advises that you start with 30 minutes (possibly in separate sessions) of activity four or five days a week at a level that makes you slightly breathless. Build up gradually to more strenuous exercise as you feel stronger.

 SELF-HELP

Lift your mood ...
to get through the dark days

Improving the way you feel can help you deal with the cancer itself and the side effects of treatment. Here are some suggestions to help you manage anxiety, stress and uncertainty.

Relaxation using simple breathing exercises, such as the one described on page 250, can help relieve stress and tension. You can easily learn relaxation techniques from a book or CD or by joining a course or group.

Meditation has been shown in scientific studies to reduce stress and anxiety levels and to lower blood pressure and pulse rate. It can also help with pain and sleep problems. Some cancer centres offer Mindfulness-Based Stress Reduction, an eight-week course based around meditation.

Visualisation or guided imagery involves learning to picture soothing images in your mind's eye. According to Cancer Research UK, a review of six studies in 2005 suggested that guided imagery may help people with cancer to manage stress, anxiety and depression.

Yoga may contribute to improved sleep and emotional wellbeing, according to a review carried out by Complementary and Alternative Medicine Evidence Online (CAMEOL).

Laughter can stimulate the circulatory and immune systems and may increase pain tolerance through the release of endorphins in the brain. It can also reduce stress and enhance quality of life. Look online for a 'laughter clinic' near you.

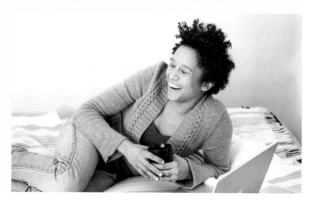

Exercise may also improve your chances of recovery. A study of 40,000 Swedish men over the age of 45 found that the more exercise the participants took, the less likely they were to die from cancer. Another study, involving nearly 3,000 American women with breast cancer, showed that those who walked for between 3 and 5 hours a week were less likely to die of their cancer than women who were physically active for less than an hour a week.

HOW EXERCISE HELPS

There is some evidence that certain cancers are more likely to return in people who are seriously overweight; exercise helps to control weight. Taking exercise may also reduce high levels of certain hormone and growth factors that, when present in the blood in excessive amounts, appear to fuel some types of cancer. When you feel up to it, aim for at least $2^{1/2}$ hours of moderate exercise a week, working up to more vigorous exercise over time. Some hospital cancer centres run exercise programs.

REASSESSING YOUR PRIORITIES

Confronting serious illness can help you work out what really matters to you and the parts of your life you would like to change. 'These are intensely personal matters and only you can sort out what needs doing (if anything) and when,' says clinical psychologist Dr Peter Harvey, who worked with cancer patients for 15 years. 'Whatever you do, take it slowly and gently, making sure that you have enough energy and commitment to carry things through.' Here are some questions you could ask yourself:

- Do you enjoy your job? If not, how could things improve?
- What about your relationships? Cancer can be a chance to put things right in families. But it can also put a huge strain on partners, and at some stage you may benefit from professional counselling.
- Do you take too much responsibility in the family? This may be your chance to share the load. Close friends and family are usually keen to know how they can help at a time like this.
- Have you always meant to do something for others? Volunteering brings many mental and physical benefits. It can make you feel better about yourself and add a sense of value to your life.
- Do you have unfulfilled ambitions, things you would like to do or places you would like to visit? Now is a good time to prioritise them and work out what you can manage, when and how.
- Cancer can allow you to take risks; in the words of one expert, 'to identify your heart's desire and see how it can be met'.

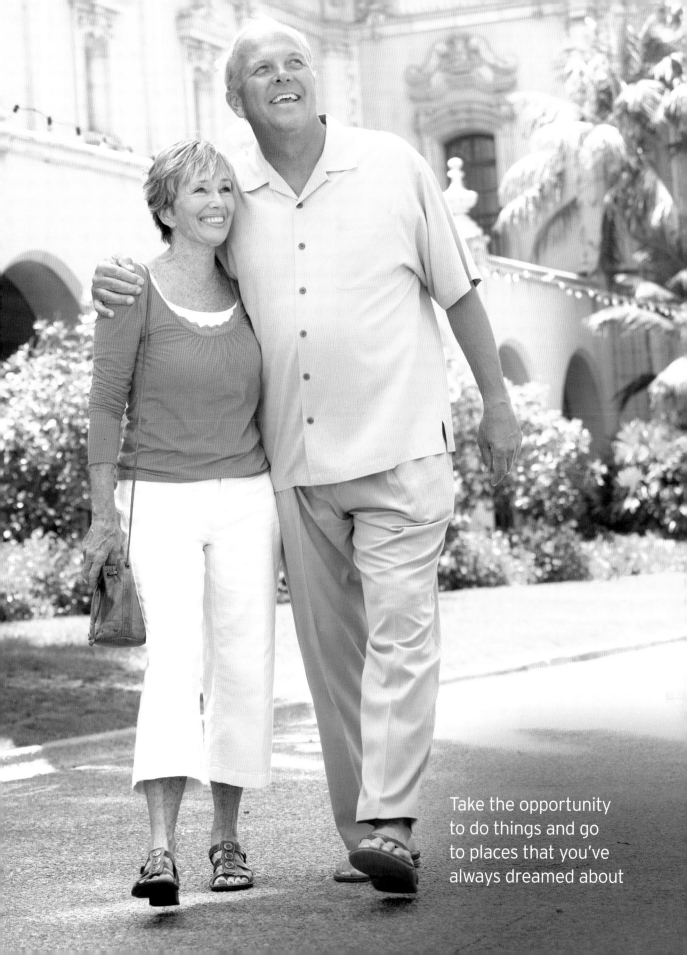

Take the opportunity to do things and go to places that you've always dreamed about

Getting through the treatment

Cancer treatments are widely thought to be almost as challenging as the illness itself. This is much less true than in the past, and there is plenty you can do for yourself to contribute to the success of whichever therapy you are receiving.

Share any concerns you may have with your surgical team

The three main treatment strands – surgery, radiotherapy and chemotherapy – are constantly being refined to increase their effectiveness and reduce the side effects. The choice is largely governed by the type and stage of your cancer, but you should always express any preferences or misgivings you have about any therapy. Often your views can be built into your treatment plan.

Cutting out cancer

Surgery remains a major weapon in the medical arsenal against cancer, with nine out of ten patients undergoing some form of surgical procedure. If the cancer is restricted to a single site, it may be the only treatment needed. If it has spread, surgery may be used in conjunction with other therapies. As well as tumour removal, surgery is also used to take a tissue

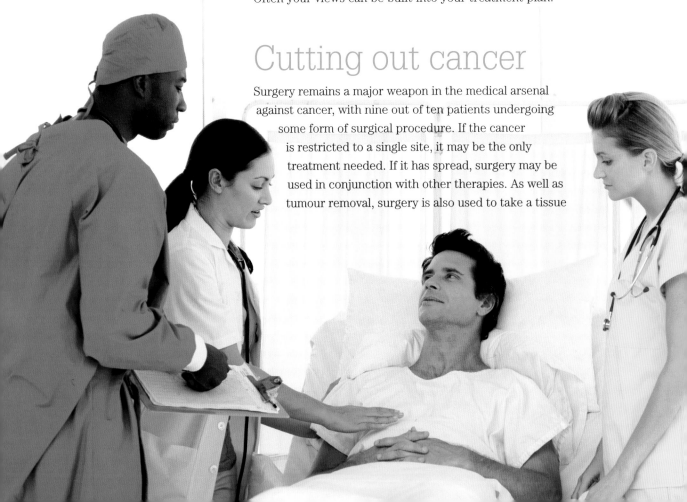

sample to find out more about the tumour; to discover how far the cancer has spread; to reduce the size of a tumour (debulking) before chemotherapy or radiotherapy; to relieve symptoms; and to reconstruct tissue that has been damaged during earlier surgery.

WHEN THE DOCTOR GIVES YOU A CHOICE

Doctors used to make all the necessary clinical decisions for their patients. But times have changed. If two or more treatments are equally successful – for example, radiotherapy or surgery for prostate cancer – your oncologist may ask which you would prefer. This can be empowering – if you feel the cancer has taken you over, it can be good to be given some choices. But some people are just not strong enough, emotionally and physically, to make that kind of decision after a cancer diagnosis.

To help you make up your mind, get as much information as you can from your oncologist or specialist nurse, including side effects, possible complications and ease of treatment. Visit reliable websites – for example, the Prostate Cancer Foundation of Australia (www.prostrate.org.au) describes the pros and cons of the different types of treatments for prostate cancer – and, if possible, speak to patients who themselves have made the decision. Online forums may be useful. If you are still uncertain, your oncologist may be willing to take the decision for you.

Questions to ask

If you are about to undergo surgery for cancer, ask your surgeon the following questions. As with other important consultations, you might want to take a relative or friend with you to ask the questions or write down the answers:

- *What is the operation called and why am I having it?*
- *What will you be removing and why?*
- *Could I have a less invasive procedure?*
- *Are there any alternatives to surgery?*
- *How long and complicated is the operation?*
- *Will you be checking for spread? If the cancer has spread, will you carry out further surgery at the same time?*
- *How will my body be affected by surgery – will it look different or function less well?*
- *Is there any preparation I can do before my operation?*
- *Will I need reconstructive surgery and, if so, can this be carried out at the same time?*
- *When will I know if the operation has been successful?*
- *Will I need to have other treatments before or after surgery?*
- *Am I likely to need further surgery?*
- *How likely is the surgery to cure my cancer?*

BODY IMAGE

Cancer surgery can save your life, but it may change your body and with it, the way you see yourself. The difference may be obvious – for example, the amputation of a limb – or seen only by those closest to you, such as a mastectomy or the removal of a testicle. It may also be totally invisible as in a hysterectomy or the removal of a kidney.

Surgery can leave you feeling disabled in other ways – for example, the need to have a colostomy bag following surgery for bowel cancer or difficulty in achieving an erection after radical prostatectomy. In all these cases the psychological effects can be profound, but there are ways to help yourself come to terms with your altered body.

Coping with your loss ...
facing body-changing surgery

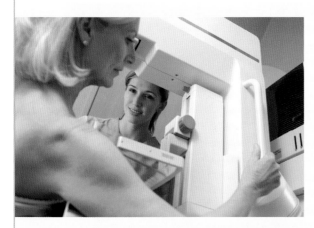

It may take a long time to accept the loss of a body part, but Maria Leadbeater, a nurse specialist with the British charity Breast Cancer Care, has some suggestions for people who face this challenge. She is referring to mastectomy, but her ideas also apply to other kinds of body-altering cancer surgery:

- Find out what to expect from your operation. With appropriate support and preparation, you can start to come to terms with the effects of surgery well before it is carried out.

- Ask about the benefits of reconstructive surgery. Should this be done at the same time or later? Find out about prostheses.

- Talk to somebody who has been through the same procedure. Breast Cancer Care tries to match callers with trained 'buddies' who have had a similar experience. Other cancer charities have similar schemes for people with different types of cancer. Encourage your partner to talk to others, too.

- You may not be able to predict how body-altering surgery will affect you. It can, for instance, challenge an individual's femininity or masculinity. Talk to your partner, family and close friends about any personal concerns. They will be anxious to help you regain any loss of confidence.

- Your health-care team should be able to support you through both your physical and emotional recovery. Charity helplines are a good source of impartial advice.

- Remember, your feelings about yourself and your body will change over time, and your anxieties will diminish as you regain your health and are able to look forward to the future.

WHY REMOVE LYMPH NODES?

The lymphatic system helps the body fight infection and drains away excess fluids. It is made up of vein-like vessels, which carry the lymph around the body, and groups of nodes or glands. Cancer cells sometimes spread from the original site into nearby lymph nodes and, if left untreated, to other parts of the body.

If doctors know or suspect that cancer cells have spread to nearby lymph nodes (a common concern with breast and prostate cancer, for example), they will remove them. The nodes are then examined. Because the local lymph system can no longer function, swelling can occur.

Sometimes, just a few nodes are removed. If any are found to contain cancer cells, the rest may need to be removed later. Sentinel node biopsy is a newer, less invasive procedure, with less risk of swelling, used to treat breast cancer. The surgeon removes the first lymph node that filters fluid draining away from the affected area of the breast. If it is clear, it is unlikely that other lymph nodes are affected. Studies show that after five years, women who had only the first (sentinel) node removed were as likely to be cancer-free as those who had more nodes removed.

The radiotherapy experience

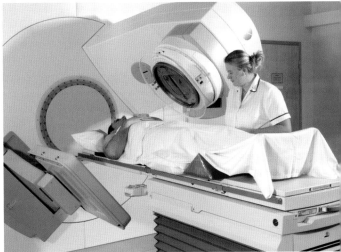

For many forms of cancer, there's a strong likelihood that you'll be offered radiotherapy – the use of radiation to destroy cancer cells. There are many different ways of delivering radiotherapy, including some recently developed methods that have speeded up treatment, improved its accuracy and reduced side effects. The type of radiotherapy you are offered will depend on the type and site of your cancer, what other forms of treatment you are having and on your general health.

EXTERNAL RADIOTHERAPY IN ACTION

Radiotherapy is carefully supervised to ensure that you receive the correct dose in the correct location. The machine, known as a linear accelerator, fires X-rays, which wrap around the exact shape of the tumour, minimising damage to surrounding tissue. It can be noisy while in operation, but you will be able to communicate with the nurse via an intercom system. The treatment is painless.

WHAT TO EXPECT

There are two main types of radiotherapy. In external radiotherapy, beams are fired at the tumour from outside the body. The treatment is usually given every weekday for two to six weeks in small doses known as fractions. Before you start your course, the radiographer will work out how to position the radiotherapy machine and may mark up your body so that the radiation can be correctly focused.

In internal radiotherapy, a radioactive substance or object is placed inside your body. This takes the form of either a liquid (radioisotope treatment) – which you drink or take as an injection – or implanted radioactive seeds, wires or tubes (brachytherapy). If you have either form of treatment, you will be in isolation for some time to protect hospital staff and visitors from radiation exposure.

Being aware of potential side effects (see page 184) and how to deal with them may help make you feel more in control. Of course, everyone is different and you won't necessarily experience all the potential side

Cutting-edge treatments

Some of the newer types of radiotherapy are listed here. However, the equipment used is very expensive and may not be available at your local hospital:

Radiosurgery or **gammaknife radiotherapy** is used for small brain tumours. The cancer is blitzed from many angles in a single, high dose of radiation.

Cyberknife uses computerised scans of the tumour to control robotic arms that deliver radiation using a linear accelerator (see previous page). The machine adjusts continuously to the body.

Proton beam radiotherapy delivers a beam of atomic particles called protons, which can be focused very precisely so that the tumour receives a high dose of radiation while the surrounding healthy tissue remains unaffected.

effects. You may also experience side effects specific to particular areas of the body. For example, head and neck radiotherapy can cause a sore mouth and problems with swallowing. Abdominal radiotherapy can cause diarrhoea, sickness, bladder problems and pain. Ask your doctor or specialist cancer nurse for advice and solutions specific to your case.

THE LONG-TERM EFFECTS

Although modern radiotherapy techniques aim to cut long-term side effects to a minimum, you may notice certain changes in the treated area. For instance:

- Your skin may look darker or feel different.
- Your hair may not grow back or, if it does, it may be a different colour or its texture may have changed.

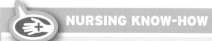 NURSING KNOW-HOW

Radiotherapy ...
managing the side effects

Here are some tips to help with the most common side effects of radiotherapy. If you experience other troubling side effects or a severe reaction, always seek the advice of your medical team:

Fatigue Pace yourself and try not to do too much. If the hospital is a long way from home, try to stay with somebody you know who lives nearer, or ask friends to give you a lift. Allow yourself time to rest but do some gentle exercise, such as a short daily walk. According to Cancer Research UK, some evidence about treating fatigue shows that exercise may be more helpful than rest.

Poor appetite It is important to have a healthy diet and to drink plenty of liquids while your body is under assault from radiotherapy. Eat little and often. The dietitian at your hospital may be able to help.

Sore skin Avoid hot baths or showers, use unperfumed soap and pat the treated area rather than rubbing with a towel. Do not use any creams on sore areas unless recommended by your health-care team. Choose soft, loose clothes that do not chafe. Cover the treated area to provide protection from sun and wind.

Depression It is not unusual to feel depressed or weepy during and after a course of radiotherapy. See *Getting the right support*, page 172.

- You may have spidery red marks from small broken blood vessels.
- Your internal body tissue may be less elastic – for example, if your lungs have been treated, you may be short of breath; if your abdomen has been treated, your bladder may fill more quickly and you may need to use the toilet more often.
- Radiotherapy may affect fertility. See *Fertility concerns* (page 188).

As effects vary, depending on the part of the body being treated, ask your specialist nurse what other changes could occur.

Coping with chemotherapy

Chemotherapy uses powerful drugs to destroy cancer cells by interfering with the cell-division process. There are over 100 different agents for the treatment of cancer and you may receive more than one.

Chemotherapy can be given alone, before or after surgery and with radiotherapy and other treatments. It is usually administered by injection or 'drip' into the bloodstream. But it can also be given in other ways – for example, as a tablet or capsule or through a pump that you wear.

Each cycle of chemotherapy consists of treatment and a rest period. This pattern makes the drugs more effective and allows the body time to recover. The drugs that are used, how they are given and the number and length of your treatment cycles will depend on the type of cancer you have, where it is, whether it has spread, how well you respond and the side effects you experience.

PREPARING FOR CHEMOTHERAPY

Chemotherapy damages cells when they divide – and cancer cells divide more often than most. But there are other tissues in which cells divide at a rapid rate – for example, those in the hair, skin and nails, the mouth, the lining of the digestive system and the bone marrow. As a result, these are the healthy parts of the body most likely to be adversely affected by chemotherapy treatment.

Chemotherapy weakens the immune system, so it makes sense to be as fit and well as possible before you put your body under assault from its powerful drugs. See *Be chemo clever*, page 187, for tips on how to deal with the side effects of treatment. Tell your doctor what medications you take – including food supplements and herbal medicines – as they may interact with chemotherapy drugs.

Top Tips

Your pre-chemo plan

Do as much as you can within your limits to help your body deal with the powerful effects of chemotherapy:

- Visit your dentist and tell him or her about your cancer. Brush up on your dental hygiene to keep teeth and gums free of bacteria to reduce your risk of picking up an infection during treatment.

- Eat as healthily as you can (see page 22), drink plenty of water, cut down on alcohol and give up smoking. Iron-rich foods, such as meat and dark green, leafy vegetables, may help to prevent anaemia.

- Plan your diary so you can rest in the days following your treatment.

- Find out about possible side effects and how they will affect you. For example, if you are likely to lose your hair, you might want to cut it short before treatment or order a wig that matches your usual cut and colour.

- Ask your doctor or nurse which complementary therapies might help. Are any available at your hospital? See *Complementary not alternative*, page 192.

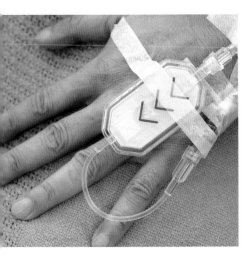

ADMINISTERING THE DRUGS

Most chemotherapy is administered intravenously, often through a drip into the hand or arm.

SURVIVING THE SIDE EFFECTS

Many people experience an array of side effects. These vary according to the type of drug, and it is important that you ask your doctor about any specific problems you experience. Knowing what to expect can actually make you less fearful, and if you can prepare yourself mentally in advance, you may well cope better with the treatment. Different people react differently to chemotherapy, and each person has an individual threshold for certain symptoms, such as pain, so it is possible you may experience only a few side effects.

WHEN TO WORRY

Most chemotherapy side effects are unpleasant rather than serious. But make sure your chemotherapy team give you a 24-hour emergency number to call if you have worrying symptoms. Call a doctor if you have:

- shivering or a temperature of 38°C or above
- breathing difficulties
- flu-like symptoms
- bleeding gums or nose
- bleeding from other parts of the body that does not stop after applying pressure for 10 minutes
- mouth ulcers that prevent eating or drinking
- vomiting that continues despite taking antisickness medication
- four or more bowel movements a day or diarrhoea.

KEEPING UP APPEARANCES

Losing your hair, eyebrows and eyelashes can feel like the final straw on top of the diagnosis, but the lost hair usually grows back within six months. It isn't vain to worry that chemotherapy will change the way you look, and you should not be afraid to discuss your anxieties with your nurse specialist.

Not all chemotherapy drugs make your hair fall out and, even if you are on one that does, you can ask about wearing a cold cap. This reduces the blood flow in the scalp by lowering the temperature, so less of the drug reaches the hair follicles on your head. Cold caps are suitable for only some chemotherapy drugs and some cancer types and, even then, they don't work for everybody. Some doctors don't like them because they worry that they may make treatment less effective.

NON-MEDICAL HELP

A number or organisations can offer non-medical support. Look Good… Feel Better (www.lgfb.com.au) is a free community service program that teaches cancer patients how to manage the appearance-related side effects of cancer treatment. It offers free workshops for women, men and teens being treated for cancer, run by volunteers from the cosmetic, hairdressing and beauty industries. Pink Sisters sells wigs and scarves and the proceeds go to cancer research (www.pinksistersparties.com.au/products). The Cancer Council has a wig service, which also lends wigs.

Men may also have problems with their body image during cancer treatment. A bald head looks less startling on a man than on a woman, but losing eyebrows and lashes can be traumatic for both. The website www.Lookgoodfeelbetterformen.org has advice on hair and skin care, including how to shave safely. It suggests using an electric razor rather than wet shaving, to minimise the risk of cuts that could become infected. It also advises that you avoid products that contain alcohol, menthol or strong scents.

NURSING KNOW-HOW

Be chemo clever ...
dealing with the problems

Here are some tips to help with the most common problems. If you experience a severe reaction or unexpected symptoms, seek the advice of your medical team.

Feeling or being sick Modern anti-emetic drugs are usually effective. Take them even if you are not feeling sick at the time. Research suggests that acupuncture, hypnotherapy and relaxation can reduce nausea caused by chemotherapy. Travel sickness wristbands can also be effective. Don't have a meal just before treatment or prepare or eat food when you are feeling sick. Avoid hot, fried or spicy food if it makes your nausea worse. Have several small meals throughout the day and plenty of soft drinks. Many people find that mint or ginger tea or pastilles help to reduce nausea.

Fatigue You're likely to feel exhausted during chemotherapy. Get plenty of rest but don't be afraid of gentle exercise such as walking or yoga. If your energy levels suddenly plummet, tell your doctor – you might have become anaemic.

Sore mouth Try a mouthwash recommended by your medical team. Clean teeth thoroughly but gently morning, evening and after meals with a soft brush, and floss daily to prevent infection. Drink plenty. Macmillan Cancer Support suggests: rinsing regularly with boiled, cooled salt water; avoiding spices, spirits and acidic drinks; and keeping lips moist with Vaseline or balm.

Infection Chemotherapy can lower your resistance and make you more prone to infection. Your doctor may give you antibiotics to protect you. Help yourself by keeping hygiene standards high. If possible, avoid people with infectious illnesses, large crowds, public transport and swimming pools.

Fertility concerns

One of the most distressing aspects of cancer is the thought that the treatment may affect your fertility, but the picture is not as bleak as it was. There are now many ways to circumvent this problem so that you can look forward to having children in the future.

If you have been diagnosed with cancer and may want to have children, be sure to discuss this with your consultant. Chemotherapy, surgery, radiotherapy and hormone therapy can all affect your ability to have children. But there are steps you can take if you plan ahead.

Egg and sperm storage, and developments in infertility treatment, mean that even if you do become infertile, you may still be able to have a child. You – and your partner, if you have one – should discuss the options with your doctor before treatment starts. If you find yourself facing the prospect of childlessness as well as cancer, seeing a counsellor may help.

If you're a woman

Fertility is a major concern for many women with cancer. Generally speaking, the outlook is better the younger you are. But certain chemotherapy drugs can prevent the ovaries from producing eggs, temporarily or permanently. The lower the dose of drug you have, the less likely it is that any infertility will be permanent. It's reassuring to know that about a third of women resume normal periods and start producing eggs after the chemotherapy ends.

Most radiotherapy treatment does not affect fertility. But if your ovaries are treated, then temporary or permanent infertility is likely. Surgery can also prevent you from having children.

If your womb is removed, you will not be able to carry a child; and if your ovaries are taken out, you will be unable to produce eggs in the future.

Knowing that you may or will become infertile after your treatment can be very hard to deal with. But there may be steps you can take before you have cancer treatment to make it possible for you to have children in the future.

OVERCOMING INFERTILITY IN WOMEN

Fortunately, techniques for overcoming cancer-induced infertility are improving all the time, and many women who have had cancer manage to conceive after treatment. If infertility is a risk, you may want to consider egg or embryo storage. Discuss this possibility with your oncologist, as he or she may not want you to delay treatment. If you have a partner, you can ask for *in vitro* fertilisation (IVF), in which eggs are removed from your ovaries and mixed with your partner's sperm. The resulting embryos can then be frozen. Roughly one woman in six who has a frozen embryo implanted after IVF gives birth. If you do not have a partner, you can have eggs removed and frozen for later fertilisation and implantation. Success rates, however, are lower than for frozen embryos. Ovarian transplantation is an emerging option.

EARLY MENOPAUSE

Removal of the ovaries and treatments such as hormone therapy, radiotherapy and chemotherapy can bring on early menopause. You may have unwelcome symptoms such as hot flushes, disturbed sleep, mood swings, low libido and vaginal dryness. If these effects are caused by hormone therapy, they may be temporary.

Hormone replacement therapy (HRT) relieves the symptoms but is not appropriate for everybody, including breast cancer patients, and it will not restore fertility. Other treatments for menopause symptoms are available; discuss them with your doctor.

If you're a man

Less talked about but often just as traumatic is the risk of infertility in men, which occurs with certain cancers and treatments. If you have prostate or testicular cancer, discuss with your doctor the implications of treatment for both your sex life and your ability to have children. Surgery for prostate, testicular and bowel cancer can interfere with your ability to have an erection. Radiotherapy to the pelvic area can also cause temporary or permanent erection problems (impotence) and may cause infertility. Chemotherapy for any kind of cancer can affect fertility – temporarily or permanently – depending on the drug used, its dosage and your age.

OVERCOMING INFERTILITY IN MEN

If there is a risk that your treatment will make you impotent or infertile, sperm banking may be an option, unless your doctor does not want to risk delaying treatment. This involves giving sperm samples over a few weeks, which are then frozen and can later be used to fertilise your partner's eggs.

IVF can help those who may face infertility as a result of cancer treatment

Chemotherapy and contraception

A woman may become pregnant and a man can father a child while on chemotherapy. However, because these drugs could damage an unborn baby, experts advise the use of contraception while undergoing chemotherapy and for some months afterwards.

Other ways of treating cancer

Some of the finest medical minds in the world's top institutions are working on new treatments that may be more effective, less invasive or have fewer side effects than the well-established approaches.

BIOLOGICAL THERAPIES

These work with the body's immune system to help fight cancer and are used on their own or with other treatments. This is a fast-evolving field, producing all kinds of new drugs, some of which target cancers with a particular genetic signature.

- Monoclonal antibodies (MABs) target abnormal proteins on cancer cells and stop the cells from growing. Some MABs trigger the immune system to kill cancer cells: this is known as immunotherapy. Monoclonal antibodies seem to destroy cancer cells with less damage to healthy cells – trastuzumab (Herceptin), for breast cancer, and bevacizumab (Avastin), originally for bowel cancer, are two examples. Side effects vary from drug to drug, but the most common is an allergic reaction such as fever.

- Cancer growth blockers interfere with the growth of cancer cells by targeting several specific molecules that are abnormal in cancer. They are often called smart drugs.

- Immunotherapy with interferon and interleukin, which are made naturally by the body, can be given to boost the immune system. Cancer 'vaccines' work in a similar way. These strategies can be used for kidney cancer, malignant melanoma and certain leukaemias.

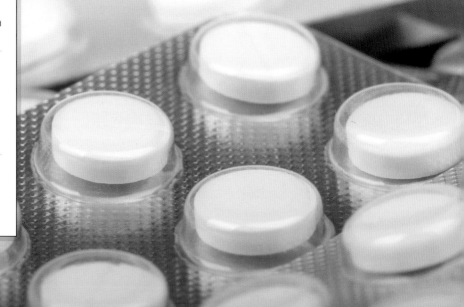

HORMONE THERAPIES

Some tumours – those known as 'hormone sensitive' – need hormones in order to grow. Hormone therapy either blocks hormone production in the body or prevents the hormones from reaching the tumour. It is used in breast, prostate and endometrial (womb) cancer. Tamoxifen, for breast cancer, and goserelin (Zoladex), for prostate cancer, are hormone therapies. Side effects vary from drug to drug but can include fatigue and hot flushes (in men too).

BONE-MARROW AND STEM-CELL TRANSPLANTS

Transplants are used in the treatment of various cancers, including leukaemia and lymphoma (cancer of the lymphatic system). For a bone marrow transplant, bone marrow is harvested under anaesthetic before high-dose chemotherapy that would destroy these cells. The harvested bone marrow is put back through a drip afterwards. If the doctor thinks that there is a high risk of the cancer returning if the patient's own marrow is used, a donor match must be found – this could be either a relative or a stranger.

Stem cell transplants work in a similar way to bone marrow transplants, but you do not need an anaesthetic when the cells are harvested. Many of the side effects of both types of transplant are similar to those of chemotherapy, but they may be more severe. It is especially important to guard against infection following one of these transplants, because your white blood cell count will be low, leaving you at greater risk of infection. The normally harmless bacteria everyone has on their skin and in their digestive systems can pose a risk, as can bacteria found in food. During this time, there may be restrictions on patient visits, and visitors may need to wear precautionary clothing that minimises the risk of infection.

 NURSING KNOW-HOW

Avoiding infection while immunosuppressed

These tips can help prevent infection while you are vulnerable:

- Use a mouthwash 3 times a day.

- Wash your hands thoroughly before eating, after using the toilet and if you've been in contact with other people and pets.

- Shower every day.

- Make sure friends and family always wash their hands before seeing you.

- Have your room cleaned every day.

- Eat only freshly prepared and thoroughly cooked meals.

- Wash and peel all fruit and avoid eating salads.

- Do not eat fresh cream or soft cheese or raw or lightly cooked eggs, or dishes or sauces containing them, such as homemade mayonnaise.

Complementary, not alternative

Around a third of people with cancer use complementary therapies in conjunction with the mainstream treatment for their condition, largely to combat the frequently unpleasant side effects associated with these often radical measures.

There is plenty of evidence to show that complementary approaches can help you deal with cancer symptoms, including pain, as well as the side effects of treatment. They can also make you less anxious, more relaxed and more in control of things at a time when you may feel that the rest of your life is being dictated by your medical team. However, there is no conclusive scientific evidence that any complementary or alternative therapy can cure cancer. Stay well away from any practitioner who claims that with their help you'll recover from the disease, or who advises you to stick to their treatment and ignore conventional medicine.

CHOOSING A THERAPY AND THERAPIST

Always talk to a member of your medical team if you are considering using a complementary therapy, to make sure it will not conflict with other treatments you are having. Some doctors recognise the benefits of complementary medicine but others are hostile to the idea. You may find a cancer specialist nurse more sympathetic and helpful. Some hospitals, hospices and cancer charity clinics offer therapies that they have found useful. You'll also find information about research into different therapies online on the websites of cancer charities (see *Helpful organisations*, page 340). The Cancer Council helpline (13 11 20) can also answer questions.

Anybody can set themselves up as a complementary therapist, so it is vital to choose one who is fully trained and who belongs to a recognised professional body that has a code of practice and ethics. Ask people you know if they can recommend somebody – but always check the therapist's professional credentials yourself. The Cancer

Acupuncture can reduce vomiting caused by chemotherapy

Council recommends asking the following questions about any treatment you are considering:

- Is this therapy specifically used for cancer patients or for people with other diseases as well?
- Are there any side effects?
- Who will be involved in delivering the therapy?
- What are their qualifications and are they registered with a professional organisation?
- What are the costs of the therapy and are they covered by my health insurance provider?
- What does the therapy aim to achieve?
- Will this therapy affect my conventional medical treatment?

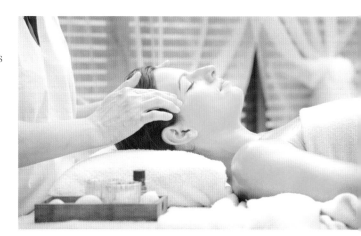

Relaxation induced by massage with aromatherapy oils can help to reduce anxiety

RECOMMENDED THERAPIES

These therapies have been shown to help cancer patients in different ways, including reducing anxiety and aiding relaxation:

Acupuncture A recent review of acupuncture-point stimulation for drug-induced nausea – using pressure, electro stimulation or needles – showed that the treatment reduced vomiting but not nausea.

Aromatherapy Many cancer sufferers report feeling relaxed, pampered and empowered by aromatherapy massage, according to Penny Brohn Cancer Care. This UK charity (formerly known as Bristol Cancer Help Centre) says, 'The balance of research evidence is supportive of aromatherapy as an effective treatment for anxiety.'

Herbal medicine Up to six in ten people with cancer turn to herbal medicine. There have been many claims that various herbs can cure cancer, but none has been backed up by scientific research. However, evidence does show that herbal medicines can improve quality of life, lift mood and help with the treatment of side effects.

Massage According to Penny Brohn Cancer Care, good trial data suggests that massage can help sleep, improve the immune system and decrease fatigue and nausea.

Reflexology In a 2007 study of 86 people with cancer that had spread, patients' partners either read to them or gave them reflexology. The group that received reflexology reported less anxiety and less pain than the other group.

Reiki healing According to the American Cancer Society (www.cancer.org), some cancer patients undergoing active treatment have reported an increased sense of wellbeing, reduced pain, and reduced nausea and vomiting after Reiki sessions.

When treatment ends

Completing treatment and being discharged by your cancer care team sounds like a cause for celebration, and often it is. But you are not alone if you feel less than euphoric when your cancer treatment comes to an end.

I t can be a difficult time', says Celene Doherty, Cancer Information Nurse Specialist with Macmillan Cancer Support. 'You are used to being supported by your medical team and suddenly you don't have that so frequently any more. People say it can take a lot of adjusting to that change, and they often describe that they feel lost, abandoned and frightened during this transition.'

But there are organisations that offer information and support even after treatment has ended. These include the Cancer Council (www.cancer.org.au), the Australian Cancer Survivorship Centre (www.petermac.org/cancersurvivorship) and the NSW Cancer Survivors Centre (www.nswcancersurvivorscentre.org). But the best place to get a referral is from your cancer nurse specialist towards the end of treatment.

YOUR TREATMENT IS OVER – WHAT NOW?

When your treatment has finished you will find yourself facing one of three situations:

- There may be no further sign of cancer. This is called complete remission. You will still have check-ups. After five years without any relapse, you will normally be considered cured.
- The cancer may have shrunk but not disappeared. This is called partial remission. Your cancer may recur. Some people – notably those with breast and prostate cancer – can live many years in partial remission with no symptoms and die in old age of something else.
- The cancer may not have responded to treatment.

Ask your doctor to explain what the long-term outlook is for you – if you want to know, and not everyone does. These are the core questions to ask, but you may have more specific personal concerns:

- What are the chances of my cancer recurring or spreading, or of another cancer developing?
- What follow-up appointments and tests will I need?
- Who should I call if I have health concerns?

- What symptoms should I look out for?
- Are there any long-term side effects that might develop from my treatment, and when might these occur?

IF CANCER RETURNS

Being told that your cancer has recurred can be even more devastating than the initial diagnosis. You may feel that you do not have the resources to cope a second time, though some people say they feel stronger and better prepared.

To help you get through this difficult period, Macmillan Cancer Support offers the following tips:

- Be aware of how you feel. Powerful emotions are natural and normal when your life is turned upside-down by illness.
- If you can, find someone you can talk to. If you feel uncomfortable discussing these things with someone you know, you may prefer to join a support group or to see a counsellor.
- Remind yourself of ways in which you have dealt with other difficult situations in the past. Remember the strengths you had then, and see if you can use them again now.

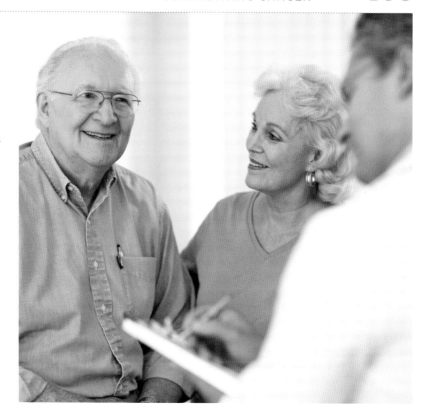

Being given the all clear is likely to bring smiles of relief

IN REMISSION

Even if your treatment has been completely successful, you may be left feeling different physically, emotionally or both. Physically, you may have to come to terms with an altered body and the long-term side effects of treatment. Emotionally, you may feel more anxious than before and fearful that the disease will return. On a practical level, you may have concerns about work and finances. Things may be made worse because those around do not seem to understand how you feel.

With the right help, you can work through these problems. This can be a good time to see a counsellor, have some complementary therapies or to visit a local cancer support centre. It's also important to follow as healthy a lifestyle as possible, so that you give yourself the best chance of staying well.

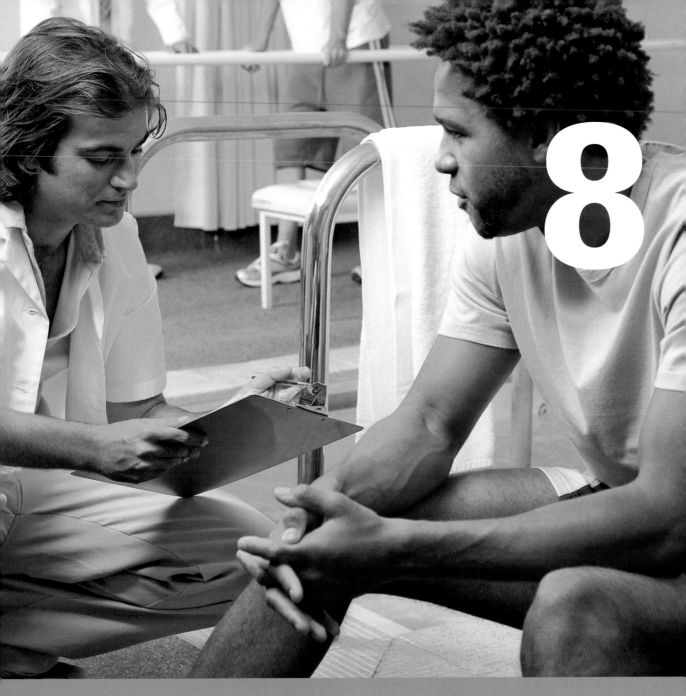

8

Before and after surgery

Advance preparation and a positive strategy for the days and weeks that follow can help to ensure a full, speedy recovery

Understanding your operation

There's a wealth of evidence showing that being prepared for major surgery – both physically and mentally – can affect the outcome. Any big operation that requires one or more nights in hospital will have a significant impact on the body so it's advisable to make sure you're as fit as possible. That means achieving a healthy weight, stopping smoking, eating a balanced diet and taking regular exercise (see *Getting fit for theatre*, pages 200–201). The stronger you are, the better your body will cope with the surgery itself and the quicker your recovery will be.

Less obvious perhaps are the benefits of preparing yourself psychologically. Although it's normal to worry about a forthcoming operation, it makes sense to confront these anxieties rather than bottling them up and fretting. There's solid scientific evidence that achieving a calm and positive outlook can improve the outcome of surgery and help recovery. A 2006 review published in the *Journal of the Academy of Orthopedic Surgeons* found evidence that psycho-social factors (including attitude and mood plus the level of social support) can play a significant role in post-operative recovery.

ASK THE RIGHT QUESTIONS

You'll almost certainly feel better if you enter the operating theatre confident that you're doing the right thing and that you can trust your surgeon and his or her team. Research your operation online for the most up-to-date information about the procedure and the questions you may need to ask. There are a large number of helpful websites (for example, www.surgery.com).

It's worth starting to write a list of questions that you'd like to ask your surgeon as soon as your GP decides to refer you for possible surgery. Far from being offended, the surgical team will welcome your interest – knowing that the more involved you are in your care in hospital, the better you'll manage your care at home afterwards.

Questions to ask

Your pre-surgery appointment is your best, perhaps only, chance to get your questions answered by the expert. Don't be embarrassed to ask about any issue that is worrying you. Here are some questions you may want to ask:

- *I'm feeling unsure about my operation. Should I seek a second opinion?*
- *What is your experience of this operation?*
- *Is there a more conservative non-surgical approach? And how successful would it be?*
- *How urgent is the operation?*
- *How long will I need to recover from the operation and when am I likely to be mobile?*
- *What can I do now to prepare myself for rehabilitation post-op?*
- *What are the specific risks of this operation – and what will you do to reduce them?*
- *If a trainee surgeon is likely to be operating, what kind of supervision will be given?*
- *Will I need medications to reduce the risk of blood clots (venous thromboembolism) around the time of the surgery?*
- *What kind of scar is this going to leave and is there anything you can do to minimise it?*

Before your operation

Once you know when you're having surgery, you should start to make practical arrangements for your post-operative recovery at home, as well as preparing mentally and physically for the operation itself.

Day surgery

Many operations, such as cataract surgery, that can be done in a matter of minutes under a local anaesthetic may seem to require little interruption to your routine. But you'll need to arrange for someone to drive you home or arrange for hospital transport. Be sure to take plenty of rest for at least a week, as well as keeping any wound dry and protected from exposure to dirt and contaminants.

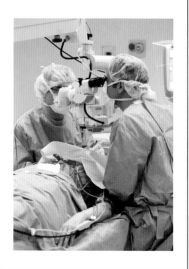

Preparing for your recovery

The time spent recuperating in hospital after even quite major operations is much less today than was the case even 20 years ago. This has the advantage of allowing you to recover in the comfort of your own home, without the inconveniences and risk of infection that a prolonged hospital stay entails. But it also means that you will have to manage many aspects of your recovery away from 24-hour nursing care.

With a planned operation, you are likely to have time to think about what help you will need and what adaptations to your home may be necessary when you return. Make sure you find out how the operation will affect you physically by getting as much information as possible from your doctors and from friends who've had similar procedures. You can discover how other people manage by taking a look at the health website www.healthtalkonline.org, where patients talk on video about their experiences of various health issues, including those requiring surgery. Here is a four-step plan to help ensure the early post-operative days are plain sailing:

1 Visualise how your life will be during recuperation to identify hidden problems. Will you be able to get around your house by yourself? You may need to consider putting your bed in a different room to allow easy access to a bathroom. If getting to the toilet is likely to cause problems, consider hiring or borrowing a commode. Your GP can advise you on where to get a commode, or you can locate companies that sell or rent disability aids using the Yellow Pages or Google. If you are dependent on car transport, you may also need to consider how soon you will be able to drive – factoring in the effects of pain-relieving medication as well as the impact of the surgery (see *When can I drive again?*, page 211).

2 Ask the surgical team about any exercises you'll be expected to do after surgery. As long as your surgeon approves, practise them regularly before you go into hospital. Working your muscles and joints beforehand will speed your recovery.

3 Find out from your surgical team about any walking aids (crutches or a walking frame, for example) that you may need after your operation if you're having hip or knee surgery. Confirm that these will be supplied by the hospital.

4 Allow plenty of time to install secure handrails and grab bars in your shower if you've been advised that you'll need them. Also, make sure you have a comfortable and stable chair with a firm cushion, back and two arms for your living room. These adaptations are sometimes available through your local hospital occupational therapy department (see also *Caring for others*, pages 266–283).

ACCEPT HELP GRACIOUSLY

You'll need support at this time, and in the run-up to your operation don't be embarrassed to ask friends and family for help – most people are happy to step up when needed. Here are some suggestions for ways to make the most of other people's kindness:

- Arrange for someone to clean the house for you. A messy environment will only increase your stress while you're recovering.
- Make a list of what help you'll need after your operation, whether it's shopping, laundry, cooking or childcare. Ask each volunteer helper to pick one or more items from your list.
- Arrange a rota of visitors post-surgery. You'll probably want your partner, children or closest friends nearby soon after surgery. After a week or two, you may well welcome new faces. But be ready to cancel, if you don't feel up to it.
- Stock up on healthy foods before you go into hospital. If you are well enough, make and freeze meals to reheat for yourself or your friends when they come to see you after you return home.

THE BEST PREPARATION FOR YOUR OP

Tailoring your pre-op preparations to your particular operation and being aware of your specific risks and recovery requirements will help you get the best outcome. In some cases, you'll need to take preparatory steps in the weeks leading up to the operation, but in other cases the main preparation occurs only in the days and hours before you enter the operating theatre. The following list will give you an idea of what you'll need to consider.

Abdominal surgery You'll have to empty your bowels and stop eating and drinking according to a strict timetable if you're having an operation on your abdomen. This also applies to hernia surgery. Pay close attention to the instructions provided by your surgical team.

Cancer surgery This type of surgery often requires several hours of anaesthesia. To recover safely, you may need a minimum of two nights in hospital. If your doctors suggest you stay longer, do as they say – there will be a good reason for this.

Hysterectomy As well as preparing yourself physically, take the time to manage the strong emotions that hysterectomy frequently evokes. Make sure you're well-informed about the subject and are fully convinced that this surgery is the best alternative. Talk to your doctor about the pros and cons of taking HRT (hormone replacement therapy) after the operation.

Orthopaedic surgery Excess weight is your worst enemy if you're having a knee or hip replacement - adding extra risk to the operation and making recovery longer and more problematic. Your surgeon may refer you to a hospital dietitian. If not, see your GP about getting expert help.

Stent or bypass surgery Eating healthily, quitting smoking and having a dental check are all recommended before stent or bypass surgery. And being psychologically prepared is also important. See *Bypassing problems*, page 132.

Getting fit for theatre

Instead of worrying about your forthcoming operation, put all your energy into making sure you're as fit as possible. You really can make a difference to the outcome of your surgery if you take action in the time remaining before your admission date.

Quitting smoking is the best way to improve the outcome of your operation at a single stroke. Stopping the habit at least six weeks before has been shown to bring about a significant reduction in health problems resulting from surgery (see also *Countdown to your operation*, pages 202–203). For quitting advice, see *Clearing the smoke*, page 136. You're three times more likely to quit if you get help from your local Stop Smoking Service. Make an appointment today.

EAT WELL

Most people think that getting fit means losing weight, but that's not necessarily the case when you're preparing for surgery. 'What's important is to become as well nourished as possible by the time you have the operation through eating a healthy, balanced diet,' says Julie Ann Kidd of the British Dietetic Association (BDA). 'You can be overweight and still be poorly nourished if your diet lacks essential nutrients. People with

A SMOKER'S STORY

How a couple's joint approach led to successful cessation for both of them

Michael was 60 years old, and had been smoking 30 cigarettes a day since he was a teenager, when he suffered two heart attacks. His wife Josie tells their story:

Michael was told that only heart surgery could relieve his symptoms and reduce his risk of an early death. Although he'd tried and failed to stop smoking several times previously, this time he asked me, also a smoker, to take part in a quit-smoking program with him, organised by a local health authority. As well as receiving nicotine therapy and individual counselling, we joined a support group.

By the end of the program we classed ourselves as non-smoking. I went through hell and back when Michael was in hospital. It was horribly stressful but I never thought about smoking. Nor did he – and we're just delighted to be looking and feeling better than ever.

cancer and other health problems ... are frequently underweight and will have a better outcome if they put on a few kilograms.'

For people whose weight loss is due to illness, the best advice is to build strength by eating a balanced range of nutritious foods (see *Preventing weight loss*, page 273). The Dietitians Association of Australia has information on diet on its website http://daa.asn.au/for-the-public/ smart-eating-for-you/nutrition-a-z. Ask your GP for a referral to an accredited dietitian for personalised advice.

LOSE IT GRADUALLY

If you are carrying extra kilos, depending on the time available before your operation, losing excess weight can be one of the most worthwhile contributions you can make to your health before surgery – especially if the operation involves weight-bearing joints. But don't crash diet just before you go into hospital. Gradual, healthy weight loss (no more than 1 kg per week, preferably under medical supervision) should be the most you should aim for.

If you and your doctor agree that you have a weight-related problem that might affect your forthcoming surgery, it's advisable to consult a registered dietitian either through your hospital or your GP. A dietitian can help you manage the move to healthy eating. Your priority should be to increase your nutrient intake. If your daily diet consists largely of food with a high-fat and high-sugar content, incorporate more vegetables, fruit and fish in your daily diet, while cutting down, for example, on fried foods, cakes and sweet drinks.

GET FIT – GENTLY

If your physical condition before your operation permits it, it is a good idea to get into the habit of gentle exercise. Your doctor will confirm what type of activity is safe for you to do. For those who are largely sedentary, regular strolls in the park or in your neighbourhood will have a beneficial impact on fitness for surgery.

ADJUST YOUR ATTITUDE

Being relaxed has many benefits, including soothing your nervous system, boosting your immune system, balancing your heart rhythms and promoting healing. In the period before your operation, focus on positive thoughts and your goal of a full and speedy recovery. You can continue to use these strategies during your recuperation. If you have specific fears about your surgery, set your mind at rest by talking to your GP or the surgical team at the hospital.

Only try to lose weight if your doctor agrees it's a good idea

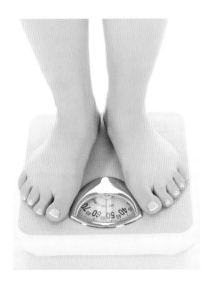

Countdown to your operation

Going into hospital can be daunting, and understandably your anxiety is likely to be increased by the prospect of surgery. For many, the best way to cope is to make careful practical preparations.

Follow the simple timetable on the facing page to help you prepare for surgery in the weeks and days leading up to your operation. Your hospital may give you a list of items to bring with you, but if not, the list to the right is a useful guide. Pack your belongings in an easily stowed soft bag. You will be advised not to bring valuables into the hospital, but you may want to have your mobile phone with you. Discuss this with the ward staff on arrival and follow their guidance.

Good preparation for surgery will help you face the operation with optimism

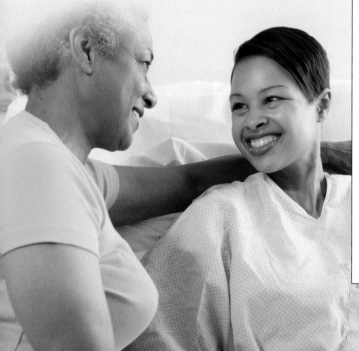

What to take to hospital

For a hospital stay of more than one night, take the following items:

✔ two sets of nightwear and a dressing gown and slippers (not slipper socks)

✔ one set of day clothes and spare underwear

✔ a small hand towel and toiletries, including soap, a toothbrush, toothpaste, deodorant and shampoo, plus sanitary protection (pre-menopausal women) and a razor and shaving materials (men)

✔ a comb or hairbrush

✔ things to occupy you (books, magazines, MP3 player, etc.)

✔ a small amount of money to buy things such as newspapers, phone calls and anything you may want from the hospital shop or ward trolley

✔ your usual medications, including eye drops, inhalers and creams

✔ antiseptic hand wipes

✔ a notebook and pen to write down any questions you have when the doctor is not available

✔ healthy, non-perishable snacks to eat between meals (nuts, dried fruit)

✔ your address book and important phone numbers, including your GP's contact details.

THE BEST PREPARATION FOR YOUR OPERATION

Two months before

Review your diet Check that you are eating a nutrient-rich diet and aim for gradual weight loss if your doctor recommends it (see page 201).

Get moving If your health allows it, start a routine of regular, gentle exercise (see page 201).

Have plenty of sleep Try to establish a regular sleep pattern. If you can't sleep for any reason, talk to your GP. See also pages 30-33.

Quit smoking Get support to quit the habit now. Giving up will help to prevent complications post-surgery. These include a higher risk of wounds failing to heal properly and of long-term heart, circulation and lung problems. Some surgeons are reluctant to agree to operate on smokers.

Limit your alcohol consumption Cut your intake to no more than a unit a day (1 small glass of wine). If you have a problem with this, talk to your doctor about getting support for reducing your drinking.

Think about home Consider adaptations you may need to make to your home when you return from hospital (see page 198) and start fitting whatever aids you may require.

One month before

Continue to follow the advice above. If you've only just been told of your surgery, it's not too late to start.

Get help in place Talk to your friends and family about the help you'll need when you get home from hospital. If necessary, start work on a rota of visitors and helpers (see page 199).

Review your commitments Make sure your employer is aware of the time you are likely to be absent. Also look at your diary to reschedule any important appointments that are booked for the time you're in hospital and during your recovery.

One week before

Adjust your alcohol intake Even if your alcohol consumption is within the recommended limits (see page 26), reduce it to a maximum of one unit a day. But if you are a heavy drinker, do not suddenly cut down, or stop, close to the time of surgery. Your reaction to alcohol withdrawal could cause life-threatening complications. Before your operation make sure your anaesthetist is aware of the level of your drinking.

Check your instructions Review pre-surgery instructions from the hospital, especially with regard to food and drink intake. Also remind yourself about the date and time you need to arrive at the hospital.

Pay up Make sure you have paid any bills that may become due while you're away and, if you're leaving an empty house, cancel deliveries.

Go shopping Buy any items that you need for your hospital stay (see facing page). Stock up on non-perishable food for your return home.

Be kind to yourself Now is the time to allow yourself to relax and be pampered. Have relaxing, fragrant baths or book a massage.

The day before

Pack your bag Refer to the instructions from the hospital and the suggestions in the panel (facing page) for appropriate items to pack.

Stop eating and drinking Be sure to observe the precise timings stipulated in your instructions from the hospital.

Make sure you're hydrated While observing the instructions you have been given (see above), have about 2 litres (4 pints) of fluids in the 24 hours before you go into hospital.

Confirm your travel Book your taxi or ask a friend to take you to hospital in good time.

After surgery

Just a generation ago, patients were made to rest for several days, or even weeks, while recovering from surgery. Today that's all changed and you'll be encouraged to get active as soon as possible.

The super-speedy recovery times achieved after surgery by elite sportsmen and women in recent years have shown the benefits of a swift return to mobility. That message has been underlined by research showing that achieving normal levels of activity as quickly as possible is the best way to prevent the onset of venous thromboembolism (VTE), one of the most serious post-operative health risks.

Modern surgical techniques, including 'keyhole' (laparoscopic) surgery, which avoid the need to cut through muscle and flesh, have also speeded recovery. In turn, this is reflected in current health-care thinking, which encourages patients to take control of their recovery from day one.

 SELF-HELP

Keep moving...
even in bed

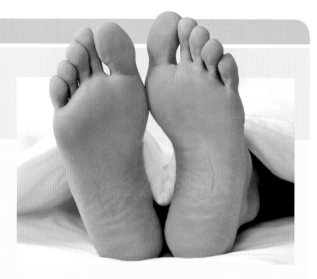

After an operation, while lying on your back, every hour you are awake:

- Take five deep breaths; fill your lungs down to the bottom of your ribcage. Try to avoid lifting your shoulders. Watch your stomach move forward as your lungs inflate.

- Move your feet up and down, pull your toes towards you, and then point them away from you. Repeat this cycle 20 to 30 times. You can also make circles with your feet, also 20 to 30 times. These movements encourage your blood to flow and prevent clots developing in your legs.

- Tighten your buttock and thigh muscles. Working each leg in turn, extend your leg straight out in front of you, tighten the muscles at the front of the thigh, and push the back of the knee down onto the bed. Hold for 3 seconds and repeat 10 times.

FIRST STAGES

You've woken up after your operation. What should you do next? The following six-point early-recovery plan comes from Louise Bland, physiotherapy manager at the Yorkshire Clinic in Bingley, UK.

- Aim to become independent as quickly as possible. Moving your legs to get out of bed, sitting, standing up from a chair and walking to the toilet are your first 'mountains to climb'. Be sure to wear your slippers whenever you get out of bed to avoid picking up an infection.

- Pace is everything. When you start exercising, follow the 'do a bit and rest a bit' rule. Listen to your body and stop whenever you feel pain. At this time, the 'no pain, no gain' mantra does not apply. Exercise that causes you excessive pain will slow your recovery.

- Pay attention to the advice of your health-care team. Your surgeon and physiotherapist will give you written or verbal instructions to support your recovery. Don't rely on anyone to chase you to make sure you're doing what you're told. Today's health-care teams expect to share care with their patients and that means that individuals need to accept a large measure of responsibility for their own recovery.

- Don't worry about how other people are managing their recovery or compare your progress to theirs. Your ability to return to mobility depends on your age and your state of health generally, as well as the operation you've had.

- Try to keep calm and relaxed during your hospital stay. With busy nurses and large numbers of visitors coming and going, hospital wards are often far from peaceful. Do your best to focus on the positive – including the many health-care staff who communicate well and offer compassionate caring. Create your own island of calm by doing deep breathing exercises, meditation and, when necessary, wearing earplugs.

Guard against infection

Don't be afraid to challenge hospital staff who don't appear to be cleaning their hands regularly. Handwashing is the most important thing everyone can do – nurses, doctors, hospital visitors, in particular – to protect against the spread of MRSA (Methicillin-resistant *Staphylococcus aureus*) and other infections such as *Clostridium difficile*. Many wards now have dispensers for alcohol-based hand rubs, which are a quick and efficient way to rid your hands of most bacteria. One hospital in Northern Ireland revealed that MRSA bacteria had been found widely on mobile phones used by doctors and nurses, showing how easily the bacteria can spread unless strict hand hygiene is observed. A useful tip is to bring a supply of antibacterial wipes into hospital with you and use them to clean any surfaces you come into contact with.

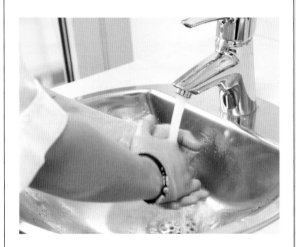

ASK THE TEAM

If you have outstanding questions about your recovery, your stay in hospital is a good time to get answers. Write a list of any questions that are still niggling you. You can then bring out the list when your consultant, physiotherapist or nurse comes to see you and get the answers you need.

Try to get as detailed a timetable as possible for your return to normal activities. These include walking, driving, playing sports, going to the gym, doing housework and having sex. They may not seem a priority now – but the information could prove useful later on. Find out in advance what will happen when you're discharged from hospital – and how you can access support services, including physiotherapy.

IF YOUR MOBILITY IS RESTRICTED

Being immobile for any length of time can cause problems, not least because you're not using many of your muscles. The following steps will help ensure you don't experience any lasting effects:

- If you have to spend a substantial amount of time in bed, you'll need to wear anti-embolism stockings and follow an exercise routine to make sure the blood keeps flowing properly through your veins.
- If you can't move your knee following knee replacement or cartilage surgery, many hospitals will put your leg on a machine that will bend it for you. As your knee becomes more mobile, you'll be given exercises to strengthen the affected muscles.
- If your foot is immobile and in plaster – for instance, after having a bunion removed – make sure it's always slightly raised, perhaps on a cushioned stool. It doesn't have to be too high up, just slightly raised to stop the blood accumulating in your foot.
- As soon as you can, use crutches to maintain mobility, which accelerates healing following surgery to the knee or foot. It will help if your crutches are comfortable to use; your physiotherapist will adjust them. Find out from your surgeon how long you'll need them.

EXPERT ADVICE WHATEVER THE OPERATION

'Keyhole' or laparoscopic surgery Frequently used for gall bladder operations as well as hernias and abdominal surgery such as the removal of ovarian cysts. This type of surgery avoids the need to make

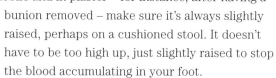

NURSING KNOW-HOW

Abdominal wound care

Abdominal wounds can be uncomfortable if you cough – or even breathe deeply. Here are some tips from a perioperative nursing expert:

- Keep a small folded towel to hand and press it onto the wound when you need to cough or when doing breathing exercises.

- If the wound makes it painful to lie flat on your back, place a pillow under your lower legs to keep your knees bent, take the pressure off your abdomen and allow the wound to heal correctly.

large incisions through muscle and flesh and therefore speeds recovery. But you've still had an operation that involved cutting soft tissue, which takes four to six weeks to heal. It's vital that you don't engage in vigorous activity including heavy housework until that tissue has had time to heal.

Vaginal and abdominal surgery Be very careful when lifting for the first six weeks after the operation. If you do have to lift something, brace your tummy and pelvic floor muscles, then raise yourself up using a smooth action without jerking.

Shoulder surgery Take care to maintain good posture, and resist slumping forward. This is vital for speedy recovery.

Knee surgery As soon as you're mobile, avoid keeping your knee in one position for any length of time as this can lead to stiffness, pain and swelling. Get up frequently and move around. On long car journeys, make a habit of stopping every hour or so and walking around for 5 minutes before continuing. Similarly, if you're travelling by train or air, get up and walk around at regular intervals.

Ankle and wrist surgery For optimum recovery, be sure to get regular exercise prescribed by a physiotherapist to ensure that the joints regain their strength and mobility. Don't worry too much about swelling during recovery. Be sure to rest the joints between exercises.

Foot or toe surgery Don't walk unaided until your physiotherapist has given you the all clear. Try to avoid standing for too long as it will cause pain and swelling in your foot.

Heart surgery Cardiac rehabilitation in the form of weekly exercise and information sessions is available from hospitals. If you've had heart surgery, you'll be invited

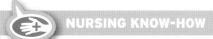

NURSING KNOW-HOW

Be clever with pain relief

Time the doses of your painkilling medication before an activity that may cause discomfort in the days and weeks following surgery – for example, before you do rehabilitation exercises, have a bath or shower or get dressed. But pain exists for a reason, so don't use painkillers to allow you to do more than you should.

Special rehabilitation programs are available for heart surgery patients

True or False?

The application of vitamin E can minimise the appearance of a scar

Unproven Anecdotal reports that the application of vitamin E oil to an existing scar or to a recently healed wound can reduce scar tissue have not been supported by scientific studies. In fact, there is evidence that it can cause local skin irritation (contact dermatitis).

to participate. The aim is to start you on an exercise program to get you fit after surgery. For further information, see *Bypassing problems*, pages 132–133.

WOUND CARE TO MINIMISE SCARRING

Most people who undergo surgery are concerned about the scar that might remain. What you want ideally is a flat, narrow scar that you can barely see – at least when you've allowed 12 to 18 months to pass by, which is sufficient time for your skin to make a full recovery.

In the days and weeks following your operation, there's a great deal you can do to ensure that your wound heals well and to reduce the risk of infection and of significant scarring:

- Before you go home, be sure to get advice on wound care from the nursing staff. In particular, you'll need to know if you should keep the wound dry (for example, when you bath or shower) and, if so, for how long.
- Dressing the wound is essential to keep it moist and prevent the formation of a scab, itself a barrier to healing. This will be the responsibility of the nursing staff in hospital. If your wound needs a new dressing when you have left hospital, a community nurse will be asked to visit you at home.
- If the wound area starts to swell, ask your doctor or nurse for advice. The use of an ice-pack or a bag of frozen peas may help reduce it. Leaving the dressing in place, cover the area with a towel and place the ice-pack on top of that. Hold the ice-pack in place and leave for no more than 5 minutes.
- Avoid touching the stitches or any threads that emerge on the skin surface from internal stitches, because this can transmit infection into the wound.
- Once the wound has healed and you remove the dressing, start to massage moisturiser around it. This will aid the release of scar-making collagen in a balanced way. Bio-oil is commonly recommended, but anything from Nivea and E45 cream to baby oil can be used as long as you're not allergic to it.
- Cortisone tape or cream reduces the risk of the development of a keloid – a raised red (hypertrophic) scar. Your GP can prescribe it.
- Silicone gel or spray (also available on prescription) traps moisture in the wound, keeping the scar from becoming rigid. You can also try elasticised Kinesiotape (www.kinesiotaping.com.au), which may improve the circulation of the blood around the wound while also preventing movement that impedes healing.

Eating for recovery

Depending on the type of surgery you've undergone, you may have to change your diet during your recovery and perhaps beyond. Equip yourself with information about the best foods for your condition, including the type of surgery you're facing. For example, if you've had a colostomy or ileostomy there may be some foods that are best avoided until you know how they affect you. Advice on these conditions can be found at www.iasupport.org and www.colostomyassociation.org.uk. After some types of surgery, you may even need to adopt a new dietary approach for the rest of your life. Ask to see a hospital dietitian for further advice, if necessary.

WHEN YOU DON'T FEEL LIKE EATING

It's common for people to lose their appetite after an operation, but poor nutrition can have a major impact on the rate and success of recovery. You need to be as well nourished as possible at this time when your immune system is low and your body faces major demands. Hospital food isn't always appetising and nutritious so ensuring good nutrition when you return home after surgery is key to recovery. Light nutritious meals that are beautifully presented are likely to tempt you into eating again.

If you live on your own, eating regularly and healthily is often a challenge even in normal circumstances. And after surgery it's all too easy to skip meals altogether if you have nobody to prepare food for you, especially if you've had an operation that makes it difficult to move around. Easy-to-prepare nutritious and energy-packed snacks such as beans on toast or chicken breast in a bun with some salad are ideal. Prepared food and tins of soup are also useful stand-bys.

WHEN YOU'VE LOST WEIGHT BEFORE SURGERY

The biggest risk for some patients, including those having cancer surgery, is losing too much weight – a pattern that might have started before the operation and may continue afterwards. As long as your doctor approves, you should eat whatever you fancy in the early days after surgery – whether it's chocolate or tubs of ice cream. Prescribable supplements can also be added to make sure your diet includes sufficient protein. GPs can also prescribe fortified drinks and custard as well as protein-rich sachets that can be dissolved in food such as mashed potatoes, vegetables or sauces. For more ideas on diet during illness, see *Caring for others*, pages 266-283.

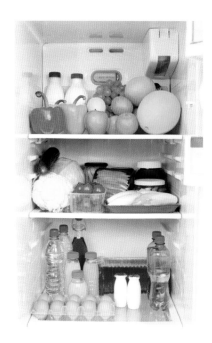

Ask a friend or relative to stock up your fridge with easy-to-prepare foods that are high in vitamins and protein

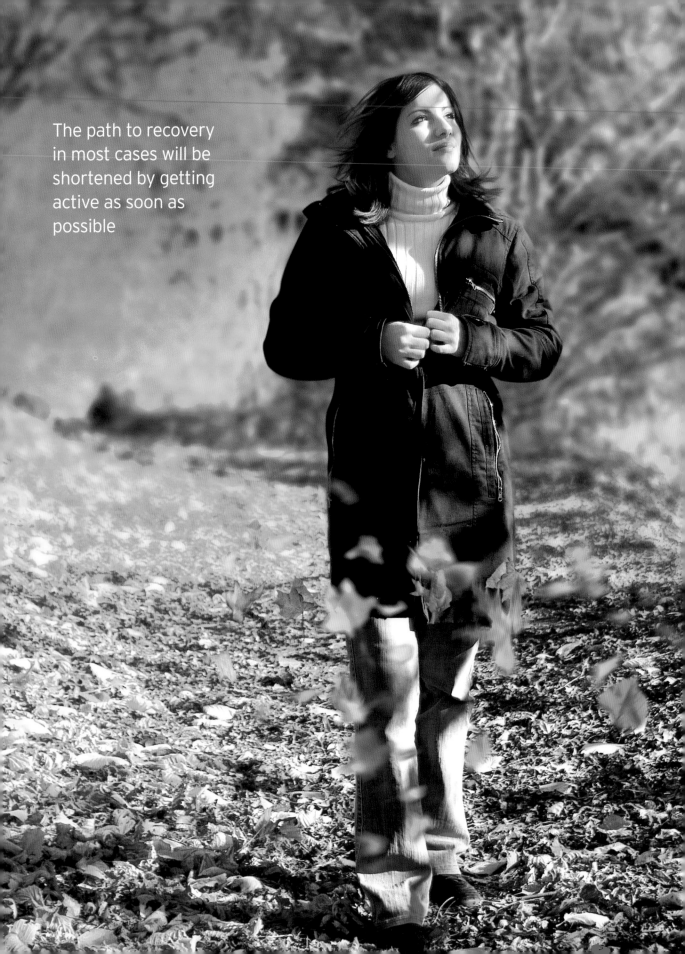

The path to recovery in most cases will be shortened by getting active as soon as possible

Getting back to normal

Recovery is rarely a straight road from A to B. More often, it's a tortuous route where progress can sometimes seem slow or even non-existent and with a series of endless hurdles ahead. But never doubt for a second that persistence will pay off in your journey back to good health.

ON THE ROAD TO PHYSICAL HEALTH

Even minor surgery involves a degree of physical trauma. You've been through a form of assault and you need to make time to take the measures necessary for effective healing. Here are four key ways to help you regain your physical health after you've had an operation.

- Soft tissue takes four to six weeks to heal. Until that time, gentle activities including walking, cycling, swimming, yoga or Pilates are helpful. But hold off on long-distance running or high-impact sports such as football until you've been given the okay by your surgeon. This is particularly important if you've had abdominal surgery.

- At home, avoid heavy household chores, though you'll be encouraged to undertake light housework and cooking – making sandwiches, for instance, rather than preparing a roast dinner for six. And start going for walks, perhaps arm in arm at first, even if you have to push yourself to take a 5-minute stroll.

- If you've had surgery on your hip, knee or ankle, you'll benefit from gait re-education under the supervision of a physiotherapist to correct faults that have crept in post-surgery and may cause problems later on. Ask about such programs before you leave hospital or ask your GP to refer you for physiotherapy once you're home.

- Keep up the recommended exercises even after you think you have got over the operation. 'Don't assume that once you're walking normally after orthopaedic surgery, you've reached your recovery goal,' says Helen Harper Smith, a clinical specialist orthopaedic physiotherapist and a member of the Chartered Society of Physiotherapists, UK. 'Exercises given to people post-orthopaedic surgery target vulnerable muscle groups that are essential to functional activity and which need extra attention following surgery. People should continue these exercises for at least four months and probably for a lot longer.'

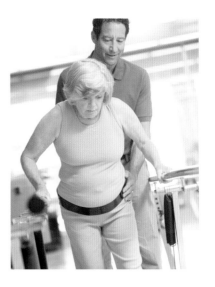

The hospital physiotherapist will provide support and reassurance

When can I drive again?

How soon after major surgery you are fit to drive is different for each patient, and is dependent on several factors, including the type of surgery, your age and your general health. You should refrain from driving for at least 24 hours after a general anaesthetic. Legally, you're allowed to drive again when your doctor agrees that your physical condition does not adversely affect your ability to control the vehicle or imperil the safety of others. When you feel ready to get back behind the wheel, talk to your doctor and follow his or her advice. It is important to tell your insurance company about your surgery and inform them that your doctor has given approval for your resumption of driving.

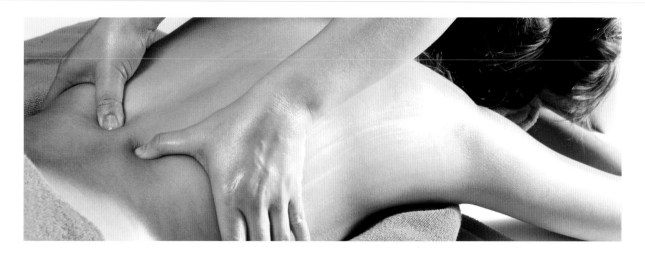

Having a therapeutic massage can both relax and energise you as you recuperate from surgery

REGAINING YOUR EMOTIONAL HEALTH

It's not unusual to suffer depression in the post-operative period – often several days or even weeks after the crisis of surgery has ended. In some cases depression may be severe or persistent enough to require treatment. 'There's a lot about surgery that patients find painful and frightening,' explains the writer John F. Lauerman in the *Harvard Public Health Review* magazine. 'It can shatter the image of our bodies as somehow intact. And the resulting feelings of mortality, of loss and of vulnerability can be profound,' he says. Such feelings can be worsened by lack of sleep due to post-operative pain as well as loss of energy and a falling off of appetite.

If you're feeling in low spirits following your surgery, talk to your GP. Once diagnosed, depression can almost always be successfully treated with talking therapies and medication where necessary.

Here are suggestions for how to take care of your emotional self in the days and weeks after your surgery:

- Try not to panic or feel guilty if you feel depressed following surgery. It's normal. Give yourself permission to cry and talk about it. Just being able to express your feelings goes a long way towards helping you feel better.
- Make sure you drink plenty of water. It's good for you anyway but will also flush out the large amounts of medication pumped into your body in a short period of time, which may be affecting your mood.
- Rest. Having been through surgery, your body needs every available resource to heal what it perceives as 'injuries'.
- Relax. Ask someone to give you a foot massage, hand massage, back rub or a shoulder and neck rub. Do what you can to pamper yourself and allow others to pamper you.

Case Study

AN EXPLORER'S STORY

Bypass surgery needn't signal the end of participation in physical challenges

Explorer Ranulph Fiennes had a double bypass heart operation in 2003, aged 59, after suffering a heart attack during training to complete the Land Rover Challenge – seven marathons on seven continents in seven days.

Having a heart attack can cause great fear and worry about what the future might hold. After the bypass, I was told that for eight weeks I shouldn't drive or take hard exercise. At first I would get out of breath after just a few steps and had to sit down. Walking was more like lurching. But within two weeks, I was jogging for an hour – and after a month for 2 hours. It took time to regain even a reasonable amount of fitness. But four months after the operation, I did complete the Land Rover Challenge. Not everyone has been as lucky as I have been. Some people will be disabled from their heart attacks. And some will lose their confidence or find it difficult to recover emotionally and physically. But many people, like me, will continue to have the lives they had before.

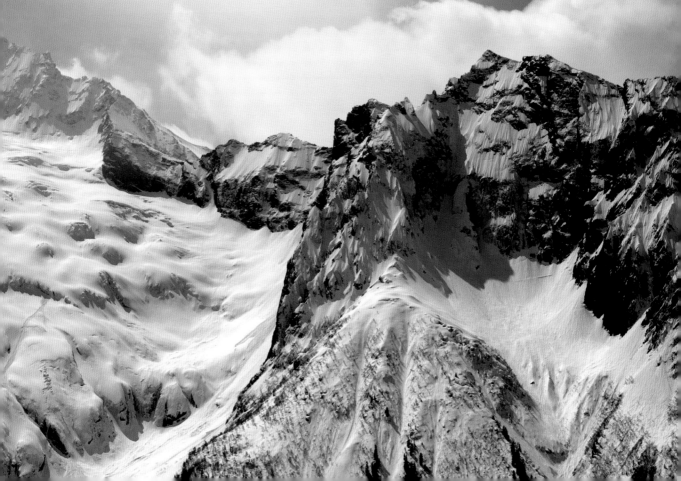

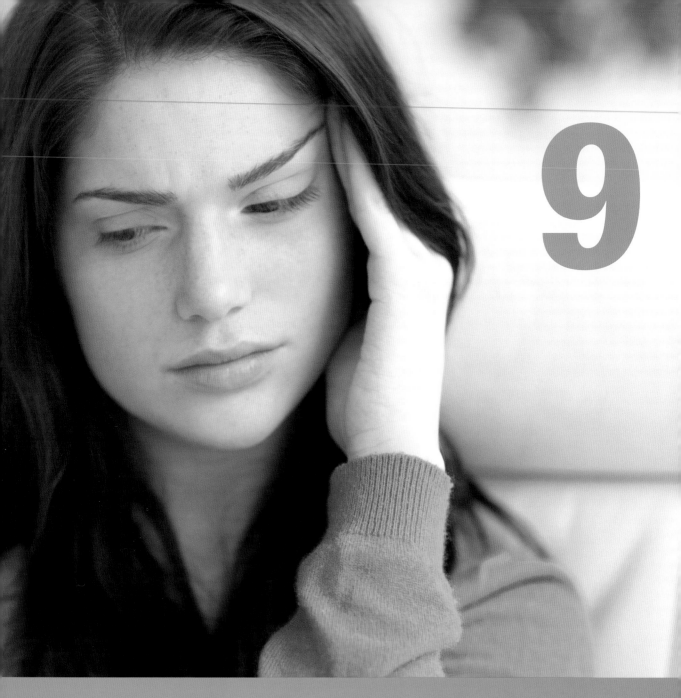

9

Relieving pain

Medical advances and a greater understanding of the benefits of complementary therapies mean that most types of pain can now be eased or controlled

A fresh approach

In the past few years, medical scientists have made great strides in understanding pain and how it works. The good news – even if you're affected by chronic pain – is that you don't have to suffer in silence. There's much that can be done to ease the problem.

If you've ever experienced even a headache, you'll know how debilitating it can be. And lasting pain of any kind can make life unbearable and affect your relationships with family and friends. Addressing the underlying problem should bring relief, but sometimes the discomfort can linger for much longer.

Because it is so individual, pain is notoriously difficult to define and treat. Only you know how much something really hurts, and the nature and degree of your suffering is often hard to convey.

A PAINFUL CONDITION

Researchers are now examining the idea that chronic pain could, in fact, be a medical condition caused by changes in the nervous system that occur in response to acute pain. As a result, doctors are being encouraged to treat chronic pain as an ailment. It has also been recognised that patients can increase the effectiveness of any prescribed treatment by adopting a range of self-help strategies.

YOUR ROLE IN BEATING PAIN

Whatever treatment your doctor or other health-care professionals recommend, you are the best judge of what works for you. In addition to medication, you may find that exercise, pacing your activity, setting goals and practising relaxation techniques also help. Even making sure you get enough sleep can be important; some research suggests that lack of sleep reduces our pain threshold, which increases our levels of discomfort. While you are taking advice and exploring new pain relief measures, you will probably find that you have better and worse days. But if you persevere, it should become clear to both you and your doctor what works and what doesn't, and, in some cases, non-drug approaches may prove as effective as painkillers.

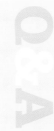

Why is pain important?

Pain is a feeling triggered in the nervous system. If you didn't feel pain, you might seriously injure yourself without knowing you'd done so, or not realise you have a medical condition that needs treatment.

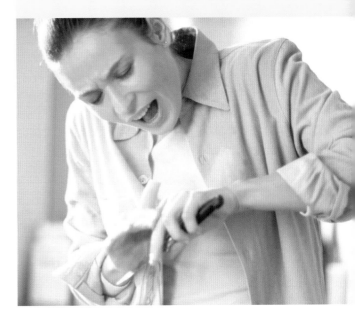

What's happening?

Whether it's the short, sharp shock of a graze to the knee or the nagging throb of an arthritic joint, pain is an unwelcome sensation, but one you can't do without. Pain is your body's way of telling you that something is wrong.

The language of pain

Doctors use different terms for different types of pain.

Acute pain is usually short-term and often caused by an injury or painful event. The cause is identifiable, and typical examples include muscle pain after exercise, pain from an accident and pain following an operation.

Chronic or persistent pain is defined as pain that lasts for more than three months, sometimes for years. It often accompanies conditions such as arthritis or backache, although the cause may not be known.

Recurrent pain comes and goes, as may happen with a headache, for example.

Referred pain is felt in one part of the body when the cause is actually in another. People with a slipped disc, for instance, often feel pain in their leg because the disc is pressing on nerves in the back that run from the spinal cord down the leg to the foot.

Pain can be difficult for doctors to get grips with because it behaves so erratically. It comes and goes according to your mood, focus, attitude and the amount of stress you're under. Sometimes even the weather affects it. You can't measure it objectively and some people are more sensitive to it than others. Most mysterious of all? Sometimes you can continue to feel pain long after the actual cause of the problem has gone.

THE CYCLE OF PAIN

The mysterious nature of pain is due largely to the complex wiring of your nervous system. When you injure your body – if you burn your hand while cooking, for example – a mass of injured tissue releases chemicals that sensitise the nearby nerve endings and send a stream of pain signals to an area of nerves at the back of the spinal cord. Known as the dorsal horn, this area acts like a router for your computer, simultaneously directing impulses to the brain and back down the spinal cord to the injured spot.

READING THE SIGNALS

The dorsal horn is much more than a passive message-processing centre. It also controls your reflexes, your automatic responses to stimuli. Your brain doesn't have to tell you to snatch your hand away if you touch a hot plate, because the dorsal horn has already done that job for you. But although the reflex takes place in the spinal cord, the pain signals also continue up your cord to your brain so that it can make sense of what has happened.

When the pain signals reach your brain, they arrive at an area deep in the mid-brain known as the thalamus, a type of sorting depot, which then directs the messages to specialised areas of the brain to be interpreted. Areas in the cortex (the thinking and behavioural centre of the brain) work out where the pain is coming from and compare it to other types of pain that you may have experienced in the past.

Q&A

Why do we cry when we feel pain?

Among the many destinations to which pain signals are sent is the limbic system, the emotional centre of the brain – this is why pain may sometimes make you cry. The limbic system is also responsible for suppressing the perception of pain in the immediate aftermath of an injury or other painful occurrence.

To make things more complicated, pain is also influenced by other factors that affect your nervous system. Your mood and memory, for example, can change the way your brain interprets pain at any given moment. If you burn your hand, your response is likely to be affected by your emotional state and previous experiences in similar situations.

CHEMICAL ALERT

In response to a pain signal, the nerves in your spinal cord and brain start to release chemicals. Some chemicals, such as glutamate and aspartate, turn up the pain, while others, such as endorphins and GABA, turn it down. Depending on the nature of the injury, your brain also sends out two messenger chemicals, noradrenaline and a type of serotonin, to calm the pain. If the pain is more serious, your brain releases other kinds of serotonin that increase the perception of pain. This mechanism is like an electric light switch in the bottom of your brain turning on or off.

'WIND UP'

As the burned hand gets better, the inflammation subsides, the pain receptors can no longer detect any tissue damage and the pain signals stop. But, in a chronic disease or condition such as arthritis, the joint is in a constant state of damage and pain signals are therefore continually transmitted to the spinal cord. The cells at the nerve endings in your spinal cord and brain may become oversensitised by the constant pain signals, making the discomfort increasingly severe. This is what pain experts call 'wind up', and it explains why chronic pain can be so difficult to treat.

Sometimes the pain continues after an injury has healed because the cause of the pain lies in the nervous system itself. It may be that the nerve fibres have become permanently 'wound up' to pain so that they transmit the pain signal, even after the original cause has gone. Inflammation – one of your body's key healing mechanisms – can also

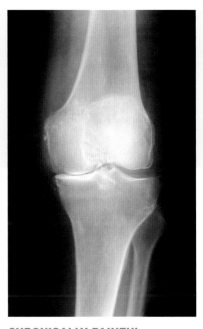

CHRONICALLY PAINFUL
The pink area in this X-ray of the arthritic knee of an 84-year-old woman shows the damage caused by narrowing of the joint space – a common cause of chronic pain in older people.

Some people never feel pain

True Although very rare, a few people are born unable to feel pain. The condition is known as congenital analgesia and those who have it are at risk of serious injury, which they cannot feel, and consequent damage.

True or False?

I should just put up with my pain without making a fuss

False There is no point in suffering unnecessarily. There is plenty that can be done to ease most forms of pain, but you can't be helped unless you seek expert pain management.

contribute to the vicious circle of pain. Usually, it subsides when the injury or damage heals. But if the injury persists, inflammatory chemicals continue to be produced, increasing the sensitivity of the area and the level of pain experienced.

Pin it down

Most people's first reaction to pain is to try to work out where it's coming from, what type of pain it is and the likely cause. If you burn your finger on the iron, the cause is obvious, but sometimes the source of pain can be harder to pinpoint. For instance, 'ice-cream headaches' can happen when something very cold touches the roof of your mouth, but the short-lasting pain you feel is in your brain.

If your pain persists and painkillers don't bring relief, it's time to see your doctor for a check-up. Don't be afraid to speak up. Only you know the nature of your pain and how it affects your quality of life. However, you may not get an instant diagnosis, because pain can't be measured in the same way as, for example, blood pressure.

For short-term pain your doctor may prescribe medication or refer you to a physiotherapist or other health-care professional. If your pain is ongoing – for example, if it is related to a chronic condition such as arthritis – your doctor may prescribe painkillers and talk to you about other ways to manage it. These can include setting goals, a gentle exercise regime and diversions, such as a new hobby.

KNOW YOUR PAIN

It can often help to understand the medical jargon you may hear from your medical team or encounter in material you read. Doctors classify pain into the following types:

Type of pain	Where you feel it
Nociceptive pain	Skin, muscles, ligaments, joints, bones
Inflammatory	Injured tissue
Neuropathic	Nerves
Visceral	Internal organs
Mixed	A combination of the above

ASSESS IT

It's a good idea to take the time to think through the answers to the following questions before you see your doctor. This information may help your GP to identify the origin of your pain and its cause:
- When did the pain start?
- What do you think is causing the pain?
- What are its main symptoms?
- Does anything make it better or worse?
- If you are taking a painkiller, how effective is it and how long do the effects last?
- Does it come on immediately, or a few minutes or hours after you've been doing something specific?
- Does it stop you from sleeping or wake you up during the night?

- Does the pain stop you from doing anything – for example, work, exercise or eating?
- Has the pain affected your mood – do you feel depressed or stressed?
- Have you experienced this type of pain before and, if so, under what circumstances and how long did it last?

Chart it

Because everyone reacts differently to pain, what you find agonising someone else might regard as merely irritating. Charting your pain can help you – and your doctor – to work out how severe it is and the best way to manage it.

- *Think about your pain and note down how bad it is on a scale of 1–10.*
- *Keep a record of how it varies during the course of the day. For example, is it worse when you wake up or in the evening? Does resting help and does it improve after eating?*
- *Keep a chart or diary for a few days or a week to see if and how the pain changes over a short period of time. Describe your pain using words such as throbbing, crushing, darting or shooting.*
- *Note down the effect of anything you may take or do to relieve your pain – for example, whether swallowing a painkiller before the pain kicks in is more effective than having it after the pain has started.*
- *Include a record of the effects of exercise – if walking makes it better or worse, for example, or if one activity causes more pain than another.*

Keeping a diary can help you focus on the things that make you feel better

Treating pain

Highly specific painkilling medications have been developed in recent years and there are many other effective treatments, ranging from self-help measures to machines that disrupt pain signals.

Using medication

Painkillers help with short-term pain, such as headaches, and certain long-term conditions, including some forms of arthritis. In many cases, the relief they bring will enable you to become more active.

While mild versions can be bought over the counter at a pharmacy, supermarket or other shop, stronger medications may be available only on prescription from your doctor. The main types of painkillers are listed below. For more information, see *Get the most from your medicine*, pages 312–339.

- Medications that work by relieving inflammation are known as non-steroidal anti-inflammatory drugs (NSAIDs). Aspirin is often considered a member of this group.
- Medications that act on specific pain receptors to alter the way your brain perceives pain are known as opioids. These are converted into small quantities of morphine in the body and should be used with caution and for as short a time as possible.
- Paracetamol is in a class of its own. How this drug works is unknown, but it is thought that it may act by blocking pain messages in the brain.

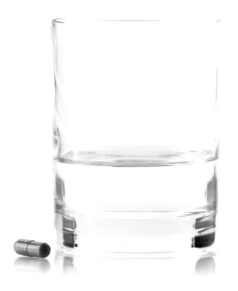

The right painkiller in the right dosage can make all the difference

WHICH PAINKILLERS FOR WHICH PAIN	
Type of painkiller	**Good for**
Non-steroidal anti-inflammatories (NSAIDs): aspirin, celecoxib, diclofenac, ibuprofen, indomethacin, naproxen	Headache, acute strains and sprains, muscle and joint pain, period pain
Weak opioids: codeine, dextropropoxyphene	Pain after surgery, broken bones, injuries, severe toothache
Paracetamol	Everyday aches and pains, such as headache, toothache and joint pain

STAYING SAFE

Don't assume that because a medicine is sold without a prescription it must be completely safe. All medicines have potential side effects. Side effects are likely only if you've been taking painkillers for longer than a week. If you start to notice any unusual symptoms, seek advice from your doctor, pharmacist or other health-care professional. Take note of the following points:

- High doses or long-term use of NSAIDs can lead to indigestion, bleeding from the gut, kidney problems, high blood pressure, fluid retention and a slightly increased risk of heart attack and stroke. They may worsen asthma in about 10 per cent of asthma sufferers.
- Aspirin must not be given to children under the age of 16 because of its association with a rare neurological disorder called Reye's syndrome.
- Prolonged use of painkillers containing codeine can lead to constipation, chronic daily headache and addiction.
- Paracetamol is generally a safe medication. But, an overdose can seriously damage the liver, sometimes permanently.

PRESCRIPTION ONLY

If your pain is severe or you are suffering from a long-term illness, your doctor may prescribe stronger NSAIDs than those available over the counter. When these don't provide adequate pain relief, you may be offered medications related to morphine, known as opioids or narcotics.

Weak opioids include:
- codeine

Strong opioids include:
- tramadol
- morphine
- oxycodone
- fentanyl
- buprenorphine
- hydromorphone.

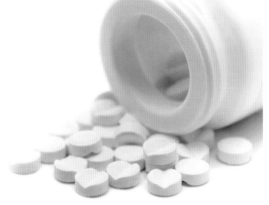

Make sure you discuss your options extremely carefully if your doctor or health-care professional suggests you try taking strong opioids. As a rule these medications should be considered only when all other methods of pain relief have failed, because they can have serious long-term

---

Top Tips

Dos and don'ts when taking painkillers

DON'T

- Take painkillers more frequently than it says on the packet or leaflet.

- Top up a prescription drug with over-the-counter painkillers without talking to your doctor first.

- Take other people's medicines or give yours to anyone else.

- Stay on painkillers for more than three days. If they're not helping your pain, ask your GP or pharmacist for advice.

DO

- Check the ingredients list on the leaflet and packet of all medicines. It can be dangerous to double up on products containing the same active ingredient, such as the painkillers that are found in many cold and flu remedies.

- If you suffer from asthma, stomach problems or if you are taking other prescription medicines, consult your pharmacist; some painkillers may be unsuitable for you.

- Take your medicines in the exact dosage and at the time it says on the packet, or as prescribed by your doctor.

side effects. People often find it difficult to reduce their dosage and may become tolerant to the medications, meaning they need more to produce the same effect. Because strong opioids often cause physical dependency, withdrawal can also be a problem. But, for those in severe pain, their benefits may outweigh the risks, especially if the medications enable them to improve their activity levels.

OTHER MEDICATIONS

Some pain, such as the pain of nerve damage (neuropathic pain), is not helped by standard painkillers. In these cases your doctor may prescribe other medications, such as antidepressants or anti-epileptics, instead of, or as well as, standard painkillers.

Antidepressant medications work by increasing the positive effects of chemicals in the brain and spinal cord that help to block pain signals.

Anti-epileptic medications work by helping to reduce the pain produced by oversensitive cells in the spinal cord – in the same way that they dampen down overactive brain cells in people who have epilepsy.

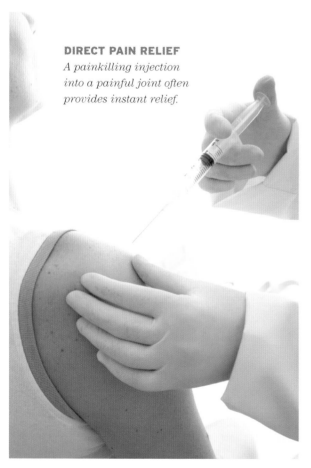

DIRECT PAIN RELIEF
A painkilling injection into a painful joint often provides instant relief.

WHEN PAINKILLERS MAKE IT WORSE

If you get frequent headaches and take painkillers to control them, you may start to experience daily headaches that can last for around 4 hours. These are known as chronic daily headaches and usually result from painkiller overuse. If you suffer from these, you need to see your doctor, who will help you to wean yourself off your medication.

TIME FOR AN INJECTION?

Injections can help with pain relief in some cases, although they are not suitable for all types of pain. Your doctor or health-care professional will be able to advise you about:

● Short-term injections of a local anaesthetic, often mixed with a steroid drug. This type of injection can be given directly into a painful joint or area, with the aim of temporarily deadening the nerves that supply the painful section.

● Epidural injections of corticosteroids. This form of injection into the space around the covering of the spinal cord may relieve pressure on a nerve root in

Why are painkillers sometimes combined?

Different types of painkiller work in different ways. Some products therefore contain more than one type so that you get the combined effects. For example, aspirin, paracetamol or ibuprofen may be combined with codeine to give you stronger pain relief.

the back that is causing sciatica (severe leg pain). The benefits can last for a few days or several months.

- A treatment known as 'denervation'. This involves having injections that partially destroy the nerves that are causing the pain.

Think yourself better

It's hard to feel cheerful if you're lying in a darkened room with a migraine or if you spend your days crippled with arthritis, but evidence suggests that a positive outlook can help to lessen the agony. Best of all, there are therapies that can help you train your brain to develop the right sort of attitude.

Some techniques, for example, visualisation, meditation and laughter therapy, encourage you to focus your thoughts away from your pain. Others, such as cognitive behavioural therapy (CBT) and hypnotherapy, teach you how to think about your pain more positively. Some have more scientific backing than others, but all have helped pain sufferers manage their symptoms better.

VISUALISE IT

Using the power of the imagination in a guided way can bring about beneficial physical, psychological and emotional changes. The technique encourages you to turn your thoughts to a place where there is no pain. It takes practice and there are experts who can explain how to use it to the full. You can find general advice on various websites (for example, www.holisticonline.com/guided-imagery.htm), and there are some helpful visualisation scripts online at www.innerhealthstudio.com.

 NURSING KNOW-HOW

Take a breather

This simple breathing exercise can often help with pain control, particularly if you are also feeling tense or stressed.

- ✔ Take slow, regular breaths. Use your diaphragm rather than lifting your shoulders.

- ✔ As you breathe, focus on the air entering and leaving your body. Try to clear your mind of all other thoughts.

CHANGE THE WAY YOU THINK

How you think about and react to any situation can make it better or worse. This is the basis of cognitive behavioural therapy (CBT), a type of psychotherapy that helps people to change unhelpful or unhealthy thinking habits, feelings and behaviours. If you find yourself thinking, 'This pain is unbearable', a typical CBT approach would be to advise you to adjust the thought to, 'If I breathe deeply, it will pass.' Research shows that if you train your mind to react differently to pain and adopt a positive attitude, you may lessen the effects. A study carried out at the University of Warwick and the University of Oxford on people with chronic back problems found that just 9 hours of CBT significantly improved their pain and stiffness. Your GP can recommend a CBT practitioner. For more information, go to www.betterhealth.vic.gov.au/bhcv2/bhcarticles.nsf/pages/Cognitive_behaviour_therapy.

SWITCH YOUR FOCUS

Hypnotherapy (the medical use of hypnosis) for pain relief comes out well in several clinical trials. According to a review carried out by the Cochrane Collaboration, which assesses the effectiveness of different treatments, it can benefit tension-type headaches.

So how does it work? A hypnotherapist helps you to focus your attention at the same time as making you feel more relaxed. He or she then focuses on your pain, why you might be feeling it and what you can do about it. The idea is to help you to control your pain yourself by using what you've learnt under your hypnotherapist's guidance. There are also many books and DVDs available from which you can learn the technique of self-hypnosis. To find a hypnotherapist, go online at www.asch.com.au.

TAKE CONTROL USING BIOFEEDBACK

Your body normally controls aspects of your body's workings, such as your heart rate and muscle function, automatically. A technique known as biofeedback shows you how to control them yourself using special equipment.

MONITORING MUSCLE TENSION

Biofeedback enables you to become more aware of the workings of different body systems and thereby learn to control how you react. Here, electrodes fixed to the skin of the neck provide feedback on muscle tension that may be causing neck stiffness and headaches.

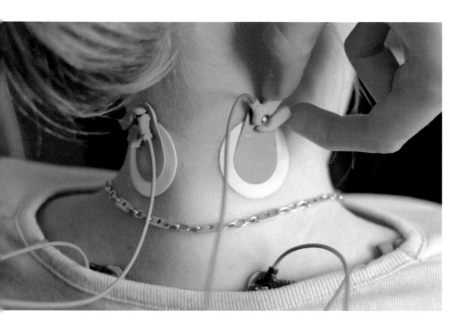

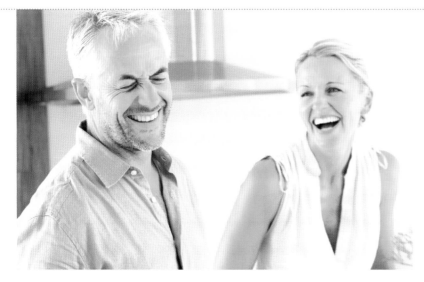

Trigger the production of endorphins – nature's painkillers – by sharing a joke with a friend

This in turn can help you to control your pain. During a session, your heart rate, blood pressure, breathing and muscle tension are monitored via electrical sensors. The results are then fed back to you on a screen or through headphones, enabling you to connect your pain to your physical reaction. You may discover that your headaches, for example, are due to tense muscles. Once you become aware of this you can consciously relax your muscles to reduce pain. The idea is that with time you can produce these responses without the help of a machine.

A review of 53 studies concluded that biofeedback can be effective for tension-type headaches, and another review of 55 studies found it to be beneficial for migraines as well. If you think this form of therapy might work for you, ask your GP for information about reputable local practitioners.

HARNESS THE POWER OF A GOOD GIGGLE

Being told that you can laugh away your pain might seem like a bad joke, but research increasingly shows that laughter really can be the best medicine. A study carried out in Japan showed that blood levels of inflammatory compounds dropped significantly after patients with rheumatoid arthritis watched comedy films. Even better, in some patients the effects lasted for 12 hours or more.

One explanation for the efficacy of laughter is that it triggers endorphins, the body's natural painkillers. Other studies suggest it could improve lung capacity and oxygen levels in the blood, low levels of which are sometimes associated with pain. Some pain

 MIND OVER MATTER

Driven to distraction

You can use the power of your imagination as well as various distraction strategies to help you conquer your pain.

- Turning down your pain on an imaginary dial may help you to feel in control of it and better able to cope with short- or long-term illness.

- Taking up knitting, doing sudoku puzzles or crosswords or joining a book group may all help to take your mind off your pain.

- Staying in touch with friends and family can benefit your health, and this is borne out by many studies. Likewise it can help to take your mind off your pain. Even if you can't get out and about, keep in touch using the phone or ask those you are close to round for a chat and a cup of tea.

clinics offer laughter therapy sessions. Alternatively, you can try to find ways to make yourself laugh more at home; thinking about what amuses you is the first step. Rent a funny film, play a game of charades, spend time with friends or family who share your sense of humour.

RELAX YOUR BODY AND SOUL
Learning to relax your body and focus your thoughts on something other than your pain can be deeply therapeutic. Various techniques can be used to induce 'relaxed awareness', the basis of the meditative state.

Meditation can slow your heart rate, reduce your blood pressure, regulate your breathing and still your mind. A study published in the journal *NeuroReport* showed that people who regularly practised transcendental meditation, one of the most popular types, had a measurable reduction of 40–50 per cent in their brain's response to pain. Try this for 20 minutes, morning and evening: kneel or sit comfortably with your eyes closed and mentally repeat a single word.

Exercise your pain away

Exercise may be the last thing you feel like doing when you're in pain, but all the evidence suggests that keeping moving is one of the best methods of pain relief. For instance, research has shown that specifically tailored exercise programs can help to improve endurance, strength and overall physical function in people with rheumatoid arthritis. The right type of exercise at the right intensity can benefit most types of pain.

Immobility increases your risk of stiff joints, weak muscles, weight gain and breathlessness. In the long term, lack of exercise may also contribute to health problems such as heart disease and diabetes.

You don't have to run a marathon or do a hearty workout in the gym to benefit. Start with something gentle such as walking, swimming, or some simple stretches, and build up gradually to something more demanding. Your doctor or physiotherapist can help you pick activities to suit you, ideally incorporating three types of exercise:
Range of movement exercises To help maintain your flexibility and strength and improve your posture.
Strengthening exercises To help build up your muscles, which support your joints.
Aerobic exercises To raise your heart rate, strengthen your heart muscle and increase your lung capacity.

Five reasons to get moving

Even if you're in pain, you'll reap the benefits of exercise. Here are just five reasons why you should get active.

1 It boosts levels of endorphins, the body's natural painkillers, while reducing levels of the stress hormone cortisol.

2 It strengthens your muscles and ligaments.

3 It helps to keep your weight under control – excess weight can increase pain and strain.

4 It helps you to sleep better.

5 It can help to take your mind off your pain.

FLEX YOUR NECK

This neck exercise is particularly good for relieving pain and stiffness in your neck; it may also help if you get headaches.

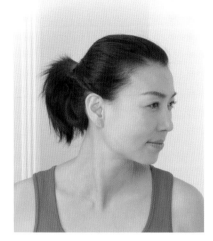 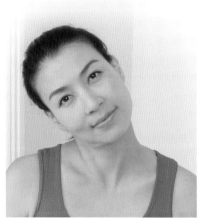

1 *Slowly turn your head to the left as far as you can and hold for 5 seconds. Bring your head back to the centre. Repeat the move to the right. Repeat 5–10 times.*

2 *Keeping your head straight, tilt it over to the right side and hold for 5 seconds (not so far that you touch your shoulder with your ear). Repeat the move to the left. Repeat 5–10 times.*

Hands-on therapies

Pain can be tiring and debilitating, especially if you and your doctors are finding it hard to pinpoint a cause. Hands-on therapies, including acupuncture and acupressure, can sometimes help. They are thought to work by stimulating the production of natural painkillers, including endorphins, within the body.

Other techniques, such as massage, can help you relax and may reduce any muscle tension in the area, which can intensify pain. The application of firm pressure to painful areas may also help to block pain signals from reaching the brain.

NEEDLING THE PAIN

Acupuncture, which involves inserting needles at specific 'acupoints' around the body, has long been used for pain relief. Traditional acupuncturists believe that this ancient Chinese therapy encourages the free flow of energy or 'chi' through channels known as meridians,

A sense of relief

Doctors at Guy's and St Thomas' Hospital, London, treat patients by implanting a pain-relief device that delivers mild electrical impulses into the spinal cord in response to movement. These impulses mask the sensation of pain. The motion-sensor technology is similar to that used in Nintendo Wii computer games.

kick-starting the body's own healing process. Many Western doctors, however, think the needles trigger the release of endorphins, making you feel more relaxed. Recent research conducted at the University of Rochester Medical Center in New York has suggested that acupuncture has a specific effect at the pain site by stimulating the production of adenosine, a natural painkiller.

Acupressure and shiatsu work on the same principles but use firm finger pressure instead of needles. For best results, consult a trained practitioner. Many people find these therapies effective for headaches, back pain and pain associated with osteoarthritis.

TINGLE THOSE NERVES

TENS – transcutaneous electrical nerve stimulation – involves applying a mild electrical current via a series of electrodes that you place on your skin at or near the site of the pain. You can get a TENS machine from your doctor or pain clinic, or you can buy or rent one from many pharmacies. Adjust the controls on the machine to regulate the strength of current until you feel a tingling sensation. Keep the electrodes in place for about 30–60 minutes.

TENS is thought to work in a similar way to acupuncture and acupressure, only in this case it is the mild electrical impulses that stimulate endorphins and interfere with the transmission of pain signals. It can be effective for low back pain, rheumatoid arthritis, menstrual or labour pain, pain after surgery and headaches.

THE PAIN RELIEF IMPULSE

A typical TENS kit comprises a hand-held control unit and a pair of electrodes that you place on the skin to transmit tiny electrical impulses near the site of the pain.

RUB IT BETTER

Massage is one of the oldest therapies in existence. There are various types of massage, ranging from soft and gentle to more vigorous. Your doctor or pain specialist will be able to advise you on which would be most beneficial. Massage is comforting, but it may also have a direct effect on the pain by helping to stimulate endorphins and soothing the nerves that carry pain signals to your brain.

Most masseurs use oils to lubricate the skin, usually a vegetable oil to which one or more aromatherapy essential oils are sometimes added. There is a huge choice available, but for pain and tension the following essential oils are thought to be especially helpful:

- camomile, eucalyptus and rosemary for rheumatic-type pain
- rosemary and lavender for headaches and muscular pain
- peppermint for headaches and migraine.

FEET FIRST

Foot massage has been used to relieve pain for thousands of years in civilisations on every continent, but reflexology, as it is known today, was refined by Dr William H. Fitzgerald, a US ear, nose and throat specialist and physiotherapist, in the early twentieth century. Reflexology is based on the principle that the body is divided into ten vertical zones or channels of energy running from the head to the feet. Reflexology practitioners believe that each organ, gland and part of the body is reflected in a corresponding reflex point on the foot.

Applying gentle pressure to these points is believed to remove blockages in the flow of energy to organs and tissues in a particular zone, stimulating endorphins and pain relief. Reflexologists sometimes use pressure on the hands instead of the feet. Benefits have been reported by sufferers from back pain, period pain, headaches and many other conditions, although conventional science cannot provide an explanation for its effects.

MANIPULATE IT

Osteopathy and chiropractic are both therapies that involve manipulating the spine and other joints and their surrounding soft tissues, to improve nerve function and circulation. Although their underlying philosophies differ, in practice there is little difference between the two, apart from the fact that chiropractors tend to use diagnostic techniques such as X-rays and scans. Osteopaths may use what is known as the high-velocity thrust – a short, sharp motion, used mainly on the spine, which may provide a dramatic relief of pain.

Both therapies have a good track record of relieving pain in a variety of conditions that affect the back, muscles and joints in general, as well as migraine and nerve pain. Your doctor may be able to refer you to a local practitioner, or you can find one yourself. You can find a chiropractor through the Chiropractors' Association of Australia (www.chiropractors.asn.au); to find an osteopath, go to the Australian Osteopathic Association (www.osteopathy.org.au).

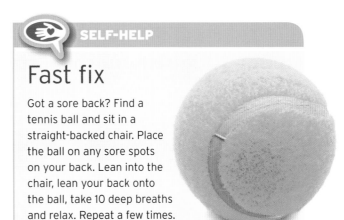

SELF-HELP

Fast fix

Got a sore back? Find a tennis ball and sit in a straight-backed chair. Place the ball on any sore spots on your back. Lean into the chair, lean your back onto the ball, take 10 deep breaths and relax. Repeat a few times.

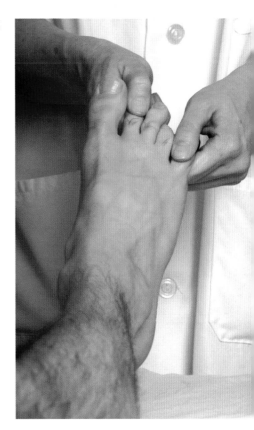

Reflexology is one of the many therapies that offer relaxation and pain relief

FOCUS

Migraine matters

Migraine is so much more than just a headache. It can affect the whole body and go on for days, as the 2 million or so migraine sufferers in Australia know only too well. Medication to prevent and treat attacks is available from your GP, but there is also plenty you can do yourself to alleviate pain.

Blurred vision, flashing lights or zigzag patterns are just some of the warning signs of an impending migraine attack. Other symptoms, known collectively as an 'aura', include confusion and pins and needles. Around 80 per cent of people with migraines, however, receive no warning at all.

During a migraine, an intense headache gradually develops on one side of the head and often becomes worse with movement. Other symptoms, often just as prominent as the headache, include nausea and/or vomiting, as well as increased sensitivity to light, sound or smell.

LOOKING FOR A CAUSE

Migraines tend to run in families, and no one knows for sure what causes an attack. Changes in brain chemistry that cause the blood vessels surrounding the brain to widen and narrow are thought to be a major factor. But exactly what prompts these changes is still under debate.

There are many triggers and these vary from person to person. Keeping a migraine diary (download one from http://headacheaustralia.org.au/headache-management/7-chronic-headache-a-migraine-diaries) can help you establish your own particular patterns or

Getting to the point

Try this acupressure move for migraine relief: press firmly on the point in the fleshy web of skin between your finger and thumb with the ball of your thumb or fingertips. Gradually increase the pressure over a couple of minutes.

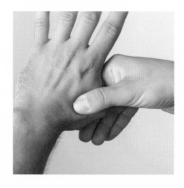

possible triggers. For every attack, note down what you ate or drank, your feelings, where you were in your menstrual cycle (if you are a woman), how well you were sleeping, the weather, skipped meals and how tired you were. If the same triggers crop up time and again, you'll know what to avoid. Common triggers include:

- red wine, cheese and chocolate
- changes in sleep patterns
- hormonal changes associated with the menstrual cycle, oral contraceptives and menopause
- stress and anxiety
- dehydration and missing meals
- environmental factors such as flashing lights, strong smells, travel and climate changes.

EASE THE PAIN

There's no magic cure for migraine but there are a variety of over-the-counter (OTC) and prescription medicines to help you manage the pain. OTC painkillers, including aspirin, ibuprofen and paracetamol, may bring relief – or you may find they don't even touch the pain. If so, your doctor may prescribe triptans – a group of medications designed specifically to cut short an attack. When taken correctly they can bring relief within 2 hours.

You need to take any medication at the first sign of a migraine, as your body systems shut down during an attack and medications are not easily absorbed.

If you have two or more migraines a month or your attacks are very severe, your doctor may prescribe other medications to help prevent them.

Don't be despondent if the first treatment option doesn't bring relief; what works for one person might not work for you. Sometimes a change of dose or medication is all that's needed, so don't hesitate to go back to your doctor.

If you're not responding to treatment, you can ask your GP to refer you to a migraine clinic for further investigation. A specialist will be able to confirm that you are having migraines, review your current treatment and suggest ways to manage your condition.

THE ALTERNATIVE ROUTE

For many people, complementary therapies can reduce the frequency or severity of migraines. Anecdotal feedback from members of Migraine Action (www.migraine.org.uk), a British research charity, shows that acupuncture, the Bowen technique (a hands-on technique that uses gentle rolling movements to loosen muscles), osteopathy, homeopathy, reflexology and chiropractic have all been found to bring benefits.

 SELF-HELP

Help yourself

Migraine Action recommends the following measures to keep migraine at bay:

● Avoid known migraine triggers.

● Keep up your fluid intake (aim for 2 litres a day), but limit your intake of caffeine and alcohol, which can be dehydrating.

● Eat regularly and avoid sugary snacks in order to keep your blood glucose stable.

● Establish regular sleep patterns.

● Take regular breaks at work, especially if you spend much of each day at a computer.

● Make time to relax and try to avoid stress.

Maintaining fluid intake is a key element of your anti-migraine plan

Finding a therapist

Some pain clinics and GP surgeries offer complementary treatments, including acupuncture and massage. If you consult a private practitioner, always check that your therapist has appropriate training and is registered with a recognised professional organisation for that therapy. Contact the professional association for your chosen therapy and ask for a list of members in your area, or ask for a referral from your doctor.

Before starting treatment, ask your doctor or health-care professional if there are any medical reasons why you should not go ahead. Then discuss with your therapist how the treatment works, what it might achieve, how long it could take and how much it will cost.

Top Tips

Write it down

To identify foods that set off your pain or make it worse, keep a food diary. Simply note down what you eat and when and any pain symptoms that follow. After a week or so you may start to see a pattern emerging, enabling you to avoid any foods that trigger pain.

Eat to beat pain

According to an Australian Government national nutrition survey, the average Australian consumes far fewer than the recommended 2 portions of fruit and 5 portions of vegetables a day (only 6 per cent of people over 19 do so). And this relatively poor diet has a part to play in the pain process. For one thing, if you're not eating fruit and vegetables, the chances are you're filling up on less healthy foods that can pile on the kilos. This in turn can put pressure on the joints, especially if you're also avoiding exercise.

But that's not all. Scientists no longer think that fat just sits around your middle doing nothing. They have now discovered that fat cells produce proteins that increase inflammation and therefore pain. And a poor diet can further exacerbate the problem. According to the latest research, the omega-6 fats found in certain vegetable oils (see below) as well as in many processed foods encourage the production of inflammatory chemicals in the body. These chemicals then mix together with the proteins produced by the fat cells in a so-called 'inflammatory soup', which excites the nerves that cause pain.

WEIGHT ATTACK

Forget diets that promise instant weight loss – they are not the answer. Choose one instead that focuses on nutrients that quell inflammation and avoids those that promote it. Here's how to get started:

Say no to 'bad' fats Steer clear of saturated fats found in animal products, omega-6 fatty acids found in corn oil, safflower, sunflower, peanut and soybean oils, and 'trans fats' – the kind of fats found in some processed foods, such as cakes and biscuits, and some vegetable oils and fats.

Say yes to 'good' fats Eat more of the anti-inflammatory monounsaturated fatty acids found in extra virgin olive oil and the omega-3 fatty acids from oily fish, fish oil, walnuts and walnut oil, linseeds and linseed oil, hempseed and hempseed oil.

Eliminate refined carbs Cut out cakes, pastries, sweets and anything else made from white flour and white sugar. These boost insulin and glucose levels, which in turn increase production of inflammation-promoting messenger chemicals.

Colourful foods can help to quell the
inflammation that leads to pain

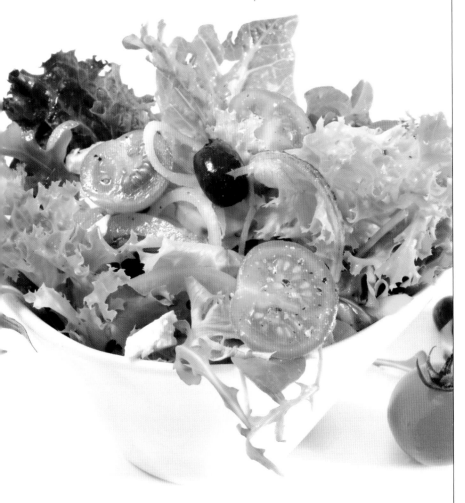

Go for colour Pile up your plate with as many differently coloured fruit
and vegetables as you can to maximise your intake of anti-inflammatory
plant chemicals such as carotenoids and flavonoids.

Spice it up Ginger, turmeric, cayenne, garlic and onions are all known
for their anti-inflammatory properties.

SUPPLEMENTARY SENSE

Many vitamin and food supplement products are advertised as having
pain-relieving properties. Treat such claims with caution. A balanced
diet provides the nutrients you need, and excessive intake of some
vitamins can cause problems.

Take care of your sex life

Perhaps you'd like to be
intimate but you're in too much
pain. Add to this the fact that
some of the medicines used
to treat pain can curb desire
and you may fear your sex life
is over for good. But sexual
intimacy is an important part
of a healthy relationship and
it might even make you feel
better. So don't give up — there
are plenty of ways to put your
sex life back on track.

✔ **Get talking** For many of us
sex can be difficult to talk
about, but talking to each
other is the best way to work
out an effective way to deal
with the problem.

✔ **Take a painkiller** Make sure
you take your painkillers
before you have sex.
However, be aware that
some painkillers can reduce
sex drive in both men and
women. Talk to your doctor,
who may be able to change
your medication.

✔ **Change positions** You
don't have to stick with the
same old routine if your
usual position is no longer
comfortable for you.

✔ **Ask the expert** Sex
therapists can often offer
helpful advice about any
problems you may be having
as a result of pain. Ask
your GP to refer you for
counselling.

Targeted pain relief for 8 common conditions

Your first reaction to pain may be to reach for a painkiller or seek medical advice, but if the pain persists, a combination of treatments and lifestyle changes often brings lasting relief.

Complementary therapies are being used more and more alongside conventional methods in hospital pain clinics – with good results. Below you'll find specific information on a range of painful everyday problems, including what to expect from your doctor, what's available on the complementary front and what you can do to help yourself. Advice on other conditions may be found elsewhere in this book. Consult the index for the relevant page number.

BACK PAIN

Ranging from a dull ache to a sudden sharp pain, low back pain affects four out of five of us at some time in our lives. Damaged discs, pressure on nerves, misalignment or inflammation of any of the 110 joints in the

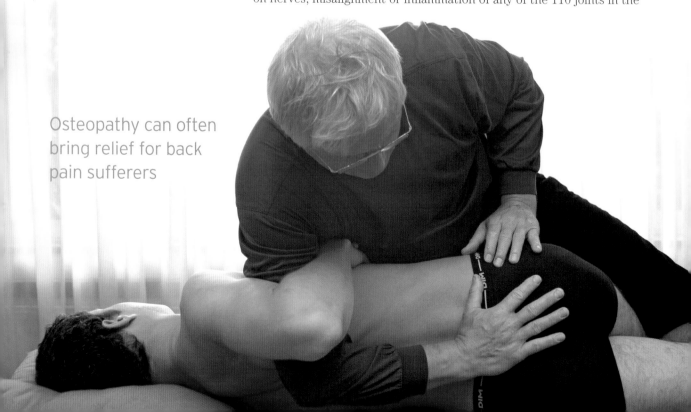

Osteopathy can often bring relief for back pain sufferers

spine, muscle spasm, damaged ligaments, injury, poor posture, wear and tear on the bones in your spine and osteoporosis are all possible causes, but in up to 85 per cent of people no cause is ever found. Advice on dealing with the immobility caused by back pain is included in *Get moving again*, pages 87–90).

Treatments that may be effective include:
Painkillers Over-the-counter medicines such as paracetamol or ibuprofen are often effective. Stronger painkillers such as codeine may be prescribed if the pain is severe. If the pain persists, antidepressants may be the answer.
Spinal manipulation and massage Your doctor may refer you for conventional physiotherapy, or may recommend that you try osteopathy or chiropractic.
TENS as described on page 228.
Yoga, Pilates and Alexander technique These exercise systems improve back strength, flexibility and posture.
Acupuncture This treatment may stimulate the release of natural chemicals that help block pain (see *Needling the pain*, page 227).
Biofeedback To help you relax (see page 224).

Help yourself:
Treat with heat or keep it cool Having a hot bath or applying a hot-water bottle or heat pack to the affected area can ease muscular pain. But in other cases the application of cold is more effective. Use a specially designed cool pack or a bag of frozen peas wrapped in a towel. See what works for you.
Weight watch Being overweight gives your body more work to do and can put pressure on your back.

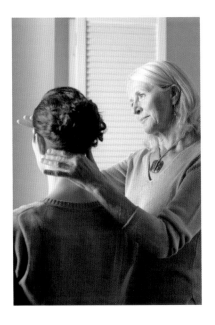

Posture correction from an Alexander technique teacher can help prevent back pain

FIBROMYALGIA
This condition causes widespread pain across the body, including your arms and legs, that lasts for three months or more. No one knows the cause, but many specialists now believe that the brain may stop interpreting pain signs properly.

Treatments that may be effective include:
Drug treatment If over-the-counter painkillers are not effective, your doctor may offer a stronger medication such as codeine. Muscle relaxants, antidepressants or anti-epileptics may be prescribed to help with muscle pain, difficulty in sleeping and anxiety.

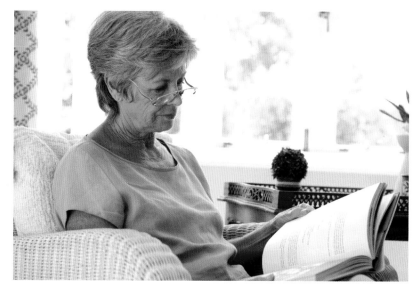

When pain affects your mobility, use the time to unwind, and perhaps relax with a good book

Physiotherapy Advice and exercise recommendations from a physiotherapist may help you to become more active. Ask your GP to refer you to a local practitioner.

Chiropractic or osteopathy These forms of manipulation may provide pain relief by helping to relax the muscles.

Help yourself:
Take exercise Walking, swimming and yoga are good choices. Aerobic exercise and strength training may also help.
Make time for relaxation Relax with a good book or DVD.

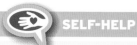
SELF-HELP

Toothache relief

Pain from a tooth can be excruciating. You'll need to see a dentist, but in the meantime try the following:

- Take an over-the-counter painkiller.

- Rub clove oil into the affected area. It contains eugenol, a natural local anaesthetic compound. Do not use this remedy if you are pregnant.

- If you have an abscess, apply a hot compress for 5 minutes every half an hour.

TENSION HEADACHE

A dull steady ache that spreads to or from the neck. It can feel as though a band is being pulled tightly around your head or a heavy weight is being pushed down on it. Stress is thought to be a major trigger. Bad posture, sitting in a draught, bright lights, too much noise or spending hours in front of a computer screen are others.

Treatments that may be effective include:
Painkillers OTC painkillers such as paracetamol, aspirin or ibuprofen may work for you. If the headache becomes chronic, your doctor may suggest an antidepressant.

Yoga and Pilates To relax muscular tension and improve posture.
Cranial osteopathy This involves gentle manipulation at the base
of the skull and top of the neck, which aims to clear tension build-up.
Acupuncture A large research review found that this could be as
effective as painkillers for tension-type headaches.

Help yourself:
Just stop If the pain persists, take some time out to relax. Get plenty
of sleep and schedule some regular 'me' time into your day.
Take a breath of fresh air Go for a walk outside to clear your head.
Keep a headache diary To pinpoint triggers. Note when the headache
occurred, what food and drink you consumed in the previous 24 hours,
your recent sleep patterns and what you were doing prior to the attack.

CYSTITIS

This condition is a urinary-tract infection (UTI) affecting the bladder that
can cause abdominal pain and discomfort when passing urine. See your
doctor, who may prescribe antibiotics (see also *UTI guidelines*, page 57).

Treatments that may be effective include:
Ibuprofen or paracetamol to reduce pain.
Potassium citrate or sodium citrate to make the urine less acidic
and therefore less painful to pass.

Help yourself:
Drink up Drinking plenty of water helps to flush out the bacteria.
It will also dilute your urine, making it less likely to cause irritation.
Hug a hottie Warmth from a hot-water bottle can be soothing.

IRRITABLE BOWEL SYNDROME (IBS)

An intermittent cramp-like abdominal pain. See *Calming an irritable
bowel*, page 55, for advice on overcoming this condition in the long
term. The following tips are for relief of discomfort.

Treatments that may be effective include:
Anti-spasmodic medications These help ease pain and bloating.
Acupuncture This may provide relief, although research findings have
been mixed according to a major review.
'Gut-directed' hypnotherapy A special sort of hypnotherapy that
teaches you how to control gut function and change the way your brain
controls gut activity.

Top Tips

Quick headache fixes

Try the following simple tips; they may be all you need to ward off a headache.

- Grasp a handful of hair at the roots and tug gently several times. Work your way round your head to release tension in your scalp.
- Apply a hot flannel to your head and neck.
- Gently massage some lavender essential oil over your temples and the back of your neck.
- Slowly sip a large glass of water to rehydrate your body and flush out any toxins that could be causing your headache.
- Soak your feet in a bowl of hot water to which you've added some mustard powder.
- Have a cup of ginger tea.

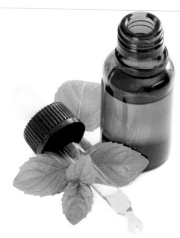

PEPPERMINT OIL

Peppermint has a relaxing effect on the muscles of the digestive tract. It can be taken as capsules or you can add a few drops of peppermint essential oil to massage oil and gently rub this into the abdomen.

Help yourself:

Cut out wheat fibre Research now shows that insoluble fibre or bran – the type of fibre found in foods such as wholemeal bread – may actually worsen bloating and pain. Instead, increase the bulk in your diet by eating a higher proportion of legumes, fruit and vegetables, which provide soluble fibre.

Keep a food diary To help you pinpoint problem foods.

MENSTRUAL PAIN

Pain or cramps in the lower abdomen just before or during a period. A build-up of hormones known as prostaglandins, which cause the muscles of the uterus (womb) to contract, is thought to be the cause.

Treatments that may be effective include:

Painkillers Over-the-counter medications, such as mefenamic acid (Ponstan), are usually sufficient. If these do not give adequate relief, a stronger medication, such as Panadeine Forte, may be prescribed.

Hormonal help If you are not trying to get pregnant, your doctor may suggest you try the combined contraceptive pill.

TENS Use of this device (see page 228) may relieve symptoms.

Acupuncture, acupressure, spinal manipulation and herbal remedies These may help to relieve pain, but the evidence for their benefits is limited.

Help yourself:

Exercise gently Try activities such as swimming, cycling or walking.

Massage Use light circular movements around your lower abdomen.

NERVE PAIN

Nerve pain (neuropathy) is often due to a trapped, damaged or pinched nerve. It can be also be caused by conditions such as shingles, diabetes or surgery. Shooting or burning pain and tingling or numbness on being touched may be symptoms of neuropathy.

Treatments that may be effective include:

Drug treatment Your doctor may prescribe antidepressants, anti-epileptics or opioid painkillers, depending on the type of pain.

 NURSING KNOW-HOW

Warm it

The application of heat to the affected area by means of a hot-water bottle is a simple but effective way of providing relief from pain resulting from muscle cramps – for example, menstrual pain, irritable bowel or back pain.

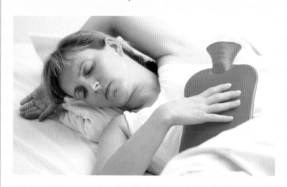

Acupuncture This seems to help some people with nerve pain.
Relaxation training and biofeedback According to research, these therapies can sometimes be useful in mild cases.

Help yourself:
Watch your glucose levels High blood glucose levels are linked with nerve pain in people with diabetes, so careful control of your blood glucose plays a part in pain control if you are a diabetic. Always talk to your doctor about this type of pain.
Try B vitamins There is evidence that taking these (often called the nerve vitamins) can help, especially if the nerve pain is linked to a medical condition such as diabetes.

PEPTIC ULCER
In this condition an open sore develops in the lining of the stomach (a gastric ulcer) or the small intestine (a duodenal ulcer). Doctors now regard damage caused by the presence of a type of bacteria, *Helicobacter pylori* (*H. pylori*), as the main cause. Long-term use of non-steroidal anti-inflammatory drugs (NSAIDs) such as aspirin and ibuprofen – for example, to control the pain of arthritis – is the second most common cause of peptic ulcers. The main symptom is a recurrent gnawing pain in the centre of the abdomen.

Treatments that may be effective include:
Antibiotics If *H. pylori* is causing your ulcer, tackling the infection can allow the ulcer to heal, bringing relief of pain.
Proton pump inhibitors A course of medications that reduce the amount of acid made by your stomach, such as omeprazole and lansoprazole, often provides effective relief in the long term.

Help yourself:
Keep it plain Avoid spicy foods and alcohol, which can trigger or worsen symptoms.
Stub out now Tobacco increases production of stomach acid, so if you smoke, give it up.
Juice it Try aloe vera juice (available in health-food shops). Some people think it helps to quell inflammation and reduce stomach-acid secretion.
Go herbal Cut back on coffee and tea, which can increase production of stomach acid. Drink herbal teas such as camomile or fennel instead.

On the horizon
Scientists are assessing the value of a new therapy, transcranial magnetic stimulation (TMS), for neuropathic pain. This involves placing a small coil over the scalp. A rapidly alternating current is then applied through the coil, producing a magnetic field that passes through the brain. Results are promising, but more research is needed to refine the treatment.

ALOE VERA
Although scientific evidence is inconclusive, drinking the juice extracted from this desert plant is claimed to be of great benefit in promoting healing in a wide variety of digestive ailments, from peptic ulcers to IBS.

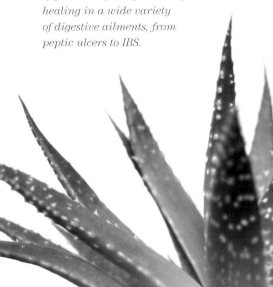

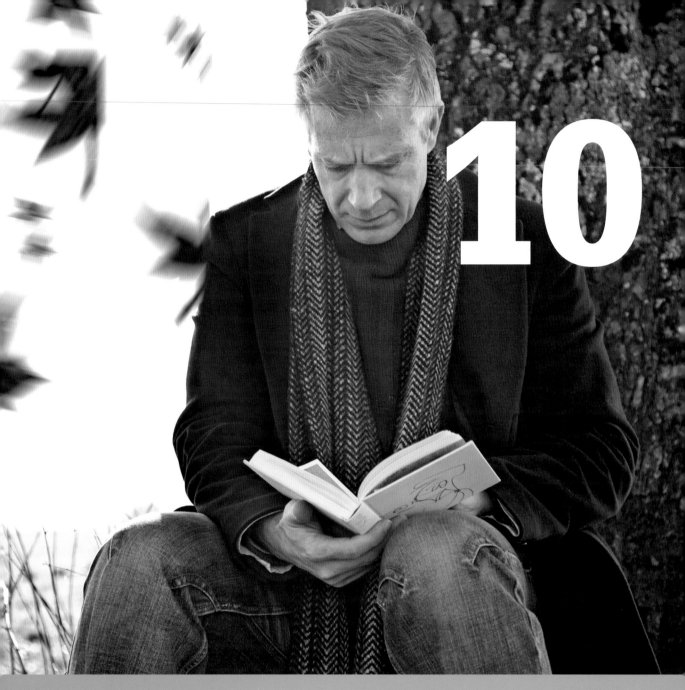

10

Overcoming mental health problems

With the right support, you can look forward to resuming a full life, often with added insight and a sense of purpose

A wide range of disorders

Mental distress can manifest itself in many ways and ranges from mild to disabling. It may affect the way you think, feel or behave and can have a knock-on effect on your work, relationships and quality of life. In more severe cases you may lose touch with reality and be unable to function in everyday life.

According to statistics, anxiety and depression are the most common mental health disorders and this chapter focuses mainly on recovery from these problems. Less common disorders, such as schizophrenia and bipolar disorder, are often lifelong problems that need continuing expert psychiatric care.

Despite being so common, mental health problems are still regarded with prejudice and stigma. This makes it difficult to admit that something is wrong. It is important to recognise it is not your fault or a sign of weakness. There is nothing to be ashamed of or feel guilty about. And with support and understanding – and treatment if necessary – it is possible to recover. The huge advances made in furthering our understanding of mental illness over the past 20 years, and new treatments – both medical and psychological – are enabling more and more people to regain control of their lives.

Seeking help is often the first step to recovery

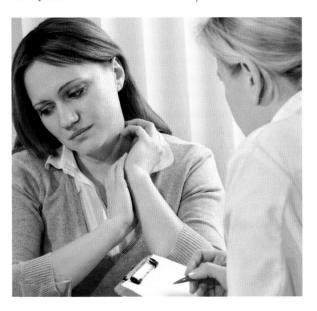

The first steps to recovery

If you or someone you care about has mental health problems, recognising and accepting the illness is the first step to recovery. This can be a hard step to take, but there is plenty of support available. For many people, talking therapies are the way forward. For others, medication may be part of the recovery process. But neither of these alone is enough – the key is a commitment to recovery. This will demand courage, strength and belief that it is possible.

Recovery is usually more successful if it is a collaborative project. Family, friends, medical or social care professionals and voluntary supporters all have a part to play. Don't keep your concerns to yourself. Make an appointment with your GP and he or she will assess your needs and make a treatment plan. This may include self-help advice and

Questions to ask

Here are some questions you may like to ask your doctor:

- *Why am I suffering mental distress and can it be treated?*
- *What kind of health professional is best qualified to help me?*
- *What are my treatment options?*
- *What can treatment offer? Will there be any side effects?*
- *What's the name of the problem I'm suffering from?*
- *Where could I find more info about my disorder?*
- *How common is my problem?*
- *What can I do to help myself?*
- *When will I start to feel better?*
- *Will I need treatment for the rest of my life?*
- *What will happen if I don't get treatment?*

information, medication and/or counselling. You may be referred to specialist services, such as a psychiatrist.

BE PREPARED

Prepare yourself for your visit to the doctor by writing some notes to take with you. Things to ask might include:

Your symptoms Note down your symptoms, when they occur and anything that makes them better or worse. Also record their effect on everyday activities such as work, school or relationships.

Recent life changes or stressful events Include events such as relationship breakdown, job loss, birth of a baby, bereavement as well as traumatic experiences you've had in the past or as a child.

Other health problems Include physical conditions and other mental health problems.

Medications Give details of any prescribed and over-the-counter medications you're taking, and be sure to include herbal or nutritional supplements. You may also be asked about your use of alcohol and recreational drugs.

LOOK AFTER YOURSELF

If you're battling with mental distress, just getting through the day can seem like an uphill journey. It can be hard even to think about starting medication, going to weekly therapy, eating a healthier diet, exercising, sleeping 8 hours a night or enjoying any of the life-enhancing activities that you suspect may be good for you in the long term, such as enrolling in a yoga class or joining a support group.

Often when struggling with mental difficulties, you feel quite incapable of facing problems and understandably try to avoid the big issues in your life. To make these seem less daunting, start by considering a few lifestyle changes that could help you feel better, then break them up into small, manageable steps. For example, to get more exercise, go for a daily walk rather than joining a gym; to eat more healthily, choose a small bunch of grapes instead of a chocolate bar; to sleep better, establish a regular going-to-bed and getting-up time. Poor health and lack of sleep can contribute to mental problems, and good food and physical activity improve mental wellbeing (see *Eat to boost your mood*, page 258, and *Exercise to keep your spirits high*, page 260). Soon these small lifestyle changes will bring big benefits and give you the confidence to do more.

HEALTHY RELATIONS

There is increasing evidence that compassion and kindness can be an antidote to mental distress and are an integral part of recovery. Close relationships with others play a major role in mental health and wellbeing, providing a buffer against the challenges of life. And talking about your problems with someone close to you is a good way to put them in perspective. Being kind to yourself is also important, and involves understanding that negative emotions such as anger, shame and fear are linked to mental distress, and addressing those feelings in a kind and uncritical manner. Research shows that the way people relate to themselves can influence their ability to get through life's difficulties.

What is good mental health?

Good mental health enables people to deal with adversity and the challenges of day-to-day problems, get on with others and have confidence and self-esteem, all of which contribute to a balanced, healthy life. To stay healthy, experts on depression at beyondblue recommend that you:

- Learn new ways to reduce and manage stress and cope with setbacks.
- Eat healthily.
- Get enough sleep.
- Get active.
- Avoid harmful levels of alcohol and other drugs.

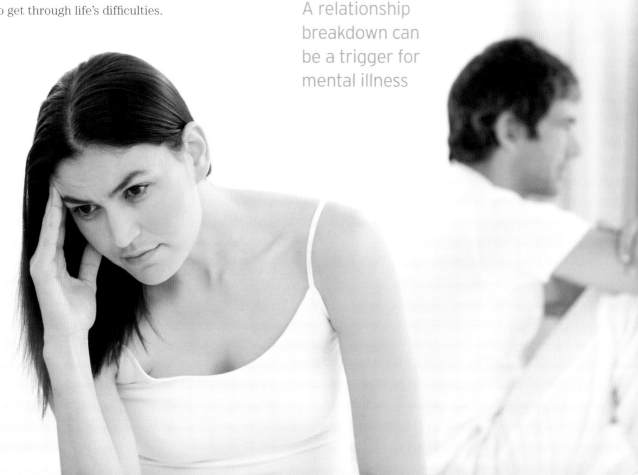

A relationship breakdown can be a trigger for mental illness

Coping with depression

One in five Australians experiences a mental illness in any year, the most common being depression, anxiety and substance use disorder. Professional help can often enable them to conquer the problem.

Am I depressed?

If at least five of the following apply to you almost every day over a two-week period, you may be depressed:

☐ Are unhappy most of the time

☐ Have no interest in life and can't enjoy anything

☐ Find it hard to make decisions

☐ Can't cope with things that you used to

☐ Feel utterly tired, restless and/or agitated

☐ Have poor appetite

☐ Take 1 to 2 hours to go to sleep then wake up earlier than usual

☐ Have little interest in sex

☐ Have lost self-confidence

☐ Feel useless and hopeless

☐ Avoid other people

☐ Feel irritable

☐ Feel worse in the morning

☐ Think of suicide.

WHAT IS DEPRESSION?

Depression is a much-misused word. You may think you're depressed when you feel miserable – for example, if you don't get a job you want, if someone lets you down or if you start to put on weight. True depression is much more severe and long-lasting than a passing feeling of being 'down' (see *Am I depressed?*, left). In extreme cases, a depressed person may decide life is not worth living and may start to self-harm or even attempt suicide. Sometimes these feelings persist for months or even years.

THE REASONS WHY

Depression varies from person to person and a combination of different factors may contribute to its development. A stressful situation such as job loss, the death of someone close or an unhappy relationship are common triggers. Women are more prone to depression than men and it can run in families. Research shows that if you have one parent who has become severely depressed, you are eight times more likely to become depressed yourself.

Scientists have also discovered changes in brain chemicals and the levels of some hormones in people with depression. It seems that three important neurotransmitters (chemicals that carry messages between brain cells), dopamine, serotonin and noradrenaline, may be in short supply. This leads to faulty communication between brain cells, which could be a cause of depression. Whatever is contributing to your illness, your doctor should be able to direct you towards the appropriate help.

TYPES OF DEPRESSION

Mental health professionals recognise different degrees of disability, which are referred to as:

Mild Depression with a negative but limited effect on daily life. Symptoms include difficulty in concentrating and/or lack of motivation.

It's possible to recover from this type of depression with self-help measures and support from your doctor and others, such as your friends and family.

Moderate Depression that has a more sustained effect on what a person can do. Symptoms include feeling low most of the time and difficulty functioning at home and at work. You're likely to need treatment from your doctor to help you get through this, but self-help measures are also key to a rapid recovery.

Severe Sometimes known as clinical or major depression, this is a serious mental illness. Symptoms include difficulty in coping with day-to-day living – eating, sleeping and many other routine activities become impossible tasks. There is a high risk of suicide. Recovery from severe depression in most cases requires long-term treatment (medication and talking therapies) under the care of a specialist. But positive changes that you can make to your diet and exercise habits can be of huge benefit after other treatments have begun to take effect.

Postnatal blues

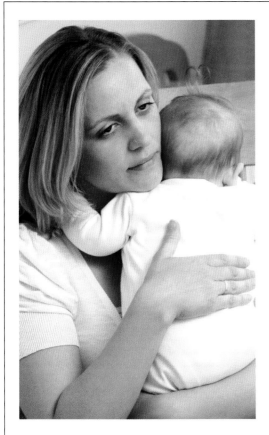

Postnatal depression (PND) occurs within a year of having a baby and affects around 10–15 per cent of new mothers. Most new mothers experience a short bout of 'baby blues' a few days after giving birth, which is the result of hormonal changes and usually passes after 10 to 14 days but sometimes lasts longer. PND by contrast may develop weeks or months after the birth.

If you think you may have PND, it is vital to seek help as, left untreated, the condition can adversely affect your relationship with your baby and partner. Your doctor can refer you to a counsellor trained in treating PND. Specific treatments may include cognitive behavioural therapy and/or medication as for other types of depression. If drug treatment is being considered, there is no need to worry that this may mean that you have to give up breastfeeding; there are several antidepressants that do not affect your baby.

While professional help is essential, there is plenty you can do to boost your own spirits and sense of wellbeing. Follow the advice elsewhere in this chapter about eating a nutritious diet and getting enough exercise, especially outside (see pages 258–261). It is particularly important for new mothers to get enough sleep. Talk to your partner about sharing the responsibility for night-time feeds. If necessary, you could express breast milk so that you can regularly have a 'night off'.

Alcohol alert

However tempted you may be, do not use alcohol to drown your sorrows. Here's why:

- Alcohol may dull your feelings in the short term, but the effects will soon wear off, leaving you feeling worse than before.

- Drinking can stop you dealing with important problems and getting the right help.

- It is easy to slip into the habit of using alcohol as a form of self-medication, which can lead to serious health problems.

- Alcohol may interfere with the helpful effects of some antidepressant medications.

- Drinking too much may also interfere with other important aspects of your life, such as work and relationships.

More specific types of depression include:

Bipolar disorder (previously known as manic depression) Characterised by mood swings between severe highs (mania) and lows (depression). Medication is usually needed in such cases.

Psychotic depression A form of severe depression requiring drug treatment, in which sufferers may experience hallucinations or delusions in addition to feelings of depression.

Postnatal depression Depression after giving birth (see page 245).

Seasonal affective disorder (SAD) Linked to lack of sunlight during the winter months. Symptoms include tiredness and lethargy and a craving for carbohydrates. Bright light therapy, antidepressants and cognitive behavioural therapy (CBT) are common treatments. For more information, visit the website of beyondblue (www.beyondblue.org.au).

Getting help

Don't suffer in silence; share your feelings with family, friends or a health-care professional. The right support and treatment can help to stop depression taking over your life.

TREATMENT FROM YOUR DOCTOR

Depending on the symptoms and their severity, the doctor may suggest self-help, medication to relieve symptoms (pages 256–257) and talking therapies (pages 252–253) to help you learn how to deal with your thoughts and feelings. Try to remember the following:

- Many people have depression and recover completely.
- You may come out of depression as a different and stronger person.
- Depression can help you see life and relationships more clearly.

HELPING YOURSELF

For mild depression, try to follow the advice on diet and exercise given later in this chapter – it is often very helpful. Guided self-help plans are available from the doctor. These may include computer-led programs that you follow by yourself or with the help of a therapist over the phone. If you are severely depressed, the GP or a specialist in mental distress will draw up a plan that includes self-help measures. Here are some self-help ideas:

Be aware of your thoughts Stand back and try to observe what's going through your head. This will allow you to spot unhelpful patterns of thinking that may be causing you to feel depressed. Don't force yourself to change them, just be aware and see what happens.

Stay in contact Talking things through with a friend or family member can help to lessen the burden of your thoughts. Sometimes they may help you to find a solution.

Join a group People who are experiencing similar problems can provide great support. Your GP should have a list of what is available in your area.

Look after yourself Pay attention to simple physical needs such as eating, sleeping and exercise, which can all help to alleviate mild to moderate depression (see page 244).

Do what you enjoy Make a big effort to do what you like doing. Buy yourself something new, listen to music, watch a movie, have a massage.

Try something new A new hobby or activity or an evening class will get you out of the house. How about joining a book club, a knitting circle or having a go at the local pub quiz? Social activities such as these can help to break the vicious circle of loneliness and spending too much time with your own thoughts.

Get active Attempt to keep yourself busy with everyday activities. If it helps, you can break these down into a series of smaller tasks. So rather than tidying up your house, you could start by clearing a desk or table, and build up from there. Completing tasks can give you a positive sense of achievement.

Think alternative Many people find complementary therapies helpful. Some, such as massage, use physical touch to help you feel better emotionally, while others, such as meditation, can help to calm you.

Put it on paper Writing down your thoughts and feelings can help prevent half-formed but emotionally powerful thoughts from getting out of proportion in your mind. The physical process of writing may help to distance you from your thoughts so you can examine them in a more detached way.

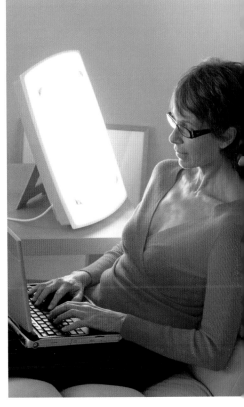

SHED SOME LIGHT ON IT

Seasonal affective disorder (SAD) is a form of depression closely related to low levels of light. Spending time outdoors in the direct sunlight during the winter months, especially in the morning, can help to reduce the symptoms of SAD. Another form of treatment is to expose yourself to bright light from a specially designed unit for several hours a day during the winter months. These can be purchased online from suppliers such as http://sleepequip. com.au/light-therapy.html.

HELPING SOMEONE ELSE

If someone you care about is depressed, you have a responsibility to watch out for him or her. Here are some guidelines:

- Listen, but be prepared to hear the same thing over and over again.
- Be careful how you offer advice; do it gently and with empathy.
- Spend as much time as you can with your friend. Encourage him or her to talk and carry on doing normal everyday things.
- Give reassurance that he or she will get better.
- Check that your friend's food cupboards are well stocked and that he or she is eating properly.
- Take seriously any talk of not wanting to live or hints of self-harming.

Dispelling anxiety

Anxiety ranges from a feeling of general unease to a serious problem that stops you from living life to the full. Fourteen per cent of Australians experience anxiety in any given year. A range of therapies can help to combat and control various aspects of this condition.

WHAT IS ANXIETY?

Feelings of unease or even fear are a normal response to challenging situations, such as a driving test, exams, financial worries or a visit to the doctor. Scientists say that anxiety evolved to help us cope with threats, forming part of the fight-or-flight response that prepared prehistoric human beings to face or run away from danger by triggering physiological changes.

Normally, when the immediate challenge has passed, the anxiety eases. However, anxiety that persists or occurs with no obvious cause can interfere with everyday activities. You may start to avoid situations that make you anxious.

If you have severe anxiety, life can become difficult. You may feel low, tired and irritable and find it hard to concentrate; you may also have physical symptoms such as sweating, palpitations (the heart beating faster than normal), trembling, dizziness and feeling faint. You may have panic attacks or a persistent non-specific sense of apprehension. The tendency to anxiety may be genetic, but major upsets, day-to-day worries and an unhappy childhood can also play a part. An imbalance in the chemicals in the brain may be another factor. Overactivity of the thyroid gland can lead to feelings of anxiety. This is treated with medication and/or surgery.

TYPES OF ANXIETY

There are different types of anxiety that can affect your life. The most common types include:

Generalised anxiety disorder (GAD) A general feeling of anxiety for most of the time. Symptoms include constantly thinking things are going to go wrong, and feeling tense and nervous without knowing why.

NURSING KNOW-HOW

Panic attacks and hyperventilation

If you start to have a panic attack or are hyperventilating, depending on where you are at the time, try one of the following methods to make you feel better:

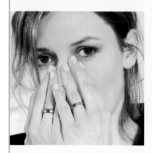

● Cup your hands over your nose and mouth for about 10 minutes, while breathing in and out as normal. This helps to raise the level of carbon dioxide in the bloodstream, which can help to relieve symptoms.

● Run on the spot.

● Distract yourself by switching your focus onto what is going on around you.

Phobia An intense irrational fear of something or a situation that actually poses little or no threat and which most people do not find frightening. Common phobias include: agoraphobia (a fear of public places, from where you feel there is no quick escape, such as crowds, queues, buses and trains); claustrophobia (fear of confined spaces); social phobia (an intense and persistent fear of being watched and judged by others in social situations); and specific phobias – for example, fear of spiders, flying or heights.

Obsessive compulsive disorder (OCD) Obsessive thoughts that lead to compulsive behaviour, such as continual washing of hands.

Panic attacks Sudden attacks of extreme anxiety that occur without warning and for no apparent reason. Typical symptoms include palpitations, sweatiness, faintness or dizziness.

Post traumatic stress disorder (PTSD) A stress reaction that usually occurs after a traumatic event, such as a road accident or a major disaster. Symptoms include re-living the experience in your head, dreaming about it and getting upset in similar situations.

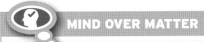

MIND OVER MATTER

Sing yourself happy

Singing familiar songs in a group can have a remarkable effect on the way you feel. For people with mild or moderate mental problems, the value of singing is undisputed. It can improve your self-esteem and confidence, reduce stress and lighten mood, it allows communication and sociability, and makes you feel part of something. Other benefits include improved breathing, better memory, feeling more alert and being generally more positive.

If this kind of activity appeals to you, see if there is a community choir in your neighbourhood – you don't necessarily need to have a great voice or musical training. Alternatively, look into the possibility of taking singing lessons.

Breaking the cycle

It is better to seek help sooner rather than later. Left untreated, anxiety can seriously disrupt your life. For example, it may prevent you from getting or holding down a job, or cause you problems in making friends or even in leaving the house and going to the shops.

Make an appointment with your doctor if:

- You feel anxious most of the time.
- Your anxiety is starting to affect your work, interests and relationships.
- You have an intense fear, compulsion, sense of panic or stress that won't go away.

WHAT WILL YOUR DOCTOR DO?

If your doctor decides you have an anxiety disorder, you will be given various treatment options, depending on your specific symptoms. For generalised anxiety disorder, treatment usually involves medication

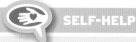

SELF-HELP

Breathe ...
your troubles away

Try this quick and simple exercise if you start to feel tense and anxious. Keep your breathing smooth and regular throughout:

1 Sit or lie in a comfortable position with your arms and legs uncrossed and your spine straight.

2 Breathing from your abdomen, inhale through your nose slowly, to a count of five.

3 Pause and hold your breath for a count of five.

4 Exhale through your mouth or nose to a count of five

5 When you have exhaled completely, take two breaths in your normal rhythm then repeat steps 2 to 4.

Repeat the exercise for at least 3 to 5 minutes.

(pages 256–257) and talking treatments (pages 252–253). In some instances, your GP may refer you for specialist help. This could be through a local therapist, using a Mental Health Care Plan, or through your local hospital's psychiatry department.

HOW TO HELP YOURSELF

There's a lot you can do to help keep your anxiety under control. It may be some time before you start to feel better, but facing up to anxiety and thinking about how your thoughts make you feel and behave can be the first step to breaking the cycle of fear and insecurity. Here are some ways to help yourself:

Join a group Support groups often involve face-to-face meetings where you can talk about your difficulties and problems, and develop coping strategies together. Many support groups also provide guidance over the phone. Ask your GP about support groups in your area.

Talk about it It can help to share how you are feeling with family and friends. You may find that they have been through something similar.

Read about it Some people find that reading about anxiety can help them deal with it. There are many books and articles based on the principles of cognitive behavioural therapy (CBT).

Write it down Making a note of any negative thoughts and the feelings and behaviour they trigger can help you to become more aware of what might be setting off your anxiety. Being able to identify triggers, and therefore make changes, can help to reduce the impact of your fears.

Refocus Distracting yourself by paying attention to what is going on around you can be an effective coping strategy. For example, if walking down a crowded street or sitting in a packed train makes you anxious, try looking for certain objects in shop windows or the passing countryside.

Relax Physical relaxation allows your mind to relax and let go of what is troubling it. Choose a quiet time of day and a place where you won't be disturbed. Sit or lie down and consciously work your way up from your toes to your head, first tensing then relaxing each group of muscles. Activities such as yoga or Pilates can also help you unwind.

Face it It can seem like the last thing you want to do, but there is evidence to show that if you expose yourself to the situation or thing

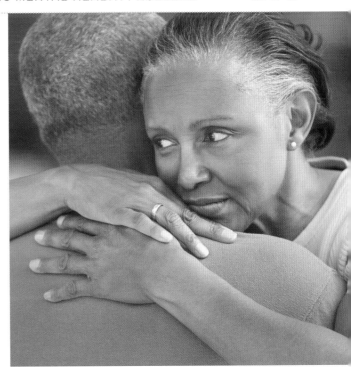

you fear in small doses, however scary that may feel, your fear will gradually reduce. Exposure therapy sessions are available for many of the more common phobias, such as fear of flying or of certain animals. Ask your doctor for advice on what's available locally.

Be alternative Yoga, meditation, aromatherapy, massage, reflexology and herbalism are just some of the complementary therapies that may help you relax, sleep better and deal with anxiety.

Stay in touch Don't let worries isolate you from loved ones or enjoyable activities. Social interaction and caring relationships can help to keep your worries in the background rather than letting them dominate your thoughts.

Record it Keep an anxiety diary. Rank your anxiety on a 1–10 scale. Note the event during which you felt anxious. Jot down any feelings or thoughts you had just before you got anxious. Keep track of things that make you more or less anxious.

Stay positive Try to replace 'negative self-talk' with 'coping self-talk'. When you catch yourself thinking something negative such as, 'I can't do this, it's just too hard', try changing it to a more positive thought, such as, 'This is hard, but I can get through it'.

Look after yourself Eat healthily, get regular exercise and try to keep a regular sleep pattern. Avoid alcohol and recreational drugs.

Physical reassurance can sometimes be more effective than wise words of comfort

HELPING AN ANXIOUS PERSON

Think about how you feel when you're anxious. This can help you to understand a friend or family member who is going through a similar experience. Here are some ideas to help an anxious person:

Balance it Be there, but don't be overprotective. This will help your friend to build up self-confidence and feel in control.

Strike a bargain If your friend agrees to go to a relaxation class, for example, you could arrange to take him or her there and then meet up again afterwards.

Reassurance Make it clear that you understand the person's distress and that it is all right to cry or to show emotions such as anger.

Be physical Physical closeness such as a touch or a hug can be comforting when a person is in distress. A gentle neck or shoulder massage may also be reassuring. Bear in mind, however, that not everyone responds positively to touch.

Your road to recovery

Recovery from most mental health problems comes about as a result of a mixture of professional help and self-help through lifestyle changes. Working closely with your doctor or counsellor to find the right strategy for you is usually the key to success.

Talking therapies

Counselling and psychotherapy can help people to understand the factors that may underlie anxiety and depression. Working with a therapist can enable you to develop coping strategies and ways of interpreting feelings to make them more bearable.

Your doctor will be able to advise you on the various options for talking therapy for a range of mental health problems including anxiety, depression and schizophrenia, available in groups or one-to-one sessions. Painful experiences can be hard to talk about, but professionals understand this. Be as open as you can so that you can receive the best help.

Learning that others share similar feelings is a valuable aspect of group therapy

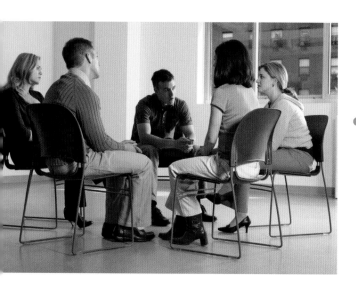

- Cognitive behavioural therapy (CBT) works by helping you to identify unhelpful and unrealistic thoughts and shows you how these can lead to problematic emotional and behavioural patterns. Once identified, you can learn to replace unhelpful thoughts with more realistic and balanced ones. This can help you react more positively to situations that may cause anxiety and depression. Treatment usually involves a 1 to 2 hour session, once a week. If you are eligible for a Mental Health Care Plan, Medicare will help pay the cost of therapy. CBT may be delivered as individual or group therapy.
- Computer cognitive behavioural therapy (CCBT) is a form of counselling that is appropriate for the treatment of mild-to-moderate depression. There are now a number of interactive CBT programs that can be used at home. A popular one is called 'Beating the Blues' (www.beatingtheblues.co.uk), usually available free through your GP. FearFighter is a program for panic or phobia (www.fearfighter.com) that is also available through your GP.

- Psychotherapy looks into past experiences to find their relevance to present difficulties. Different forms of psychotherapy include interpersonal therapy (IPT), which focuses on relationship and communication problems; family therapy, in which the therapist works with the whole family; and couples therapy, which involves both partners.

FINDING SOMEONE TO HELP

Ask your GP if the practice provides any mental health services directly. If not, ask to be referred to a therapist. You could also look at registers of practitioners at your local library or on the internet. Being on a register does not ensure quality, but it does mean that if you have a problem, you can take the matter up with the organisation. Registered psychologists can be found through the Australian Psychological Society (www.psychology.org.au/ FindaPsychologist). And if you know someone who has seen a therapist, ask for a recommendation.

Online CBT programs include THIS WAY UP (https://thiswayup.org.au), Mood GYM (https:// moodgym.anu.edu.au/welcome), and eCentreClinic (www.ecentreclinic.org).

WHAT HAPPENS NEXT?

It may be worth seeing several people before you choose a therapist. The key question to ask yourself is, 'Do I trust this person and can I communicate with him (or her)?' Ask the therapist the following:

- Could you explain what type of talking treatment you provide and how do you think it could help me?
- What are your qualifications?
- How much do you charge?

Who's who in mental health?

GP Many mental health problems are dealt with by family doctors. If specialised help is needed, your GP can refer you to a mental health professional.

Mental health nurse Mental health nurses have had postgraduate training in mental health and deliver a wide range of care, from giving medications, to assessing the needs of acutely unwell people, to empowering patients to care for themselves. Nurses often act as 'case managers' for people with complex mental health needs, coordinating their care.

Counsellor A counsellor does not have to be a psychologist; the type of training they have undergone (and how much and what quality) varies widely. They usually provide a service by being good listeners.

Psychologist Psychologists have had extensive university training and can offer a range of psychotherapies, such as cognitive behavioural therapy.

Clinical psychologist These are psychologists who have undergone more extensive postgraduate training.

Social worker Like nurses, social workers can do a number of different jobs. This may include providing psychotherapies, such as cognitive behavioural therapy, or assisting people with everyday activities, such as managing their money. They may also be case managers.

Dealing with eating disorders

FOCUS

If you or someone you love has an eating disorder, it should be confronted and resolved. There is plenty of help available, even though it can sometimes be difficult to know who to turn to.

At least nine per cent of Australians are believed to have a serious eating disorder such as anorexia, bulimia and binge eating, and it's thought many more may be suffering in silence. Eating disorders can seriously affect physical and emotional health and can be fatal if left untreated. But recovery is possible if you pluck up the courage to take the first step.

'Many young people phone our helpline and say they fear something is wrong but they don't want to worry their families … by seeking support, sufferers can be helped to live a normal, healthy life,' says Emma Healey of Beating Eating Disorders, UK (www.b-eat.co.uk).

A QUESTION OF CONTROL

A person with an eating disorder has distorted thoughts about food and his or her weight, size and shape, and becomes obsessed with food and eating, while at the same time often feeling out of control.

Eating disorders can affect both males and females at any age, but young women aged 15–25 are especially at risk. Experts believe the disorders are a symptom of inner emotional pain – for example, feelings of helplessness, sadness and anxiety. Abnormal eating behaviour becomes an (inappropriate) way of taking control, and is often linked to feelings of perfectionism, shame or self-dislike.

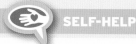

SELF-HELP

If you think you have an eating disorder ...

There are different routes to recovery but the first step is to get information and to trust others to help. Here are some tips to start with:

✔ Accept you have a problem and seek professional help. The first step could be to talk to someone you know who cares about you or make an appointment with your GP.

✔ Try to work out what the eating disorder is telling you. Is it disguising your feelings over a difficult relationship, a divorce or events in your past that have affected how you feel about yourself?

✔ Challenge your thoughts. Recognise that although you see yourself as overweight, others do not. They like and accept you for who you are, not what you weigh.

✔ Develop a healthy, varied pattern of eating. A dietitian can help you work out a balanced diet.

✔ Accept and respect your body. No matter what your shape or size, learn to value yourself and try to be aware that your body is not the same as your identity.

For more information, contact the Butterfly Foundation (http://thebutterflyfoundation.org.au).

In anorexia, sufferers are often in a deep state of denial about the weight they have lost, says Janet Treasure, Director of the Maudsley Hospital's Eating Disorder Unit, London. 'Sufferers become so afraid of gaining even half a kilogram that they are terrified of seeking treatment. But left untreated, anorexia can dominate their lives indefinitely and can be fatal.'

Bulimia, which can occur on its own but often precedes or follows anorexia, may go unnoticed as people with it maintain a normal or near normal weight – bingeing uncontrollably and then inducing vomiting, using laxatives, diuretics or other medication, fasting or exercising excessively.

There are also a host of less well-known eating disorders. The most common is binge eating disorder (BED), which involves eating uncomfortably large amounts of food without attempting to rid the body of it afterwards. Sufferers often get caught in a cycle of bingeing, guilt and restraint followed by more bingeing.

HELPING SOMEONE ELSE

If someone you love develops an eating disorder, it's important not to ignore it.

Broach it Let the person know that you are concerned about their eating and health but be prepared for them to deny they have a problem.

Don't nag Never try to persuade the person to put on or shed weight.

Encourage the acceptance of professional help
If the person refuses to get help, you may need to alert the professionals yourself.

Encourage with support and praise Phrases such as: 'You can do it' or 'You are doing really well' help show that you understand and are supportive of the effort involved.

Look after yourself Don't let the eating disorder take over your life too. Recognise your own limits and make sure you make time to do things that you like to do.

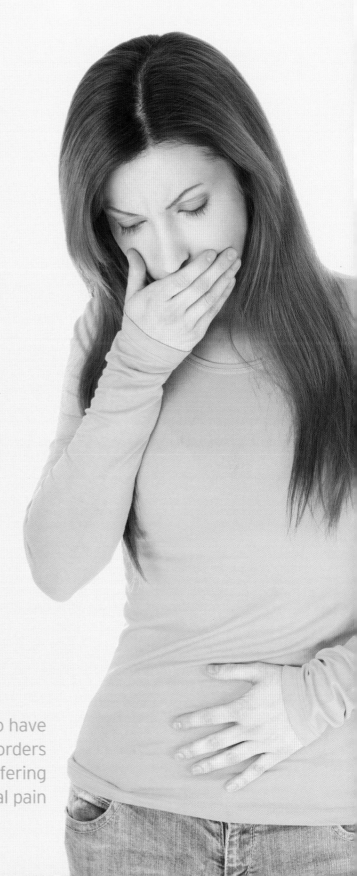

People who have eating disorders are often suffering emotional pain

Using medication

Prescribed medications can be an important part of your recovery process, particularly if your mental health problems are severe or long term. There are many medications available and it can take a while for your doctor to find the right one for you. You'll need to be patient because it may also take time for the benefits to be felt. For example, antidepressants take at least two weeks to start working and up to six weeks to be fully effective, though you may feel less anxious and be able to sleep better after only a few days. It is very important to continue a prescribed dose, and you should on no account stop taking the medication because you feel better. This is a sign that the medication is working and stopping it may cause a relapse. If you are worried about how a medication is making you feel or think, go to your doctor or hospital as soon as you can. You may also find it helpful to talk to a friend or family member about your medication so that they can alert you to any changes in your behaviour. For further information on medications, see *Get the most from your medicine,* pages 312–339.

see *Get the most from your medicine,* pages 312–339.

> ## ! ALERT
>
> ### Be alert
> Some medications for mental problems can cause drowsiness. Beware of driving or operating machinery until you know how your medication affects you.

Use with caution

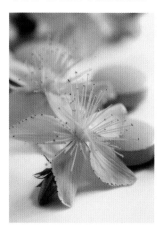

Sometimes known as the sunshine herb, St John's wort (its botanical name is *Hypericum perforatum*) is a yellow flower that was first used by the Ancient Greeks to relieve anxiety and depression. Several research studies have found it helpful in the treatment of depression. However, it has a potential for interaction with a number of medicines, including prescribed antidepressants and several drugs used in the treatment of disorders of the heart and circulation. It should also be avoided by women who are pregnant or breastfeeding. This herb should be taken only after consultation with your doctor.

ANTIDEPRESSANTS

There are four main types of antidepressant medication that your doctor may prescribe. Each type is used for different forms and degrees of severity of depression:

Selective serotonin reuptake inhibitors (SSRIs) are the first choice for mild depression. They can also be used for particular types of anxiety, such as panic attacks, social phobia and obsessions.

Serotonin-noradrenaline reuptake inhibitors (SNRIs) are among the newest classes of antidepressants. Your doctor may prescribe these if SSRIs don't have the desired effect within a reasonable time.

Tricyclic antidepressants (TCAs) were the most commonly prescribed antidepressants but are used less often now due to the risk of serious side effects. They are sometimes still used in cases of moderate-to-severe depression.

MAOIs (monoamine oxidase inhibitors) are used only when other medications have not worked, because they can cause severe adverse reactions with some types of food and other medications. If you are prescribed an MAOI, ask your doctor for details of what you can and cannot eat.

ANTIPSYCHOTICS

This class of drugs includes medications, such as chlorpromazine and haloperidol, that were originally developed to calm patients before surgery. They are used mainly to treat serious mental illnesses such as schizophrenia as well as psychotic depression and bipolar disorder (manic depression).

ANTI-ANXIETY MEDICATIONS

These medications tend to be prescribed for the short-term relief of anxiety, especially if there are no symptoms of depression.

Benzodiazepines, such as diazepam and temazepam, are very effective but they can cause dependency and should be used only as a temporary measure for severe or disabling anxiety.

Beta-blockers can reduce some of the physical symptoms caused by anxiety, rather than anxiety itself. For example, they can reduce shaking (tremor) and a fast heart rate.

Buspirone is sometimes prescribed for feelings of anxiety, tension and fear, but it can take longer to work than some other medications.

COMING OFF MEDICATION

Deciding when and how to stop taking medication is an important step in the recovery process. You should never stop taking your medication without first talking to your doctor; neither should you alter your dose without advice. Discuss with your doctor whether it is the right time for you to stop the medication. Some medications, especially those, such as benzodiazepines, that carry a risk of dependency, need to be tapered off over a period of weeks or months to avoid side effects. Make sure you keep in touch with your doctor as you are coming off medication to monitor any problems that may arise.

How do antidepressants work?

Experts are still arguing about how antidepressants work. Most believe that they act by making one or more of the neurotransmitters (chemical messengers) in the brain more available and that this improves communication between neurons (brain cells), which in turn reduces depression. The relationship between neurotransmitters and depression is still not fully understood and a minority of experts even suggest that the effect of these medications has nothing to do with the action of neurotransmitters and is due to the placebo effect (thinking they are going to work).

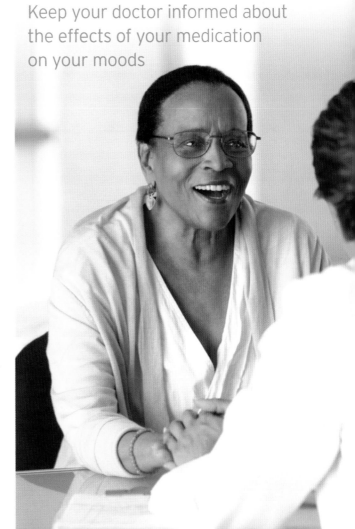

Keep your doctor informed about the effects of your medication on your moods

Lift your mood ... naturally

Lemon balm - taken as a tea, a tincture, or rubbed on the skin in the form of an essential oil - can significantly improve calmness and increase memory and brain function. Research shows that it can help people suffering from anxiety and depression, and can even improve the emotional and mental state of those with dementia. Unsurprisingly, it has been known for centuries as the 'calming herb'.

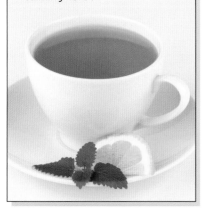

Eat to boost your mood

People turn to comfort food in moments of distress and without doubt feel better as a result, but do specific foods really have the power to lift the spirits or bring them down? Although the precise cause-and-effect relationship between different foods and mood has yet to be scientifically established, the answer seems to be 'yes'. Studies link poor diet with a host of mood problems including depression, anxiety, bipolar disorder and attention deficit hyperactivity disorder (ADHD) in children.

Research published in *The American Journal of Psychiatry* in June 2010 found that, of a randomly chosen group of 1,046 women aged 20–93, those who consumed a typical Western diet – high in processed or fried foods, refined cereals, sweet foods and beer – were more likely to suffer depression, anxiety and other mood problems. By contrast, those who ate a diet rich in vegetables, fruit, meat, fish and whole grains had much better mental health. Numerous other studies back this up.

WHY THE BRAIN NEEDS A HEALTHY DIET

A healthy diet supplies amino acids, from protein foods, such as fish, meat, eggs and pulses, which are the building blocks of brain messenger chemicals (neurotransmitters), such as serotonin and dopamine. It also provides the vitamins and minerals necessary to drive the enzyme reactions that convert amino acids into neurotransmitters. Poor eating habits can have a negative effect on the brain. Low blood glucose levels can produce psychological disruption and food intolerance can cause a range of behavioural difficulties.

10 WAYS TO BOOST MOOD WITH FOOD

1 **Balance up** A healthy balanced diet is the best way to ensure that you get all the nutrients you need for good mental health.

2 **Eat more wholegrain cereals** Foods such as brown rice, wholegrain couscous, wholemeal pasta, buckwheat, oats and other so-called slow-release carbohydrates give your brain a steady supply of glucose – the brain's main fuel. Whole grains also contain B vitamins – linked with better mood.

3 **Always eat breakfast** A nutritious breakfast will ensure that your brain has nutrients and glucose to see you through the morning. Try eggs with wholegrain toast and some fruit, or a bowl of wholegrain breakfast cereal, such as muesli with fruit.

4 **Eat regularly** Regular meals are vital to prevent mood-lowering dips in blood glucose.

5 Eat protein at every meal Protein, for example from meat, fish, lentils, beans or tofu, supplies the building blocks for brain messenger chemicals – neurotransmitters – that affect mood.

6 Eat more oily fish Omega-3 essential fatty acids found in oily fish, such as salmon, mackerel and sardines – as well as walnuts and linseeds – appear to be especially important for a healthy brain.

7 Eat your seven a day Seven portions of fruit and vegetables provide the vital vitamins and minerals needed for all the enzyme reactions needed to drive chemical processes in the brain.

8 Steer clear of processed foods Trans fats (also known as hydrogenated or partially hydrogenated fats) found in some biscuits, pastries and ready meals can interfere with the brain's uptake of healthier fats. Processed foods are also high in sugar, which can cause fluctuations in blood glucose, triggering a mood roller coaster.

9 Boost your tryptophan intake Include bananas, walnuts and turkey in your diet. These are rich in tryptophan, which the body uses to make serotonin, a mood-boosting neurotransmitter.

10 Drink up Dehydration can cause loss of concentration and irritability. Drink plenty of fluids, but don't overdo caffeinated drinks such as tea and coffee; these can increase agitation.

 SELF-HELP

How can I tell if my diet is affecting my mood?

If you think your diet may be affecting your mood, keep a food-and-drink diary for at least a week. Write down in it everything you eat and drink, when you consume it and how you feel emotionally and mentally at the time and afterwards.

Look for patterns See if this record shows any correlation between your mood and diet. According to the mental health charity Mind, the biggest troublemakers are alcohol, caffeine and sugary foods, artificial additives and foods containing trans fats (see 8, left), most of which come from processed foods.

Food intolerance If you experience digestive upsets after eating certain foods (common culprits are wheat, dairy products, yeast, corn, eggs, oranges, soya and tomatoes), you may have a food intolerance that could also be affecting your moods.

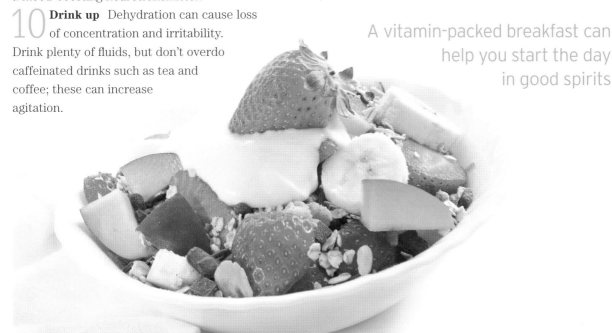

A vitamin-packed breakfast can help you start the day in good spirits

Yoga can help schizophrenia?

True It has been found that exercise and physical activity can also benefit people with severe or long-lasting mental health problems, such as schizophrenia. Studies have shown that exercise can reduce the perception of 'voices', increase self-esteem and improve sleep and general behaviour. A Cochrane Review published in 2010 found that regular exercise improved both the physical and mental health and wellbeing of individuals with schizophrenia. Yoga, in particular, was reported to benefit mental state and quality of life.

Exercise to keep your spirits high

Even thinking about exercise when you are mentally distressed can seem out of the question, but research shows that regular activity can help increase wellbeing, alleviate stress, lift depression, ease anxiety and enhance mood and self-esteem.

WHY GETTING ACTIVE CAN HELP LIFT MOOD

Understanding how activity can improve your mental health may help motivate you to get moving. Here are some very positive reasons to start exercising:

Boosts levels of feel-good brain chemicals For years exercise was thought to improve mood by causing the release of relaxing chemicals called endorphins. The latest research, however, suggests that exercise also increases the availability of brain messenger chemicals such as serotonin, dopamine and noradrenaline, which are lowered in depression and other mood disorders.

Increases self-esteem According to research, exercise can improve self-confidence and reduce depression. The improved muscle tone and weight loss that may come about with regular exercise can also make you feel good – an extra boost if you have negative feelings about your body.

Takes your mind off things Distraction can lead to a greater improvement in mood than more inward-looking activities such as journal keeping or reading.

Warms up your body The rise in body temperature – both the core temperature and that in certain regions of the brain, such as the brain stem – following exercise helps to reduce muscle tension and aids relaxation, a factor that may be especially useful in alleviating anxiety, according to some research.

Helps you sleep better Regular exercise can help ease insomnia and other sleep problems that often accompany emotional distress.

GETTING STARTED

Depression, anxiety and other mental health problems can sap motivation and make it hard to get active. The key is to pick an activity you enjoy and that you are likely to stick with. A good start might be to aim for a 20-minute brisk walk or swim three times a week. Once you're happy doing that, step up the amount you do until you are exercising for 30 minutes most days, and start to vary your activities.

If that still seems like a lot, break it down into 10-minute chunks. You will still benefit. The intensity of the exercise is not in proportion to its effect on your mood. Moderate-intensity exercise such as vigorous housework or gardening, brisk walking, swimming and dancing is just as good a mood lifter as high-intensity exercise. Examples of high-intensity exercise include fast cycling, aerobics and running. However, even low-intensity activity, such as walking to the shops, can lift mood.

In some areas of the country your doctor may be able to prescribe exercise classes at a local gym at a reduced cost. According to a report called *Moving On Up* published in 2009 by the Mental Health Foundation, 21 per cent of GPs prescribe supervised exercise as one of their three most favoured treatments for mild-to-moderate depression.

MAKE YOUR EXERCISE 'GREEN'

Research from the University of Essex suggests that exercising in nature is especially beneficial to mood and self-esteem. Benefits were found to be greatest after just 5 minutes of such 'green exercise', with light activities having the biggest effect on self-esteem and light or vigorous activity the biggest effect on mood. Walking, cycling, boating, horse riding, gardening and 'wild swimming' in the sea, lakes or rivers are all good options.

 SELF-HELP

Beat the blues ...
stay on course

To maintain the benefits of exercise you need to keep at it. Here are some tips:

Pick up a pedometer This small gadget that you clip to your waistband counts your steps and can be a great way to track your progress and keep you motivated.

Track progress Keep an exercise diary to keep track of your exercise progress. As well as noting down how much and how long you exercise, write down how you feel after exercising.

Listen up Listening to music while you exercise can help to lift your spirits while helping to dampen down negative feelings, according to research.

Be a groupie Exercising with a friend or in a group is a good way to stay on track, especially if you are depressed, according to the National Institute for Health and Clinical Excellence (NICE), which recommends group-based exercise as part of its arsenal of treatments for mild-to-moderate depression.

Set goals For the best chance of success make your goals SMART – specific, measurable, achievable and time-related – and reward yourself when you achieve them.

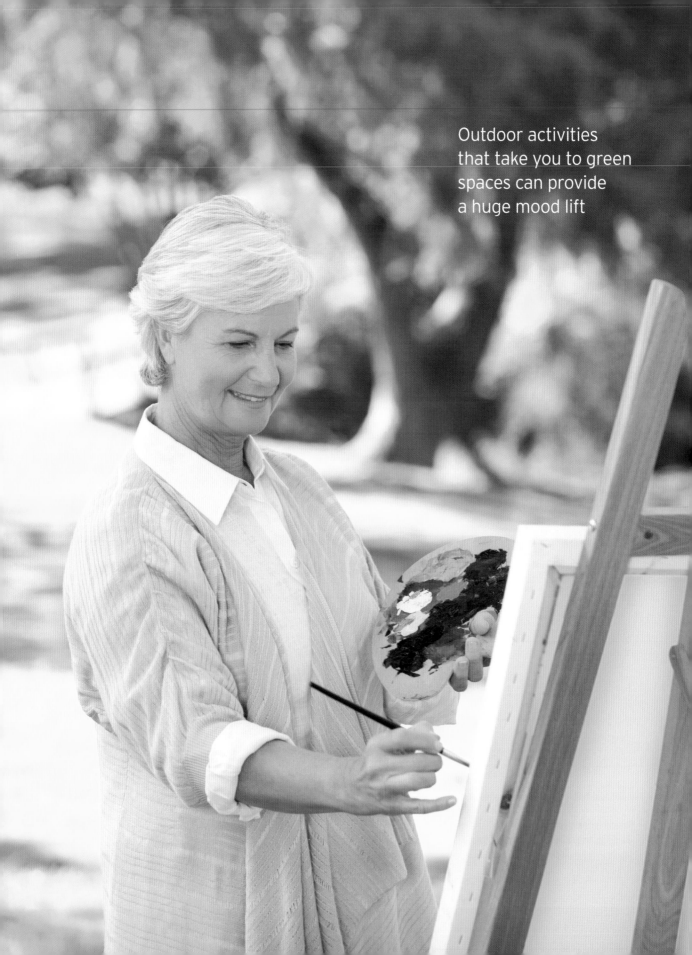

Outdoor activities
that take you to green
spaces can provide
a huge mood lift

The long view

If you – or someone you care about – has a severe mental illness (SMI), long-term treatment and support are likely to be a part of life. New medications and approaches to mental illness over the past few decades have seen huge advances in understanding and treatment.

The term 'severe mental illness' usually refers to a long-standing condition that causes significant difficulties in one or more areas of life. For example, people may find it difficult to look after themselves independently or to hold down a relationship or a job. Schizophrenia, bipolar disorder (formerly called manic depression), schizoaffective disorder (a mixture of schizophrenia and depression and/or mania), severe mood disorders and dementia are examples of SMI. For those with an SMI the key thing to remember is that it is possible to lead a full and meaningful life – working, having relationships, and enjoying activities, such as travel, exercise, art, music and dancing, even with the limitations that having a mental illness may impose. Although in many cases there is no permanent cure at present, people with these conditions can be contented and enjoy close relationships with their family and friends.

FILL YOUR LIFE

Living with a severe mental illness can be challenging, but it's important to try and live life as fully as possible without allowing mental illness to dominate each day. Here are some ideas for steps you could take:

Accept yourself Accepting you have difficulties from time to time can help you to arm yourself with the necessary skills and coping strategies to rebuild your life on a stronger foundation.

Keep taking the tablets Medication is likely to be a part of living with an SMI. Learn as much as you can about the medication you are prescribed and work with the doctor to find the right treatment plan.

Watch for changes

Bouts of mental illness or relapse are often heralded by changes in behaviour some time - days, weeks or months - before symptoms become obvious. If you notice in yourself or in someone you care for any of the following changes in your behaviour or emotions - based on a list drawn up by mental illness charity Rethink - it could be time to seek professional help:

● increasing anxiety and/or irritation

● difficulty concentrating or remembering things

● depression or suicidal thoughts

● obsession with unusual new ideas, or odd beliefs

● too much or too little sleep or none at all

● behaviour changes, such as becoming over friendly or withdrawn

● marked changes in mood

● difficulty in functioning; for example, being unable to cope with work or studies

● undue suspicion of people

● social isolation

● avoidance of activities previously enjoyed.

! ALERT

Suicide watch

Around 5 per cent of people suffering from schizophrenia and 2–9 per cent of people with severe depression take their own lives. Here is some useful advice if you fear that someone close to you may be at risk:

- If someone you care about threatens suicide, do not delay telling a health or social care professional or a mental health support organisation.

- If the person talks about feeling hopeless about the future and that there is no hope of things improving, ask if they have thought of suicide. Don't worry that you will offend them or 'put ideas into their head'. If they are thinking of suicide, it will be a relief to talk about it and it could be a life saver.

- For more information, and for support, contact Lifeline on 13 11 14 (in Australia) or visit their website at www.lifeline. org.au.

- If a life is in danger, call 000 (in Australia).

Cultivate hope Feeling hopeless can make you feel helpless. Working to regain a sense of purpose and hope can help you move forward.

Come out to play According to a US professor of psychology, Barbara Fredrickson, play helps to boost joy and creativity and cements bonds with others that can help you in the bad times. Whether playing tennis or sharing a joke with a friend, find something you enjoy and just do it!

Get creative According to a study published in 2007 in the *Journal of Psychiatric and Mental Health Nursing*, making music, painting and other creative pursuits can distract from worries or 'voices', foster hope, give purpose and help develop ways of coping and a sense of identity.

Focus on strengths Concentrate on things you can do rather than on what you can't. Take pride in your ability to survive the setbacks you have faced and think how you can use what you have learned to enhance your ability to cope in future.

Reach out Connecting to others is an important part of recovery – not just friends and family but the people you come across in your everyday life. Support groups such as those run by the mental illness charity beyondblue, in which you can share your own experiences with others who have been through similar experiences, can be invaluable, too. Visit www.beyondblue.org.au or call 1300 224 636.

BACK TO WORK

Returning to work either full time or part time after any kind of mental illness can help recovery by lifting confidence and self-esteem, but it can be daunting. Here are some practical things you can do to ease yourself back into the workplace:

Drop in Visit your workplace before going back, to say hello to colleagues and re-familiarise yourself with the work environment.

Ease back slowly Ask your boss or HR department if you can build up your hours slowly or even work part time.

Consider changes Ask if you can change your hours or job description if you think that such adjustments might help you cope.

If you are thinking of looking for a new job, Rethink has compiled a list of questions to ask yourself:

- Where do I want to work?
- What type of work do I want to do?
- What support will I need?
- Who can help me look for a job?

Your local job centre, which should have a special department for dealing with people with mental health difficulties, will be able to help you answer these and any other questions you may have. However, they may not be experienced in dealing with mental illness, so be prepared to talk about your condition and any impact you think it could have in the workplace.

SEEKING HELP FOR SOMEONE ELSE

If you suspect someone you care about might be on the point of a relapse, try to encourage him or her to seek help. Point out that stress, anxiety or other symptoms may be making it difficult to cope and offer to accompany your friend or relative to the doctor. If there is resistance but you feel professional help would be beneficial, you may want to seek help on their behalf (see below). Here are some other tips:

- Try to keep stress to a minimum.
- Recognise that he or she may be feeling afraid, confused or 'got at'.
- Listen and try to understand how he or she may be feeling.
- Do not judge or suggest snapping out of it.
- Encourage talking about feelings.
- Don't impose solutions – encourage your friend to be in control of getting better.
- Stay calm and patient and give praise for seeking help.

GETTING HELP IN A CRISIS

You may find yourself in a situation where you feel you need immediate help. Be reassured that there are several sources of advice and support:

Case manager If you have an ongoing case manager, he or she should be your first port of call and may be able to arrange an admission, a home visit or an urgent outpatient appointment.

GP He or she may be able to visit the person at home.

Emergency department If you are worried you are going to harm yourself or someone else, go to your nearest emergency department. A doctor will see you there and, if necessary, arrange for a review by the mental health team.

Mental health line Some states have a 24-hour mental health line, staffed by mental health experts. They will assess the severity of the problem and arrange help. Ask your GP for the number. In an emergency, call Lifeline on 13 11 14.

Top Tips

Ways to find hope

However hopeless you may be feeling, remember that millions of people with similar difficulties have found ways to cope and recover. Here are some ways to help you feel more in control of your destiny:

Dream big Imagine what your future could be. Paint a mental picture of how your life could look in the future regardless of your situation now.

See the good If you are in mental distress, it is easy to always see the worst side of things. Challenge your negative vision and ask yourself whether it is realistic.

Challenge yourself Try to stretch your limits and do something different, no matter how small, every day or at least once a week.

Be true to yourself Make sure the path you follow is going where *you* want to go, rather than in the direction chosen by someone else.

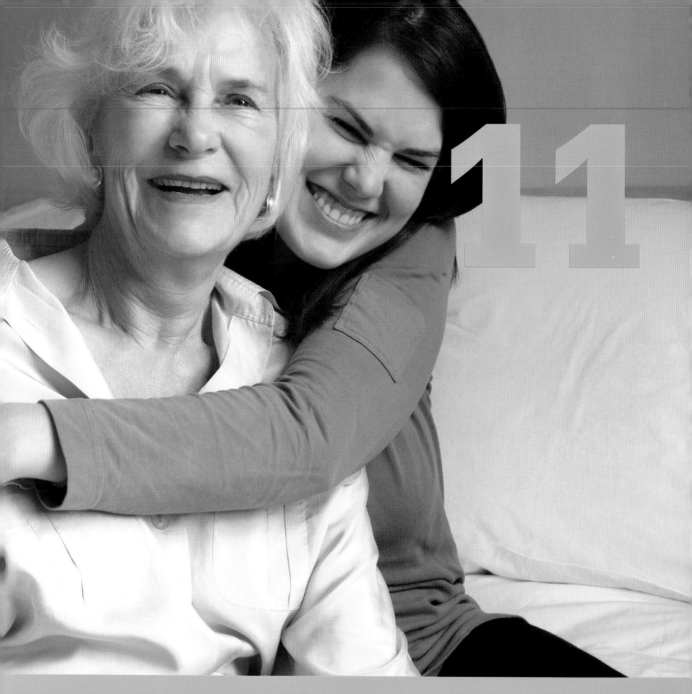

11

Caring for others

Taking on the responsibility for caring for another person may seem daunting. But having the right help and advice can give you the confidence you need to make a real difference to their recovery

Taking responsibility

At some point in life most people have to look after someone else – whether it's a period of intensive short-term care as a friend or relative recovers from an accident or illness, or a much longer-term or even full-time commitment. Knowing that your efforts can help someone you love to recover or feel better can be its own reward. But effective caring can be demanding. It often requires patience and optimism, as well as nursing know-how, which doctors and other medical professionals can help you to acquire. Having a clear idea of the way forward and the help and support of others will enable you to cope with the challenges ahead.

YOUR GOALS

You'll be able to plot the future much better if you think about the level of care that your loved one might require. This is something that you must discuss initially with the person's GP, consultant or medical team. Before taking on this new responsibility, you should consider important issues, such as how full-time the care is likely to be, whether the person can be left alone and how becoming a carer might affect your own life, especially if you have other family members who need your time and attention. You should also find out if back-up support will be available if you need it.

But there are undoubted advantages to caring for someone at home – both for you and the person in need of care:

For you
- You are less likely to worry about him or her.
- It can bring you closer to your loved one.
- Your intimate knowledge of your loved one means you can give individually tailored care that no other carer, however well trained, can provide.

For your loved one
- It's less disruptive than moving to residential care, sheltered accommodation or another more formal care setting.
- Loneliness is less likely to be an issue for someone who's in familiar surroundings with people he or she knows and loves.
- He or she will be reassured that you are there to talk to, providing support and comfort.

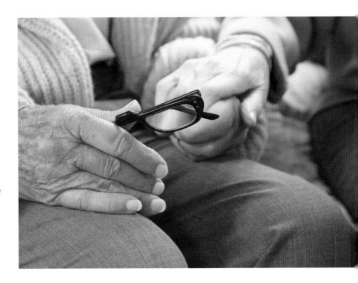

Caring for a loved one during their recovery can bring you closer

Continuity of care

Those with long-term needs should have in place a care plan that enables different health-care professionals to know what has already been done and what other arrangements are in place. In practice, however, you may find that information sometimes fails to get passed on from one person to another. Be sure to explain the relevant points of your loved one's condition and needs each time you encounter a new health professional.

DOS AND DON'TS FOR NEW CARERS

Here is some useful advice for those taking on short- or long-term care.

Do involve your GP He or she can help you to access social, mental health or other services and may be able to offer home visits, if the person you are caring for cannot easily get to the doctor's surgery.

Do get a care plan Your GP can write a care plan that summarises who will be doing what, how to contact them, what the goals are, and what the steps are along the way. The plan is not only a blueprint for care but may enable the person to receive Medicare-assisted allied health care.

Do think about work Talk to your employer about reducing your working hours or organising flexible hours for the duration of recovery.

Do get support If you are committing long-term, you're going to appreciate all the help you can get. Check out Carers Australia's website, www.carersaustralia.com.au, or call their Carer Advisory Service on 1800 242 636.

Do consider how you can maintain and demonstrate respect Treat the person as a partner in care, encouraging him or her to be as independent as possible and to take part in any decision making.

Do plan how you will handle bad news It can be difficult to be the bearer of bad tidings – a poor medical prognosis or the need to consider residential care, for example. Your GP, community nurse, counsellor or a carers' organisation may be able to help.

Do ask about respite and emergency care Carers need regular breaks and carers can also find themselves temporarily unable to do the job. Unfortunately, respite can be hard to organise at the last minute. Ask your GP or specialist whether respite care can be approved in advance.

Don't underestimate what it means to be a carer It's vital to acknowledge that caring for someone else is not necessarily easy. Enlist the help of friends and family and seek advice and support, if necessary, from your GP and local authority social services (see facing page).

Don't try to do everything all the time It's vital to take breaks and make time for yourself.

Don't miss out on financial help The benefits system may seem complicated, but it's worth persevering to find out what you're entitled to. Your GP may be able to help you navigate the system. There's also plenty of useful information on the Centrelink website, at www. humanservices.gov.au/customer/themes/carers.

Making the most of...
the help available

There's a wide range of services available to help make your job as a carer easier. Here are some sources you might want to consider:

- **Doctors** Your GP is the first port of call for your loved one's general health and acts as a gateway to hospital-based specialties such as oncology (cancer), cardiology (heart), neurology (brain and nervous system), geriatrics (care of older people) or psychiatry (mental health problems).

- **Nurses** A range of different nursing staff can offer valuable help. These include: practice nurses, based at your GP's surgery, who carry out procedures such as checking blood pressure and taking blood tests; and district and community nurses, available through your GP, who perform nursing tasks such as changing dressings. Nurse specialists can also assist with specific conditions such as diabetes, mental health issues (for dementia or emotional problems) and rehabilitation after a heart attack.

- **Physiotherapists** can suggest exercises to increase mobility and give guidance on ways for you to help.

- **Speech therapists** can help your loved one communicate more effectively.

- **Occupational therapists** provide advice on equipment and ways to adapt your home for safety and mobility.

- **Podiatrists** can attend to foot problems that may affect mobility.

- **Home care workers** Usually arranged through Home Care services, these people can help with personal care, such as washing and dressing, changing bedding and emptying commodes, supervising meals to make sure your loved one eats properly, and helping him or her at bedtime.

- **Other professionals** These may include: dietitians, who can advise on food, nutrition and issues such as a poor appetite, weight loss or gain, supplementation and much more; continence advisers, who can provide advice and treatment (your GP can make a referral); and psychologists, who can assess and offer advice on problems concerning memory, understanding and other mental skills.

- **Private personal care and companionship** It may be an option to hire someone privately to live in or come in at various times during the day to help with meals, shopping and laundry as well as providing companionship. A variety of schemes are available – ask people you know, or your GP, or check online. If you decide to hire someone privately, check his or her fees and qualifications.

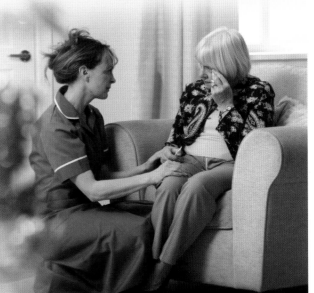

FOCUS

Changing rooms

Someone recovering from illness may need to spend many hours, or perhaps all day, in the same room - usually a bedroom. Thoughtful adaptations to create a healing environment can make a huge difference to a patient's state of mind and, in turn, to his or her recovery.

11 WAYS TO TRANSFORM A ROOM

Most people will feel better in a space that is light and airy, and free from clutter. Here are some ideas for easy ways to turn a sick room into a 'recovery room' that promotes healing.

1 **Lighten up** Draw back curtains whenever possible. Mirrors can also increase the sense of light and space, but may not be suitable for rooms used by patients with dementia or mental health problems, who can find them distressing.

2 **Bring the outside in** Adorn the room with plants or cut flowers but keep them fresh.

3 **Harness water energy** A small indoor water feature can be very soothing in a room.

4 **Be a colour therapist** Colour affects mood. Pale shades are calming. Keep brighter colours for cushions or ornaments.

5 **Keep it clean** Clean carpets at least once a week and wipe over hard surfaces, sink and taps daily.

6 **Picture it** Favourite artworks and photographs of the family or much-loved pets all add a personal touch that can raise spirits.

7 **Declutter** Keep the room free of unnecessary objects. This is not only important for fall prevention; a clutter-free environment is also a soothing place in which to spend time.

8 **Control the climate** Make sure the room isn't too hot, cold, stuffy or dry. Open windows when you can, but remember that those who are inactive may prefer the room warmer than you find comfortable.

9 **Vary it** If there's space, place a coffee table and a couple of chairs in the room so that the person can entertain visitors in a comfortable setting.

10 **Scent it** Use essential oils in a burner or spray. Be guided by the scents your loved one likes. Try lavender for calm and rosemary, thyme, peppermint or clove to kill germs.

11 **Make space for favourite things**. A bedside table for books, a portable TV, a radio or a laptop computer.

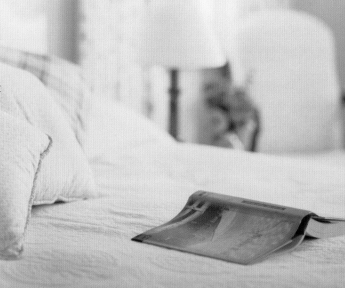

Care basics

When you're looking after someone who is recovering from illness or surgery, there are certain practical concerns that you'll need to consider. The following pages address the all-important questions of how to keep the person you are caring for well fed and clean.

A healing diet

If you're caring for someone who's ill, you'll want to provide a healthy diet that contains the right balance of nutrients needed to promote recovery and set the person on the path to better health in the long term. Medication, digestive complaints, dental problems and swallowing difficulties can all have a bearing on the amount of food consumed. Small, tasty, home-cooked meals packed with nutrients and presented attractively can help whet a feeble appetite and improve health.

THE BASICS

The best diet for those recovering from illness or the elderly in need of long-term care is based on the standard recommendations for healthy eating (see pages 22–26). However, it is worth remembering that anyone who is bed-bound may need fewer kilojoules than a physically active person. Your patient's GP or medical team will be able to tell you if there are any special dietary needs that you need to take into account. For most people, the following foods and nutrients are especially important:

Starchy foods and fibre Bread – preferably wholegrain – rice, pasta, cereals, legumes and potatoes provide vital energy, protein, vitamins, minerals and fibre to help prevent constipation and enhance digestive health. Avoid insoluble fibre in the form of bran, though, as it can hinder the absorption of calcium and iron.

Iron Red meat, offal, legumes, oily fish such as sardines, eggs, bread, green vegetables and fortified breakfast cereals are foods that can help prevent iron-deficiency. Vitamin C (see below) aids iron absorption, so offer a glass of fruit juice with meals. Avoid serving tea with iron-rich meals, as it can block absorption of this mineral.

Vitamin C This is a key nutrient for promoting resistance to infections and wound-healing. Encourage the person you care for to consume citrus fruits, green leafy vegetables, capsicums, tomatoes, potatoes,

Stay safe checklist

Older and ill people find it harder to fight infections, so good food hygiene is a must. Use the following checklist:

✔ Wash your hands and clean work surfaces, utensils and chopping boards before and after use.

✔ Check use-by dates and adhere to them strictly.

✔ Be sure to heat chilled and frozen food until it's steaming hot throughout.

✔ The food-poisoning bugs such as salmonella and listeria are a risk for anyone with reduced immunity, especially the over 60s. Avoid raw or lightly cooked eggs (or products that contain them), raw or undercooked meat, soft cheeses such as camembert and brie, soft blue cheeses and pâtés, including vegetarian options.

fruit juices and fruit drinks with added vitamin C. Smoothies are a good way to provide additional vitamin C for someone who does not feel like eating solid food.

Calcium Dairy products such as milk, cheese and yoghurt, canned fish with bones, such as sardines, green leafy vegetables (such as broccoli and cabbage, but not spinach), soybeans and tofu are all good sources of this vital mineral, which can help strengthen bones.

Vitamin D Those whose poor health or poor mobility may limit their opportunities for going outside can be short of vitamin D, which is made in the skin from sunlight and is also found in oily fish, such as salmon, tuna and mackerel, and dairy products. Try to incorporate these foods into the daily diet of the person you are caring for, or ask the doctor or a dietitian about the advisability of supplements.

Top Tips

Saving time in the kitchen

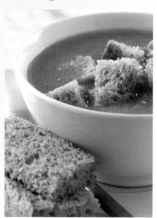

Here are some tips to help you reduce the time you spend in the kitchen without sacrificing the attractiveness or nutritional value of the meals you offer.

● **Keep it simple** Easy, familiar dishes usually go down better than haute cuisine. Soups and sandwiches are great staples for lunch or a snack. Why not try wraps, pitas or soft rolls too? Toast topped with tinned fish, beans, cheese or other favourites is another useful stand-by.

● **Stock up** Get in supplies of canned, frozen, dried and long-life foods and check out online delivery services that can bring your weekly shop to the door. Make and freeze portion-sized meals for times when you might be in a hurry.

● **If you don't feel like cooking** Fresh food is best most of the time, but if you're in a rush, don't hesitate to use ready meals. Tinned oily fish such as tuna, pilchards and sardines are useful easy-to-prepare stand-bys, as are eggs, pasta, rice and tinned fruit and vegetables.

Water A good intake of fluids is essential to hydrate the cells, maintain the tone and elasticity of tissues and ensure nutrients are absorbed. Experts advise consuming at least 1.2 litres of fluids every day (this total includes any liquid in food). Fluid requirements may be higher if there is a fever, or diarrhoea or vomiting. If the person you are caring for doesn't like plain water, offer tea, milk, juice, smoothies and soups instead.

WHEN APPETITE IS POOR

When a person is in the initial stages of recovery from surgery or illness, eating hearty meals is likely to be the last thing they feel like doing. But you'll need to provide light meals and snacks to supply the person with the energy and nutrition that he or she needs to fuel the healing process. Avoid serving large platefuls of food, which may be off-putting. Go for small portions of soft foods, and soups, which are nutritious as well as being easy to swallow. Be guided by the patient's appetite and preferences, while doing your best to include a balance of protein, healthy fats and carbohydrates in the meals you provide. Here are some ideas for someone in the early days of recovery:

Breakfast Porridge with honey and fresh berries
Mid-morning snack Milkshake or smoothie
Lunch Scrambled egg on toast; piece of fruit
Mid-afternoon snack Fruit yoghurt
Evening meal Fish pie and steamed vegetables; baked apple and custard.

PREVENTING WEIGHT LOSS

In some cases, a person recovering from a long-term illness may need to put on weight, but may not feel hungry. Rick Wilson, Director of Nutrition and Dietetics at Kings College Hospital, London, has these tips for meals when the aim is to maintain or increase weight:

- In a reversal of normal healthy-eating guidelines, make sure every mouthful contains plenty of kilojoules and protein. Fortify food with melted butter, grated cheese or cream. Add finely ground nuts or seeds to fortify smoothies and soups, or sprinkle over vegetables. Add milk and sugar to tea and coffee to provide extra kilojoules.
- Choose high-fat options such as pastry and full-fat milk. Offer a biscuit with hot drinks.
- Boost vitamin C intake to speed healing. Go for fruit juice rather than fruit, which may lead to a feeling of fullness.
- Offer six small meals a day instead of three big ones.

> **Be gadget aware**
> Check out special equipment to make it easier for the person you are caring for to feed him or herself. Try two-handled cups or cups with lids and spouts, angled cutlery and plate guards.

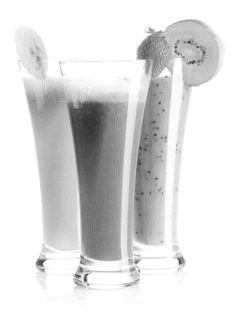

Fruit smoothies can provide a vitamin-packed treat for those with little appetite

- If weight loss continues, ask the doctor whether supplement drinks might be advisable and if you should consult a dietitian.
- Provide plenty of water but not in the 30 minutes before a meal – it will cause feelings of fullness.
- Ask the doctor if you should give vitamin supplements. Vitamin D levels may be low if the person is not getting exposure to sunshine.

Keeping clean

Those who are confined to bed, or have very limited mobility due to ill health or injury, are largely dependent on their carers for maintaining personal hygiene and for ensuring that their clothing and bedding is kept clean.

EVERYDAY CLEANLINESS

Being clean and fresh is vital to wellbeing and self-esteem. However, for short periods, no damage is done if the ill person misses a daily bath or shower. Providing soap and a damp washcloth so that the person can wash their face, hands, armpits and genital area (in that order) is adequate for a couple of days. If the person is confined to bed for any longer, you may have to give a bed bath (see instructions on the facing page). If he or she is sufficiently mobile and the doctor agrees, you may be able to help him or her to have a bath or shower. This may require safety equipment such as non-slip mats and grab rails.

A MATTER OF CONVENIENCE

A key element of caring for a sick person is to provide access to toilet facilities. This highly sensitive aspect of personal care needs to be handled with tact and respect. A basically healthy person confined to bed with a short-term illness can usually get up to use the toilet, provided it is reasonably accessible. In such cases it may still be advisable to stay close by in case of falls.

If it is not possible for the person to walk more than a few steps, you may need to consider acquiring a commode to keep in the sick room. Ask your occupational therapist, community nurse, GP or practice nurse where you may acquire one. Or you can rent or buy them privately from disability care shops found online or through the Yellow Pages. For a person completely confined to bed, a bedpan may be the best option. You'll need advice from your medical team and training for helping the person on and off the pan.

GIVING A BED BATH

If you are bathing someone who is confined to bed, make sure the room is warm and that you have everything you need to hand before you start. Here's how to do it:

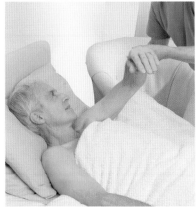

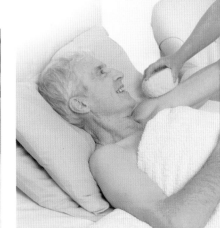

Ease the pain

Consider giving the person you are caring for a painkiller about 20 minutes before any activity he or she finds painful, such as a bath or bed change.

1 *Remove the clothing on the person's upper body, pull up a sheet to the armpits and cover this with a towel.*

2 *Wash and dry the face and upper body with a well squeezed-out sponge or washcloth, then wash and dry each side of the body from the arm down to the waist, adjusting the sheet and towel as you do so to cover the parts that are dry.*

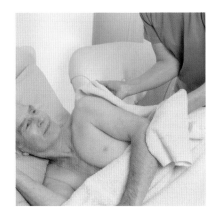

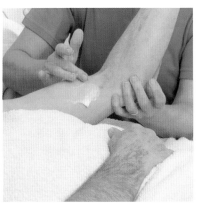

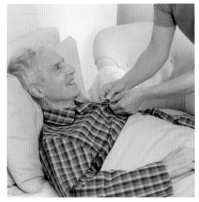

3 *Remove the lower body garments. Gently turn the person on one side facing away from you; wash and dry the shoulders, back and bottom. Finally, get the person to wash the genital area, if possible, or do so yourself. Use a fresh sponge or disposable wipes and disposable gloves.*

4 *When you've finished washing and drying each area, gently apply an emollient cream or lotion to prevent the skin from becoming dry.*

5 *Apply deodorant and help the person to dress in clean, fresh pyjamas or clothes.*

CHANGING BED LINEN

If the person you are caring for is bed-bound, you may have to change the bedclothes while he or she remains in the bed. This may seem daunting, but with practice you'll soon get the hang of it. Here's how to do it (seek professional advice first if the patient has special movement needs):

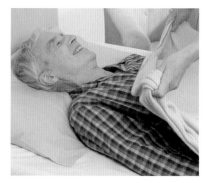

1 *Get the person to lie back and cover with a blanket for warmth and privacy. Remove the top covers (doona or sheets and blankets) to be washed.*

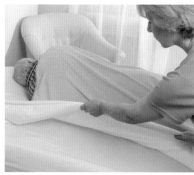

2 *Remove the pillow(s) and help the person to roll over until facing away from you. Loosen the bottom sheet and roll it forwards until it's close to the person's back.*

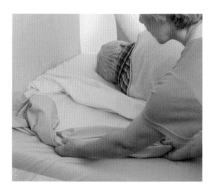

3 *Arrange the clean sheet on the uncovered side of the bed and tuck it under the mattress. Roll the remaining portion of the new sheet until the roll reaches the rolled-up old sheet.*

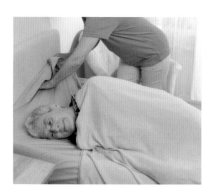

4 *Help the person to roll right back over both sheets to the other side of the bed. Remove the old sheet and unroll the rest of the new sheet over the rest of the mattress. Tuck it in neatly and smooth out any wrinkles.*

5 *Help the person to roll back to the centre of the bed and cover with clean top covers. Change the pillow case(s).*

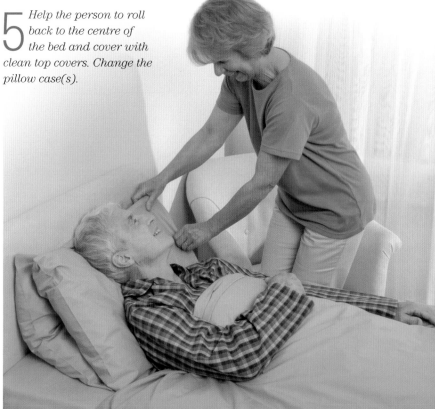

FOCUS

Surviving as a carer

Being a carer can reinforce the love you feel for the person you are looking after and provide a satisfying sense of achievement. But, especially when the need for care extends for a long period of time, it can also be physically exhausting and mentally draining. It's crucial that you care for yourself too, especially if your commitment is a long-term one.

BE A HEALTHY CARER

As a carer, it's vital to think of your own needs as well as those of the person for whom you are caring. There will probably be times when you experience negative feelings and emotions, such as helplessness, resentment, anger, guilt, anxiety and loneliness.

Taking care of your own health and wellbeing – making sure you're eating well, exercising regularly and taking time out to relax and enjoy yourself – will help you to stay on top of these feelings.

Here are some tips for keeping physically healthy and emotionally strong:

Don't try to do it all You aren't superhuman. Ask for the help you need. Friends, family or neighbours often want to help and it's up to you to tell them how. This might include housework, gardening, shopping or sitting with your loved one.

Eat a healthy diet It's tempting to eat junk food or to snack and run, but try to make time to enjoy healthy food and relaxed mealtimes.

Sleep tight Have a bedtime routine to help you wind down at the end of the day. See also pages 30–33.

Be health alert Keep an eye on your own health. Eat sensibly and make time for exercise.

Mind your back Caring for someone who is bedbound can involve lifting. Ask your doctor if you need special equipment.

Deal with stress – healthily A massage, a dance or yoga class, a walk in the country, the park or by the sea, or a visit to a spa if you can afford it, are all great ways to combat stress.

Make time for yourself Take some time out every day to read a book or the newspaper, watch TV, listen to some music or simply relax.

Find emotional support Your friends and relatives have different things to offer. Some may be hopeless at practical tasks but offer a sympathetic ear. Try to pick someone with an open mind who's a good listener. If you're religious, you may find help within your faith community.

Seek respite If you are caring for someone with a long-term condition, look into respite care. Residential care homes and nursing homes may offer short-term options. Ask your GP for advice.

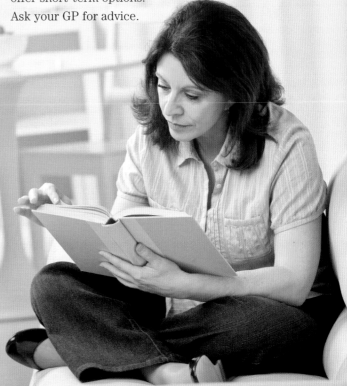

Hastening recovery

When you are caring for a loved one who is ill, you'll want to do more than simply keep them safe, well fed and clean. It's natural to want to take active steps to speed their recovery, by supporting the doctor's treatment and encouraging a return to full health.

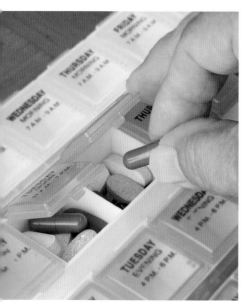

KEEPING TRACK OF TABLETS
To help you know what should be taken, when and how, it's a good idea to obtain an organiser box from the pharmacist. These have different compartments in which you can store the tablets to be taken each day or at particular times.

Taking charge of treatment

When you look after someone who is bed-bound, it is likely that you'll need to take charge of administering medicines – especially if he or she is drowsy or confused. In this situation you'll need to find out as much as possible about them. Ideally you should discuss this with the doctor. You'll find plenty of general advice in *Get the most from your medicine*, pages 312–339, but here are some useful reminders:

● Check the leaflet in the medicine box. It often has useful guidance on storage and what to do if a dose is missed or too many are taken.

● Don't guess or estimate doses for liquid medicines. Pharmacists can provide syringes, pots or spoons for precise measurement.

● All types of medicine have the best effect when taken at regular intervals. If the medicine is to be taken once a day, try to administer it at roughly the same time each day. For more frequent doses, ask the doctor if you should wake the person in the night to take medication or space the doses through the waking hours.

● If the information for a tablet says 'to be swallowed whole', it is very important not to crush these tablets as stomach acid could make them less effective. People who have difficulty swallowing may need special help to take medication safely as choking or a fatal chest infection could result if a tablet became lodged in the windpipe. The best way to take medicines is standing or sitting up, with a small amount of cool or tepid (not hot) liquid from a cup or glass. If the patient cannot take a medicine for any reason, consult the doctor.

● Never give the person medicines prescribed for someone else. This could cause a potentially dangerous interaction with other medicines or adversely affect the person in other ways.

● If the person for whom you are caring needs to go to hospital, take a copy of the most recent prescription or the medicines themselves if the prescription cannot be found so that the hospital staff are aware of what he or she is taking.

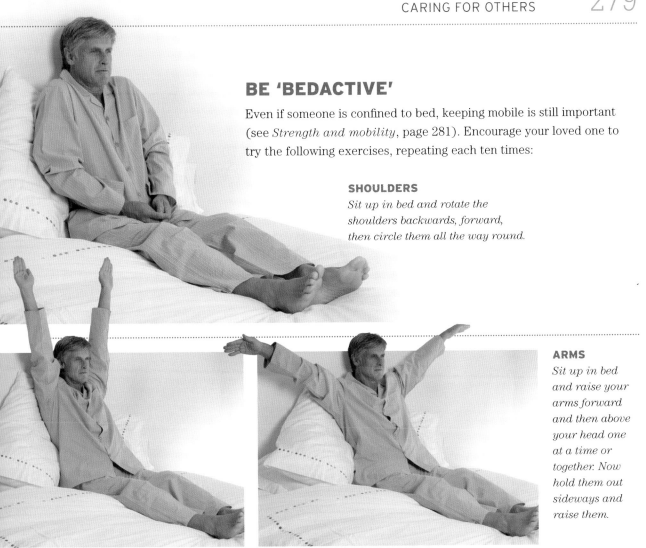

BE 'BEDACTIVE'

Even if someone is confined to bed, keeping mobile is still important
(see *Strength and mobility*, page 281). Encourage your loved one to
try the following exercises, repeating each ten times:

SHOULDERS
*Sit up in bed and rotate the
shoulders backwards, forward,
then circle them all the way round.*

ARMS
*Sit up in bed
and raise your
arms forward
and then above
your head one
at a time or
together. Now
hold them out
sideways and
raise them.*

KNEES AND HIPS
*Lying on the bed, straighten one leg, pulling your
toes towards you and tightening the front of the thigh.
Keeping the leg straight, raise your leg off the bed.
Count to 10 and then slowly lower it. If your back
arches, bend the knee of the resting leg.
Repeat on the other side.*

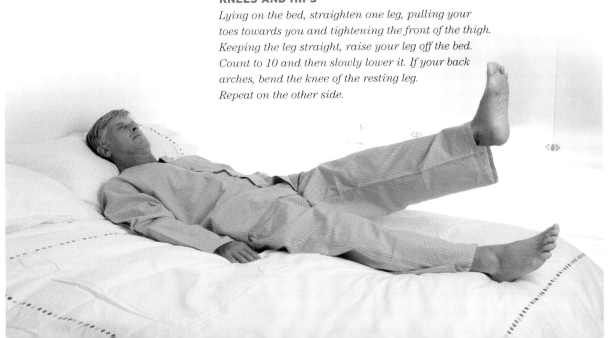

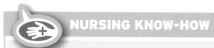

NURSING KNOW-HOW

A helping hand...
assisting someone to get out of bed

If you are caring for someone who has been confined to bed for a lengthy period, encourage him or her to get out of bed often - if only to sit in a chair. Use the method described below if the person is too weak to get up unaided. If you can't manage alone, ask another person to help if possible. Equipment such as bed raisers, grab handles, leg lifters (a reinforced strap with a loop on the end), lifting poles and mechanical lifting devices (hoists) can also help.

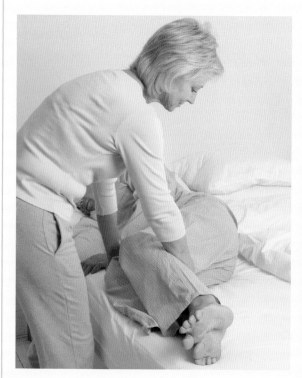

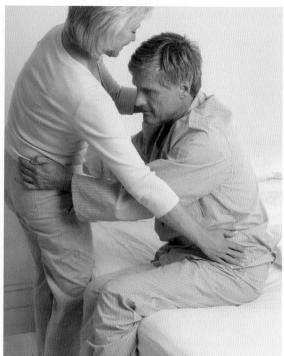

1 Turn the person onto one side, stand beside the bed, put your hands behind their knees and ease the legs off the bed.

2 Ask the person to place a hand on your waist for balance and stability, put one hand on the hip and the other on the back of the shoulder.

3 Press on the person's hip and, leaning back on your back leg, help ease him or her to a sitting position. Don't let the person use their hands to put weight on your waist.

4 Once the person is stable, you can either let go or help him or her to sit in a chair.

Strength and mobility

As little as ten days of bed rest in healthy older men and women can cause significant loss of muscle mass and with it the power and ability to perform everyday tasks, according to research published in 2007 in the *Journal of the American Medical Association*. What's more, people who remain immobile in bed for too long are vulnerable to chest infections, constipation and pressure sores.

EARLY MOVES
You should encourage the person to move around as soon as possible. As a first step, discuss with your doctor whether any medicines may be affecting the person's ability to stand or walk – for example, by causing side effects such as fatigue, muscle weakness or dizziness – and if so whether a change of medication could help. Also check how any medical conditions are likely to progress and how they may affect mobility at a later date.

If the doctor gives the all clear, the person can try the 'bedactive' exercises described on page 279, moving on to the 'chairobics' routine (page 282) as soon as he or she is comfortable sitting in a chair.

CONFIDENCE AND SUPPORT
If you think walking aids may provide the reassurance your loved one needs to feel confident on their feet, ask your doctor or physiotherapist whether a cane or walking frame might help. These are often available through local council social services departments.

EXERCISE PROGRAMS
Once your loved one has regained confidence and a certain amount of mobility, attending a course of tai chi, gentle yoga or Pilates can improve core strength and balance. Your GP, practice nurse, physiotherapist or occupational therapist can provide guidance about local exercise programs. A physiotherapist or exercise physiotherapist can also develop a personalised regimen.

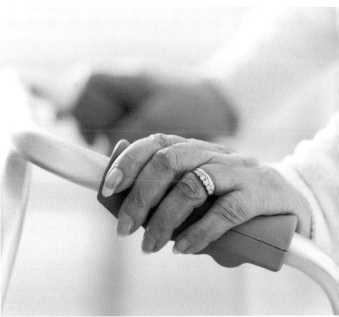

The right support will reassure a person as they regain their mobility after illness

TRY 'CHAIROBICS'

Once your patient is able to sit in a chair, it's worth suggesting some gentle exercises using light weights to help build strength. Cans or small bottles of water can make ideal improvised weights. Choose a chair that allows the person to keep their knees at 90 degrees when seated. During the exercise, it is important to sit tall and hold in the stomach muscles to maintain good posture. Each exercise should be repeated ten times.

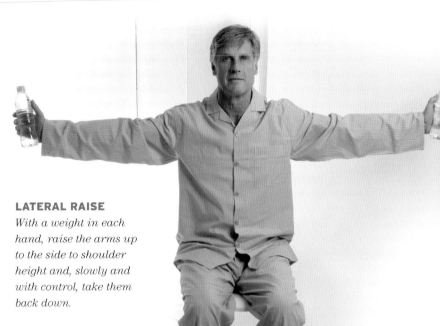

LATERAL RAISE
With a weight in each hand, raise the arms up to the side to shoulder height and, slowly and with control, take them back down.

OVERHEAD PRESS
With a weight in each hand, hold the arms with the elbows bent and the weights next to the ears. Push the weights upwards, then return the hands to their original position.

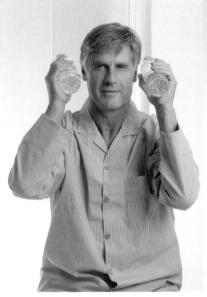

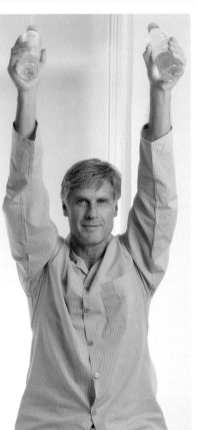

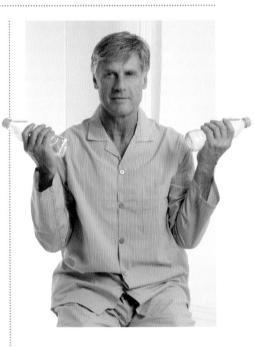

BICEPS CURLS
With a weight in each hand, elbows at the sides, palms facing upwards, curl the arms towards the shoulders, then slowly bring the hands back down to their original position.

CaseStudy

A CARER'S STORY

How a shared sense of humour helped a couple survive the journey through chemotherapy

Phil Wilson, 51, from Canberra, is a professional musician. He describes caring for his partner Sarah, during her treatment for breast cancer, below.

" When Sarah was diagnosed with breast cancer in January 2009, I clung onto the words, 'it's treatable'. I knew we had to stay positive and get through it as a team.

On the day of her lumpectomy in February, we brought along a furry blue puppet called 'Radley' to lighten the mood; he never failed to make her laugh. That set the tone for the next few months: we laughed more than we cried. Even the name of her chemotherapy drugs, 'FEC', made us laugh, because it reminded us of Father Jack in the sitcom

Father Ted. The consultants were amazed by her positive attitude and said, 'you wouldn't believe she had cancer'. But there were some tough times too. After her operation Sarah was in a lot of pain and had to do a series of exercises at home to help restore the mobility in her arm. I did them with her every single day, even when she didn't feel like it.

One of the most traumatic things we had to deal with was when Sarah lost her hair. Just before her second dose of chemotherapy it started to fall out in clumps, which was extremely upsetting. The first time we went into a wig shop, she ran outside in tears. I said, 'what happens next is up to you, but if you don't go inside now, you might never go'. That day we bought two fantastic wigs: one electric blue bob and the same in black. She looked incredible.

Emotionally, I also had my own ups and downs. There were times during Sarah's treatment when I felt very low and would take myself off for a weep. I had to stay strong for her sake.

On the final day of Sarah's chemotherapy, I decided to mark the occasion by having a special trophy engraved for her saying, 'Thank FEC it's over!'. Cancer will be in the back of our minds forever, but we know we'll be there for each other, whatever happens. "

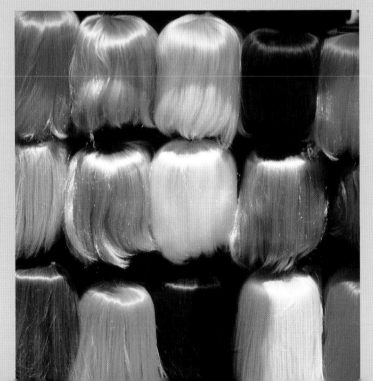

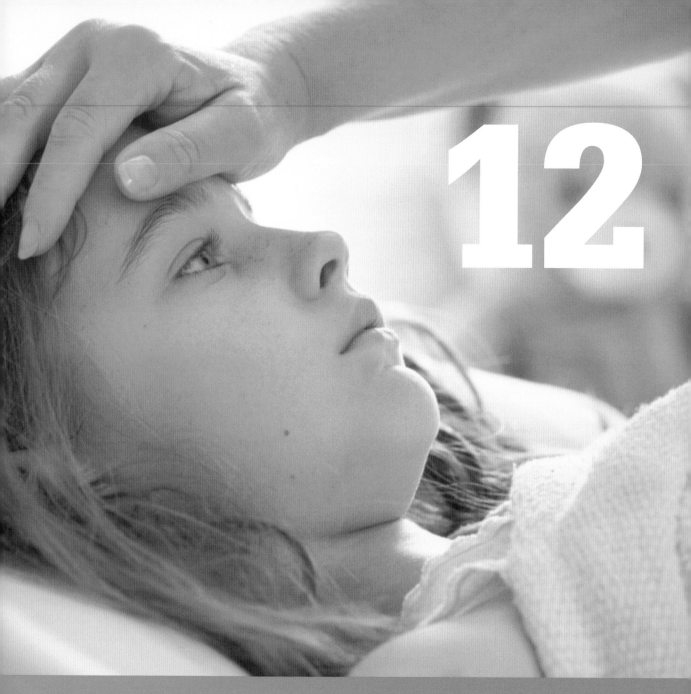

12

Make it better

While having a sick child can be upsetting, it's worth remembering that, with the right support, children have a great capacity for recovery

Natural resilience

A nutritious diet, the right amount of sleep and physical activity, as well as loving care, are all key ingredients for a healthy, happy and resilient child. But illness is a normal part of every child's life. Some illnesses come on suddenly and often get better on their own within a short time. Because their immune systems are immature, children tend to be more susceptible than adults to these acute ailments, which are often relatively minor. It's quite normal for a child to go down with a virus up to 12 times a year. In fact, catching infections is what helps your child to build up his or her natural resistance.

LONG-TERM CONDITIONS

Sometimes a child may develop a more lasting (chronic) physical or mental health problem such as diabetes, a food allergy, attention deficit disorder or depression. Such conditions can initially disrupt everyday life and will take time to get used to. Maintaining a calm, practical approach will help both you and your child adjust and live as normally as possible. In this chapter you will find plenty of tips to help you through the times when your child is unwell.

AVOIDING ILLNESS

From birth onwards, there is much parents can do to prevent a child from becoming ill. Some of the measures are similar to the general guidelines for healthy living. Others, such as immunisations, can give lifetime protection against major diseases. Here are some important steps that you can take to safeguard your child's health from birth through to adolescence:

- Attend routine health checks. These are scheduled during infancy and the childhood years with your GP or early childhood nurse. They provide an opportunity for health professionals to spot any health or developmental problems early and take necessary action.
- Give your child a healthy diet. Your child needs a balanced diet that supplies the nutrients required at each stage of development. Current National Health and Medical Research Council guidelines recommend breastfeeding exclusively for the first six months. If this is not possible, formula feeds can provide a satisfactory alternative. Then provide your growing child with meals packed with plenty of fresh vegetables, fruit and protein. Choose unrefined carbohydrates (wholegrain bread, wholemeal pasta and brown rice) and 'good fats' rather than the less healthy alternatives (see *Diet*, pages 22–26).

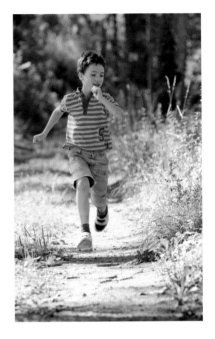

Just as children have vast natural reserves of energy, they have a huge capacity for healing and recovery from illness

Your child and your doctor

With luck, your child won't need to see a doctor very often - perhaps only for routine checks. But on the occasions when a visit to the GP is necessary, encourage your child to see the doctor as someone who is there to help him or her get better when unwell.

To help a young child get used to the idea of visiting the doctor, a teddy or doll can be brought along too and perhaps bandaged, or given an injection or pretend medicine. Most GPs are used to talking to children in a way that is not intimidating.

Don't expect a prescription every time you take your child to the doctor and make your child understand this. Most minor illnesses get better on their own and it is important to encourage your child to realise that the body has a great capacity to heal itself.

- Make your home smoke-free. Quitting smoking is good for the health of parents as well as the child. Passive smoking increases your child's risk of ear and throat infections, asthma and cot death. And the example you set is bound to have an influence on your child as he or she grows up. For advice on quitting, see *Clearing the smoke*, page 136. If you or your partner are unable to give up, try to smoke outside the house. In most of Australia, smoking in your car with children on board is illegal.
- Make sure your child has all the required vaccinations. Go to www.medicareaustralia.gov.au/provider/patients/acir/schedule.jsp for the schedule or call Immunise Australia on 1800 671 811 or talk to your GP.
- Encourage your child to get enough sleep. Babies need up to 18 hours a day and even older children need 10 to 12 hours sleep including daytime naps.
- Make sure your child gets sufficient exercise. Children need at least an hour's physical activity every day – outside whenever possible. This is key to weight control and heart health in the future. The American Academy of Pediatricians discourages TV and other media use by children younger than 2 and recommends that older children should engage with entertainment media for no more than 1 to 2 hours per day.
- Monitor your child's weight. Childhood obesity is on the increase and with it a greater risk of diabetes, heart disease, cancer, arthritis and many other illnesses. Check your child's weight against age and height on an appropriate chart, for example, from www.health.nt.gov.au/Remote_Health_Atlas/Forms/growth_charts.

On the alert

As a parent, you'll need to be alert and prepared for a range of minor ailments and some more serious conditions that may affect your child. The following are common types of problem during childhood:

Colds and coughs (see page 292).

Childhood infectious diseases (see page 295)

Developmental delay Talk to your GP or early childhood nurse if you think your baby or child is not progressing (for example, crawling, walking or talking) normally for a child of his or her age.

Hearing and vision problems These are often picked up at routine health checks, but can be easily missed by parents. Ask your GP to arrange a hearing test for your child if he or she appears to have speech problems or often fails to respond when you talk. Have your child's

WHAT IMMUNISATIONS AND WHEN?

Here's a checklist of the immunisations that are routinely offered to all children in Australia, and the age at which they should ideally be given.

Birth

- Hepatitis B

2 months

- Diphtheria, tetanus, pertussis, polio, Hib (*Haemophilus influenzae* Type b), hepatitis B, pneumococcal, rotavirus

4 months

- Diphtheria, tetanus, pertussis, polio, Hib, hepatitis B, pneumococcal, rotavirus

6 months

- Diphtheria, tetanus, pertussis, polio, Hib, hepatitis B (or at 12 months), pneumococcal, rotavirus

12 months

- Measles, mumps, rubella, Hib, hepatitis B (or at 6 months), meningococcal C

18 months

- Measles, mumps, rubella, varicella, pneumococcal

4 years

- Diphtheria, tetanus, pertussis, polio, measles, mumps, rubella

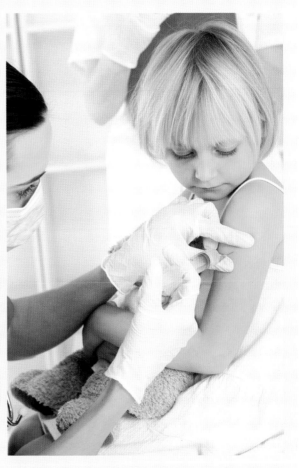

eyesight tested if he or she seems slow to acquire reading skills or always sits close to the TV.

Emotional or mental health problems Be alert for changes in behaviour or problems at school. The explanation may be an external factor such as bullying but conditions such as depression can occur in childhood (see pages 308–311). Eating problems such as anorexia, which may affect teenagers, are discussed on page 254.

Adolescent development A time of enormous change for your child both physically and emotionally, the teenage years can be a challenge for parents too. Be ready to seek advice from your GP if you are concerned about any aspect of your teenager's wellbeing.

FOCUS

The best start in life

Coming home with a new baby signals an enormous and challenging life change for both parents. But with the support of health-care professionals and a network of family and friends, the early days and weeks of your baby's life will not only be a precious and memorable time for you, but can lay the foundations of a lifetime of good health for your baby.

Every new mother should be aware that her wellbeing and that of her baby are closely linked in the early days and weeks. So looking after yourself is not selfish self-indulgence, but a necessary part of caring for your newborn. If you've had a vaginal delivery you may be in discomfort from stitches and bruising while, if you had a Caesarean section, you may have a painful wound. Your emotions will be in turmoil due to hormonal upheaval, and if your new baby has health problems or was premature, you will naturally be anxious about his or her health. The secret is to take good care of yourself, rest as much as possible, address any problems as they arise and try not to do too much too soon.

ADJUSTING TO BREASTFEEDING

One of the biggest decisions you will have to make as a new mother is how to feed your baby. Childcare experts are in no doubt that breast milk provides the best nutrition for a baby. It supplies a perfectly balanced meal at every feed, passes on a degree of resistance to some infections and its constituents change over the weeks to meet a growing infant's changing needs. Even if you are only able to breastfeed for a few days or weeks, you will have given your baby a flying start in life.

To help you get over any difficulties in the early days, your midwife will visit when you get home and can help with feeding problems. If you need additional support, contact the Australian

 NURSING KNOW-HOW

Soothing soreness

Stitches, bruising or small tears in or around the vagina are almost universal following childbirth. These can be sore and uncomfortable in the first few days, but there are things you can do to ease discomfort and speed up healing:

- Keep the vaginal area clean and look out for signs of infection such as redness, swelling or discharge. Contact your GP, midwife or obstetrician if you have problems.

- Over-the-counter painkillers may help to reduce discomfort, but if you're breastfeeding ask your GP or pharmacist for advice on what medicines are safe for you to take.

- Sit down gently and lie on your side rather than your back. Cushions or a special soft ring-shaped seat on your chair can help to ease pressure while you are sitting down.

- You may feel anxious about passing urine because of the soreness. Try sitting in a warm bath or in a bowl of lukewarm water or running a warm shower over the area as you urinate. Drinking lots of water can help dilute urine so it stings less.

- Eat plenty of fresh fruit and vegetables to prevent constipation and straining, which can put pressure on any stitches when you go to the toilet.

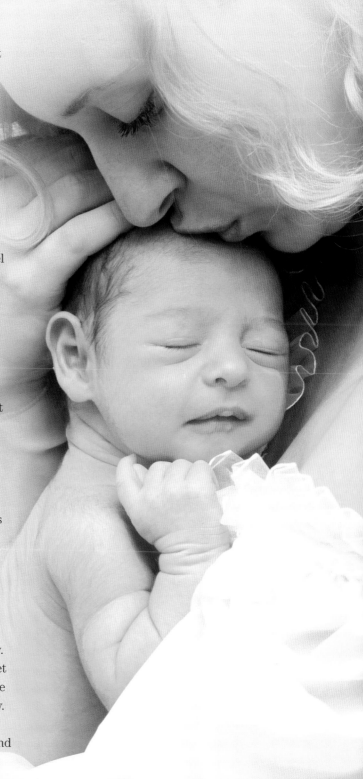

Breastfeeding Association (1800 686 268; www. breastfeeding.asn.au). If, for any reason, you cannot breastfeed, your midwife or early childhood nurse will discuss bottle-feeding options with you. Don't feel guilty; bottle-fed babies also thrive.

EMOTIONAL UPHEAVAL

It's normal to feel weepy and low a few days after giving birth – this is known as the 'baby blues'. These feelings affect around 50 per cent of mothers and are thought to be largely due to hormonal changes. Emotions usually start to stabilise after around six to eight weeks although you may still feel emotional at times. If such feelings become worse or continue for longer, you may be suffering from postnatal depression (PND) (see page 245). If you are feeling like this, be sure to talk to your GP.

CONSERVING YOUR RESOURCES

Here are some ideas to help you through the weeks following childbirth so that you can provide the best care for your baby:

Rest when you can Adopt your baby's rhythm and sleep when he or she does.

Get help Delegate household tasks to others (your partner, friends, family or employed help).

Eat well Make sure you have a balanced, nutritious diet. Regular meals are important, especially if you are breastfeeding.

Avoid caffeine Drinking caffeine-containing drinks can increase anxiety and may affect the baby if you are breastfeeding.

Stay in touch Other mums can be a great source of support and friendship when you have a new baby. Arrange get-togethers with women you may have met at antenatal classes or ask your early childhood nurse to put you in contact with other new mothers nearby.

Don't forget your partner Nurture your relationship by spending time together every day and get a babysitter occasionally so you can go out.

Taking care of your baby

If you're new to parenthood, the slightest sign of possible illness is likely to worry you. You may sometimes need the reassurance of a doctor, but will quickly gain confidence as you learn the many simple steps you can take to comfort your baby and speed recovery.

! ALERT

Emergency action

It's vital to recognise if your baby's symptoms should be treated as an emergency. Call 000 (in Australia) immediately if your baby:

- is not breathing
- is unconscious
- seems breathless, or is breathing much faster than usual
- looks very pale, or the skin is blue or dusky around the lips
- is having a convulsion (fit)
- has cold hands or feet, but also a fever (a temperature above 38°C)
- feels floppy or limp (perhaps when cuddled)
- has a raised, tense or bulging soft spot (fontanelle) in the centre of the top of the head.

TELLTALE SYMPTOMS

Knowing how to differentiate between the many variations of normal behaviour and a real cause for concern is one of the hardest things for a new parent to learn. But you should trust your instinct and contact your doctor or After Hours GP Helpline (1800 022 222) if you are at all worried. Visit www.babylifecheck.co.uk to help you to work out whether your baby is ill. In addition to the emergency signs listed left, the following are important warning symptoms to look out for:

- excessive drooling instead of swallowing saliva
- bruised or discoloured skin, or a rash
- unusual drowsiness or failure to respond to you as normal
- crying in an abnormal way (moaning, whimpering or high-pitched) that soothing doesn't help
- no interest in feeding
- severe leg pain or tenderness
- irritability and dislike of being touched
- fever (a temperature above 38°C)
- abnormal wetting or soiling.

Newborn babies often sniffle and snort especially when asleep. This often indicates that mucus has accumulated in their nasal passages as a result of lying on their back and is nothing to worry about. More persistent sniffles can be a sign of a cold (see page 292).

COULD IT BE COLIC?

Crying is your baby's way of communicating. You will soon learn whether a particular cry means that he or she is hungry, too hot or too cold, teething or feeling unwell. If babies have long crying spells at a particular time of day, won't stop crying and draw up their knees or go rigid, it may be colic. No one knows the exact cause but there's no long-term risk to a baby that has this condition. Here are some ideas to help restore calm:

Massage A gentle tummy massage, using clockwise circles can help move any trapped wind through the gut.

Walk it away Put your baby in a pram and go for a walk.

Check feeding If you are breastfeeding, make sure your baby is latching on properly. If bottle-feeding, try an anti-colic teat.

Burping/winding Try winding your baby halfway through and after a feed to help expel trapped air.

NO MORE NAPPY RASH

Nappy rash is common. Fast action will stop it getting worse. Here's how to help it to heal and prevent it from recurring:

- Let your baby go without a nappy for as long as possible. Change nappies frequently and immediately after bowel movements.
- Clean your baby's bottom thoroughly using cotton wool and water (not baby wipes) and dry well between nappy changes.
- Use a barrier cream. Preparations containing zinc oxide are good choices.
- A tablespoon of bicarbonate of soda in the bath water may help to sooth soreness. Avoid using strong soaps and bubble baths.

DIARRHOEA AND VOMITING

Proper vomiting – as opposed to bringing up a small amount of milk after feeding (possetting) – can be a sign of an infection. If your baby also has diarrhoea and a temperature, or if the vomiting ejects the stomach contents with force, consult your doctor without delay.

Keeping your baby's bottom clean and dry is the best treatment for nappy rash

Crisis point

Living with a baby who never seems to stop crying can test your patience to the limit, especially if nights of broken sleep have left you exhausted. If you feel that you can't take any more, it's vital to seek help. Ask your early childhood nurse if there is any local support for parents of crying babies. Some areas run a telephone helpline.

If your baby is crying and you feel that you can no longer cope, hand him or her to someone else to hold. If you are alone, put your baby down in a pram or cot straight away. Make sure he or she is safe and close the door. Go into another room and calm yourself down before going back. Leaving your baby to cry for a short time will not do any harm.

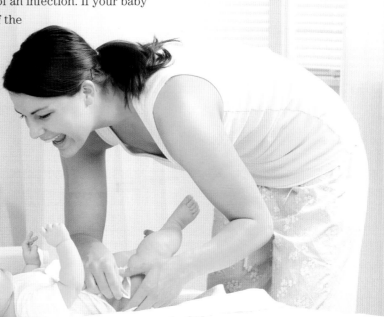

Getting better from common illnesses

Whether it's dealing with a minor illness such as a common cold, or supporting your child as he or she recovers from a more worrying condition such as mumps or chickenpox, on the following pages you'll find plenty of advice to set your child on the road to recovery.

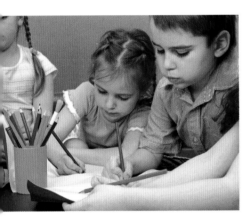

Young children do not have immunity to a wide range of infections so it's not surprising that they go down with lots of coughs and colds. In fact, infants or toddlers may have as many as 12 a year, especially if they attend daycare or preschool or if you have older children, who may bring germs home with them from school.

While a cough or cold is rarely serious, it can sometimes lead to other problems such as feeding difficulties in young babies or sinusitis or a chest infection. Colds can also trigger asthma attacks in susceptible children. Recurrent colds are sometimes blamed on infected tonsils. However, while their removal (tonsillectomy) prevents infections of the tonsils, it has no effect on the frequency of colds or other infections.

Mixing with other children is the natural way to build immunity

WAYS TO SOOTHE A COLD

Colds are caused by a virus so there is no specific medication to help, but there are plenty of ways to make your child feel better:

● Don't force a child with no appetite to eat, but make sure he or she has plenty of fluids – plain water, diluted fruit juices, honey and

 NURSING KNOW-HOW

Easing congestion

If mucus is causing your baby or child to have difficulty breathing at night or when feeding, try squeezing some saline (salt) solution (one or two drops) into each nostril before he or she feeds or settles for the night to clear the nostrils.

To loosen phlegm when an older child has a cough, sit him or her on your knee, leaning slightly forwards, and pat the child's back.

lemon in warm water, and barley water are all excellent options. (Don't give honey to a child under one year old; it can cause serious food poisoning.)

- Raise the head of the cot mattress or bed to help your child to breathe more easily at night.
- Keep air in the bedroom moist with a humidifier.
- Be patient if your child is more clingy than usual. Your undivided attention can be as restorative as any medicine.

COUGHING IT UP

A cough is the body's response to inflammation or irritation in the respiratory tract. In children, coughing is usually simply a symptom of a cold, as mucus drips down the back of the throat (post-nasal drip). Sometimes, however, a persistent cough can be the result of an infection lower down the respiratory tract, asthma or other condition. Make sure your child gets plenty of fluids to maintain hydration and reduce the stickiness of secretions.

Over-the-counter children's cough linctuses do not help the underlying condition, but – for a child over one year old – a honey and lemon drink can be soothing and comforting. (Never give honey to a child who is less than one year old.) Seek medical advice if your child also has difficulty breathing or seems distressed, or if the coughing seems unrelated to a cold.

COULD IT BE CROUP?

Croup occurs when the larynx (voice box) becomes infected, usually by a virus. It typically affects children aged between six months and four years. It causes a harsh, barking cough with a whistling sound when breathing in and usually occurs at night or in the early morning. The condition sounds alarming, but in most cases soon gets better without specific medical treatment.

If your child develops croup, the following simple measures will often ease the problem:
- Hold him or her upright to help ease breathing.
- Seek medical help immediately if your child's breathing becomes rapid or difficult, or if the lips, tongue or skin become grey or bluish.

When to see your doctor

It can be difficult to know, especially with a young baby, when to visit the doctor with coughs and colds. As a general rule, make an appointment if any of the following apply:

- Your baby cannot feed because of a blocked nose.

- Your child has a persistent cough especially at night.

- An apparent cold continues for more than ten days.

- Your child's temperature remains raised for longer than three days.

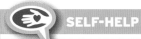

SELF-HELP

Self-help to stop hiccups

Although far from life-threatening, hiccups can be intensely annoying and children tend to get them quite often. One simple thing you can do, which often seems to stop them, is to get your child to put one finger in each ear while you pinch his or her nose, and simultaneously help the child to sip from a glass of water. However, if the hiccups last for more than 24 hours – or if your child has frequently recurring short bouts of hiccups – see a doctor to find out if there is an underlying cause.

Supporting your child's recovery

Whether dealing with a minor cold or a more serious illness, as a parent, you'll want not only to make sure your child recovers speedily, but feels secure and comfortable while healing takes place.

There are plenty of ways you can support children as they get better from either a minor or perhaps a more major illness. Try to adopt a calm, matter-of-fact attitude. This will help you avoid undue stress and will prevent your child picking up on any anxiety. Here are some tips:

- Streamline your life and cut out unnecessary tasks for the time being to enable you to give your child the time and attention he or she needs to make a speedy recovery.
- Keep your child's room at a steady temperature and well-ventilated. Change bedding frequently.
- Expect your child to revert to more babyish behaviour for a while. Be patient and make allowances for this.
- Don't worry if your child doesn't want to eat much. Drinking is more important than eating.
- Provide a treasure bag of special toys. While your child is ill, he or she may want to play with favourite toys he or she enjoyed at an earlier age.
- Watching TV or a DVD can help occupy your child for short periods and enable you to have a break.
- Your child won't be able to concentrate for long so vary activities. It can help to jot down a list of games and toys to inspire you with ideas.
- If your child's illness looks likely to last more than a day or two keep in touch with your own friends to avoid isolation. It may be possible to arrange a babysitter for a short time to enable you to go out.

- As your child begins to feel a little better, he or she can go outside as long as the weather is fine. However, don't let your child go out on foggy or cold days until fully recovered, especially if he or she has had a chest infection.

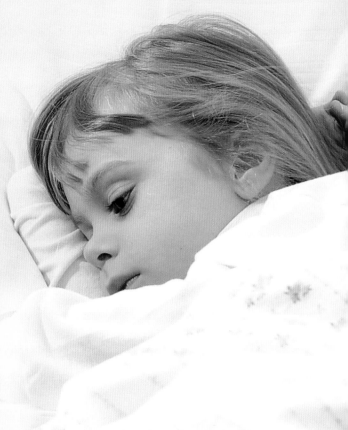

Dealing with feverish illnesses

Children's temperatures can range widely, depending on the time of day and how active they've been. A fever is a core temperature above 38.5°C (see box for how to get an accurate reading). A fever is thought to be part of the body's natural defence and healing mechanism, which is why some experts think it should not be interfered with. Here are a few simple measures you can take to reduce your child's temperature:

- Sponge your child's forehead with lukewarm water – not the whole body as this can cause shivering and goose pimples.
- Encourage your child to drink plenty of fluids to reduce the risk of dehydration, which can occur as a result of sweating.
- Give children's paracetamol or ibuprofen. Don't give both these medicines together, but you can alternate them every 3 hours if you need to, to control fever or pain. Always stick to the dosage on the bottle.
- Dress your child in light clothing and keep the room below 18°C.

FEBRILE CONVULSIONS

Febrile convulsions (fits) are relatively common in small children. Although these can be very frightening to witness, they are rarely life-threatening and do not indicate a serious problem, such as epilepsy. The convulsion is a result of the body overheating and normally stops after a couple of minutes, although for a parent it can feel very much longer. Some children appear more prone to febrile convulsions than others but most grow out of them by the age of five.

Here are some tips on what to do if your child suffers a febrile convulsion:

- Stay calm.
- Put your child on their side in a safe place, preferably on a soft surface on the floor to avoid a fall or other injury.
- Make sure the child's mouth is empty and that he or she can breathe easily. Tilt the head back slightly if possible.
- Call for an ambulance or doctor if your child has never before had a convulsion.

Taking your child's temperature

A fever is a core temperature above 38.5°C, but core readings are difficult to get without specialised equipment. To get the best approximation of a core reading, it's best to take a temperature rectally. Not only is a rectal temperature the best indicator of core temperature, rectal readings are usually more accurate than readings from other sites. Use a probe thermometer with a digital display and follow the manufacturer's instructions.

The next best options are an oral temperature or an under-arm temperature, using a probe thermometer. Use the 38.5°C cut-off for rectal and oral readings. Use a 38°C cut-off for armpit readings, to allow for the fact that the periphery of the body is about half a degree cooler than the core.

Ear and skin thermometers are easy to use but notoriously unreliable. Mercury thermo-meters are not recommended for children or adults because breakages will release poisonous mercury into the body.

CHILDHOOD INFECTIONS THAT CAUSE FEVER

Most common childhood infectious diseases are characterised by a fever. This table includes other symptoms and the home nursing measures that may help to relieve symptoms and hasten recovery. There is also an indication of how long your child is likely to remain infectious.

Illness	Additional symptoms	What to do	Infectious period
Chickenpox	● Sore throat, itchy spots that blister and then form scabs.	● Keep cool and comfortable. ● Offer warm baths with bicarbonate of soda. Apply calamine lotion. Keep fingernails short.	● From one to two days before spots appear until scabs have formed.
Rubella (German measles)	● Sore throat, runny nose, swollen glands, flat, pink rash of fine spots.	● No treatment, but keep the child away from public places and pregnant women for the duration of the rash.	● As long as the rash remains.
Measles	● Cough, sore red eyes, white spots inside mouth; after three or four days, red blotchy rash behind ears spreading to body, sensitivity to light.	● Children's paracetamol or ibuprofen. Clean away any crustiness around eyes using damp cotton wool pad (one for each eye). It's very important to see a doctor so that the diagnosis can be confirmed and the local public health unit notified.	● About five days before the rash appears to five days after its appearance.
Mumps	● Swelling in front of and below one or both ears.	● Plenty of fluids and soft, cold foods. Avoid acidic foods and drinks.	● From two days before swellings appear until they disappear.

ENCOURAGING YOUR CHILD TO EAT OR DRINK

When a child has a feverish illness, he or she may be reluctant to eat or drink. To help speed recovery it is important that your child gets enough fluids – 1 to 1.9 litres of fluid a day depending on age, but this will be greater when there are extra losses due to fever, vomiting or diarrhoea. Provide water or an oral rehydration solution (available from pharmacies). If your child is reluctant to sip from a cup, try offering fluids in an oral syringe, giving about 10 ml every 10 minutes, or an oral rehydration ice block (available from pharmacies). Here are some other suggestions for ways to keep a child nourished and hydrated:

Offer fizzy drinks that have gone flat The sugar can help boost blood glucose, providing energy, and the lack of gas is easier on the digestion. Sports drinks should never be used to rehydrate a child.

Avoid giving milk (except breast milk for breast-fed babies or formula milk for bottle-fed babies) if your child has been vomiting.

Create fun food Arrange sandwiches and small portions of fruit and vegetables to look like a face or an animal.

Serve snacks Provide small, frequent snacks and nutritious but easy-to-digest foods such as soup or fromage frais.

BE MENINGITIS AWARE

Although it is now rare, meningitis (infection of the membranes surrounding the brain) is one of the most frightening possibilities for parents dealing with a feverish child. The symptoms are not always easy to recognise and can appear in any order. They may initially resemble those of other more common illnesses including flu. Doctors always advise caution when there is a possibility of this potentially dangerous infection. If you suspect that your child may have meningitis, it is essential to seek an expert opinion without delay. A child with meningitis will usually appear ill and other symptoms may include:

- fever
- headache
- nausea or vomiting
- muscle pain, with cold hands and feet
- drowsiness and lethargy
- rash (see *Test it with glass*, right).

Contact the Meningitis Centre (www.meningitis.com.au) for more information on this illness.

⊕ NURSING KNOW-HOW

Test it with glass

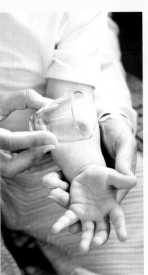

A rash that does not fade under pressure is a sign of meningococcal blood poisoning. There may also be meningitis. If your feverish child has a rash, press the side of a drinking glass firmly against the skin. If the spots do not fade, seek medical help urgently.

Home from hospital

A stay in hospital can be traumatic for a child and stressful for you. The initial cause will be worrying enough, but a separation may add to your anxiety. What is clear is that when children return home from hospital, they need special care, reassurance and nurturing.

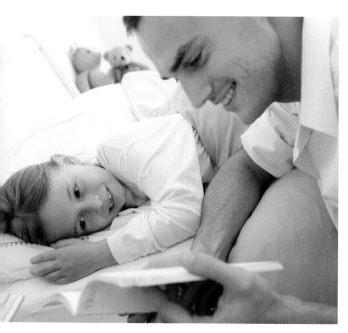

Your recovering child will relish activities such as story telling that feed the imagination

When they've spent time in hospital, as well as needing to complete their physical recovery at home, children may also feel emotionally unsettled and require extra reassurance. A toddler may be clingy and may seem angry with you. It is common for a child to revert to babyish ways and may have wetting accidents even though previously dry. Be patient and ensure that your child – of whatever age – knows that he or she is safe and cared for. The regressive behaviour will soon pass.

There are numerous ways in which you can help to speed up your child's recovery and help him or her get back to normal. Here are some general ideas but obviously your child's age and tastes will have a bearing on what is most effective. More information is available online from www.chw.edu.au/parents/stay/prepare_for_hospital.pdf.

Play along Toys and board games, movies and creative activities such as construction kits, crafts and sticking, colouring and playing with dough can help to stop boredom setting in and divert your child from thinking about his or her illness.

Read all about it Books about hospital can help children to come to terms with their experience.

Be social Children need to feel cared for and connected to their normal life, so make sure they see friends and family but keep an eye on 'visiting times' so they don't get overtired.

Stay close Talk, cuddle and sing to your child to help him or her regain confidence that may have been lost in hospital.

Get in touch with school If your child is of school age, speak to the teacher about work that can be done at home when the child is well enough. This will help a child return to his or her normal routine.

COPING WITH A FRACTURE

Breaking a limb is one of the most common reasons for children to be admitted to hospital. Once discharged with the fracture protected by a plaster or similar support, life can return to some semblance of normality. But you should be aware of potential problems to look out for:

- Some pain is normal but if it seems excessive, call the doctor, who will recommend a painkiller.
- If your child's fingers or toes turn white, purple or blue, the cast may be too tight – call the doctor.
- If the skin around the plaster looks red or raw, the plaster may have become wet inside from sweat or water – call the doctor.

While it's important to encourage a child to cope independently, you'll need to be ready to help with everyday activities and moving around, depending on which limb or area has been affected, as well as the child's age.

KEEPING PAIN AT BAY

If the reason for your child's hospital stay was an operation or injury, when he or she comes home, there may still be some discomfort. Children feel pain, and research shows it can be worse the younger they are. This could be because they are less likely to understand what is happening. Discuss the need for pain relief with the doctors and nurses before you leave the hospital and make sure you know what pain relief to give and when. Here are some tips to help keep your child pain free or at least keep the pain under control.

- Give regular doses of painkillers initially to prevent the pain becoming unmanageable.
- Be alert. A child who is feeling pain may deny it if the medicine is unpalatable. Look out for signs such as fidgeting, stillness, crying, pallor or shallow breathing.
- A reward chart can encourage children to take their medicine.
- Contact your doctor if the recommended pain relief does not seem to be working.

Top Tips

After tonsillectomy

Removal of the tonsils, sometimes along with the adenoids, is a common operation during childhood. Here are some useful tips for the recovery period:

- It's important for children to eat solid foods to speed the healing process. Surprisingly, scratchy foods such as crisps are a good choice - their abrasive texture promotes healing. Give plenty of plain fluids but avoid anything acidic, such as orange juice.
- Pain may increase during the first week after surgery, but should gradually improve during the second week. Offer pain relief if necessary.
- If your child starts to feel ill, develops a fever or has smelly breath, it could indicate an infection. You may have been given an emergency number for the ENT department, but if not contact your GP or take your child to the emergency department.
- If there is any bleeding from the throat call 000 or go to your nearest emergency department.
- Keep your child off school for two weeks to reduce the risk of picking up an infection.
- Ensure your child cleans his or her teeth regularly to help fight infection.
- Earache is common after a tonsillectomy and is no cause for concern but may require pain relief.

Adjusting to allergies

Conditions such as asthma and eczema affect around one in four people at some time in life. As many as half of all sufferers develop symptoms during childhood. Many children grow out of them, but timely diagnosis and treatment can make a huge difference to your child's quality of life.

! ALERT

Asthma warning

If your child needs to use a reliever inhaler three or more times a week, it is possible that the asthma is not being controlled properly. Ask your doctor or asthma nurse to arrange a review.

Asthma action

Asthma occurs in a susceptible child when he or she comes into contact with airborne allergens, leading to symptoms of wheezing, coughing and breathlessness. Common asthma allergens include pollen, certain foods, some medications, animal hair and dander (scales shed from animal skin). Colds and flu can also trigger an attack. Although asthma can't be completely cured, the use of medication and the reduction or avoidance of environmental 'triggers' can enable your child to have a happy, normal childhood. Work closely with the doctor and asthma nurse to develop a personalised action plan. For a downloadable plan, visit the Asthma Foundation's website at www.asthmafoundation.org.au/asthma_action_plan.aspx, which also provides useful information about the condition.

KEEPING ATTACKS TO A MINIMUM

If your child has been diagnosed with asthma you are bound to be concerned. It is a condition that can very suddenly become life threatening. The key to managing asthma and minimising attacks – or even avoiding them entirely – is knowledge of the illness in general and how it affects your child in particular. Here are some pointers:

- Learn to recognise warning signs such as sneezing or a runny nose. You may be able to stop an attack in its tracks by using the appropriate medication promptly.
- Keep a diary to identify triggers and situations that set off an attack.
- Protect your child as well as possible from known allergens.
- Rid your house of dust traps, in particular, keep your child's bedroom dust free (see *Allergy action*, page 47).
- Keep your child active – swimming and walking are good options. Anything too strenuous, however, can trigger an attack.
- Monitor your child's weight. Carrying excess weight can force lungs to work harder.

- Help your child avoid stress, which can often trigger an attack, and offer reassurance if he or she appears anxious.
- Attend regular appointments with your doctor or asthma nurse to ensure your child's asthma plan continues to meet his or her needs.
- Don't overprotect your child. Encourage him or her to join in normal activities as much as possible.

Other allergies

Common allergic reactions in childhood include allergic rhinitis (the most common type is hay fever) and skin reactions, notably eczema. Food reactions are also becoming increasingly common among children, although not all of these are true allergies.

HELP FOR HAY FEVER

The symptoms of hay fever, a form of allergic rhinitis, are caused by an allergic reaction to grass, tree or plant pollens, which is why this condition occurs during spring and summer. If your child has hay fever symptoms all year round he or she may have perennial allergic rhinitis, often a result of a dust-mite allergy. Here are some tips to help you reduce the impact of hay fever on your child:

Make a record Keep a diary to detect which particular pollen or pollens affect your child most. If symptoms are worse in spring, tree pollens may be the culprit. If he or she is affected after you have mown the lawn, grass pollen could be the trigger.

Check the pollen counts These are published in newspapers, on TV, radio and online every day during the spring and summer. Visit www.weatherzone.com.au/pollen-index.

Keep it out Reduce pollen levels inside by closing windows when the pollen count is highest: early morning and late afternoon and evening.

Get expert advice Ask your doctor about antihistamine medications and discuss whether 'desensitisation' treatment may help.

Be dust alert If you think your child's symptoms are due to a dust-mite allergy, follow the advice on page 47.

SELF-HELP

Dealing with an asthma attack

Make sure that you and anyone else who has regular care of your child - for example, other family members, childminder, daycare, preschool or school - knows what to do if he or she has an attack. Here are some key action pointers:

- Administer inhalers and other medications according to instructions you have been given by your doctor or asthma nurse.
- Encourage your child to sit upright.
- Stay with your child until the attack subsides.
- Seek urgent medical help if symptoms do not abate within 5-10 minutes.

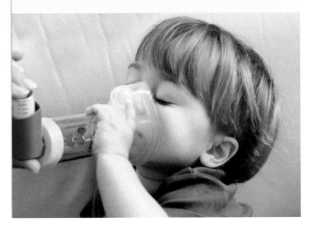

! ALERT

Allergic shock

Some children with a severe food allergy may develop anaphylaxis (severe swelling of the airways and shock) after eating a particular food. This is an emergency - dial 000 or get your child to your nearest emergency department as soon as possible.

COPING WITH ECZEMA

Eczema is a skin rash that is often linked to allergy. It often first occurs in babyhood. Symptoms include a dry, red, scaly rash that may begin on the face and head or the forearms and lower legs. Symptoms often come and go and may be exacerbated by factors such as cold, wind, stress and certain foods. Eggs, milk, seafood and peanuts are all common culprits. Many children grow out of eczema as their immune system becomes better able to deal with 'foreign' substances. Here are ways you can help if your child is affected:

- Keep skin well moisturised at all times. Look out for over-the-counter creams and ointments. Your doctor may prescribe a mild steroid cream or ointment. Follow the instructions carefully.
- Oral antihistamines can help to relieve troublesome symptoms such as itching, especially at night – they can cause drowsiness so have the added benefit of helping your child to sleep.
- Ask the doctor whether skin preparations containing 'immuno-modulators' (medications that help control inflammation and reduce immune-system reactions) are appropriate for your child.
- Keep your child's skin from coming into contact with potentially irritating products such as soap and bubble baths.
- Keep your child's bedroom cool – use cotton sheets and a light doona.
- Keep pets out of the bedroom.
- Keep your child cool. Do not overheat your home or give your child hot baths. Cotton clothing is best – avoid wool next to the skin.
- Keep fingernails short and put scratch mittens on a baby. Discourage an older child from scratching and praise their restraint.
- Try to pinpoint triggers. Keeping a diary can help but don't get stressed if you cannot track down a particular factor. To find out more visit www.eczema.org.au.
- Eczema sufferers may have low levels of gamma-linolenic acid (GLA), which is found in evening primrose oil, starflower oil and blackcurrant seed oil. Ask your doctor if it might be advisable to give your child supplements.

ADVERSE FOOD REACTIONS

Not all reactions to food are due to a true food allergy. A food allergy occurs when your child's immune system reacts to a particular food by producing IgE antibodies every time that food is eaten. Common culprits include milk, eggs, fish, nuts, citrus fruits, tomatoes, sesame and soy. Although a third of parents remove foods from their child's diet because they believe they cause an allergic reaction, only around

GETTING A REACTION

Check this chart for clues to the type of adverse food reaction that
may be affecting your child if he or she has symptoms.

Illness	Food allergy	Food intolerance	Coeliac disease
Common symptoms	● eczema – especially on the face in babies ● rash around mouth ● bumpy, itchy rash (urticaria or hives) anywhere ● swelling ● vomiting ● breathing difficulty	● irritability or crying, sleep disturbance ● abdominal pain ● vomiting ● diarrhoea ● headaches	● fatigue ● bloating ● abdominal cramps ● diarrhoea ● constipation
Age of onset	● under 2	● any age	● any age
Management	● complete avoidance of identified allergens	● diet modification with help of dietitian or clinical nutritionist	● gluten-free diet

3 per cent of children have a true food allergy. Food allergy can be
diagnosed by skin prick tests – when a small amount of the food is
placed on your child's skin and the skin is pricked to see if a reaction
develops. Other tests include blood tests to measure IgE and checking
the response when a food is withheld and then reintroduced.

Food intolerances and sensitivity are reactions caused by
food additives and naturally occurring food chemicals.
Coeliac disease – an autoimmune disease in which
gluten in food causes inflammation of the gut
– is another potential problem. Experts
often refer to all these abnormal
responses to food as adverse food
reactions. The possible symptoms
are listed in the table, above.

A food allergy or
intolerance needn't
spoil the fun of food

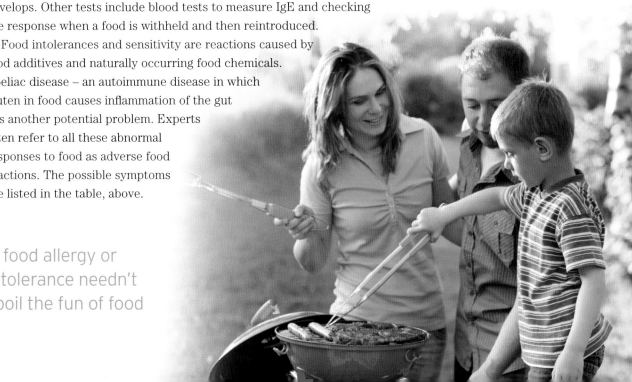

Supporting your diabetic child

Type 1 diabetes affects over 122,300 people in Australia and is one of the most common chronic diseases in children. Helping your child to accept and manage this lifelong condition will provide an invaluable contribution to his or her future health.

SELF-HELP

Injecting a baby or small child

Hold your baby or child firmly over your lap while giving the injection. Be sure to rotate injection sites - stomach, bottom, thighs and arms (see *Bear it in mind*, facing page). An insulin pen is usually easiest to manage and some have the advantage of delivering half units.

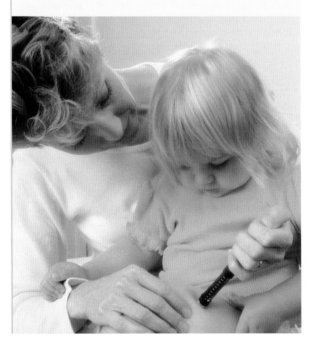

Type 1 is the form of diabetes most often linked to onset in childhood. However, today increasing numbers of children and teenagers are being diagnosed with type 2 diabetes – a phenomenon linked to the growing numbers of youngsters who are overweight (see also *Getting the better of diabetes*, pages 100–119). Other types of diabetes are secondary diabetes (caused by another disease or as a side affect of a medication); gestational diabetes mellitus (which occurs in pregnancy) and impaired glucose metabolism (sometimes called pre-diabetes).

Learning that your child has diabetes can spark a range of emotions – from guilt to fear and anger. You may mourn the loss of your child's health and wonder how you and your child will ever deal with injections, blood testing and other issues. Remember your child's diabetes care team is there to help you and support your child. Here are some tips:

- Learn as much as you can about diabetes. Contact the Juvenile Diabetes Research Foundation (www.jdrf.org.au) or Diabetes Australia (www.diabetes australia.com.au; 1300 136 588).
- Encourage your child to visit the Australian Diabetes Council's website for children and teens, www.diabeteskidsandteens.com.au.
- Involve your child with the management of diabetes so he or she is familiar with what to do when old enough to manage it alone.

- Make sure your doctor refers you and your child to a structured education program to learn how to manage diabetes.
- Other parents of children with diabetes can be supportive. Ask your doctor or diabetes specialist nurse if there are any family or children's support groups in your area.
- Talk to teachers, friends and family about how your child's condition should be managed at school and make sure they know what to do if your child has a hypo (a drop in blood glucose).

DIFFERENT AGES AND STAGES

Diabetes can be challenging however old your child. But the toddler years – when your child may not understand why he or she has to have injections and blood samples taken – and the teens can be especially difficult. Teenagers do not like to be different from their friends and may rail against the inevitable restrictions diabetes places on their life, and rebel against your attempts to offer advice and help. The physical changes of puberty can also make diabetes more difficult to control. The Juvenile Diabetes Research Foundation has fact sheets, a blog, a peer support program, and information for adults and kids (www.jdrf.org.au).

INSULIN AND YOUR CHILD

In the same way as adults with type 1 diabetes, children have to take daily insulin either by injection or insulin pump. Your child may find the first few injections distressing but as you both become used to it and relax, it will get easier. To help ease your child's anxiety:

Be positive Encourage your child to think of injections as a fact of life and give praise afterwards.

Make no excuses Don't give in to delays or excuses. If your child wants to grumble about the injection, insist this is done after the injection.

Address fears If your child has a severe fear of needles, discuss this with the diabetes health-care team. An insulin pump (see page 306) might be suitable for your child.

BEAR IT IN MIND

It's important to vary the insulin injection site to avoid small lumps building up under the skin that can impede insulin absorption. To aid rotation, children are usually shown a picture of a human figure with injection sites identified within a grid. But children often find it hard to use this kind of aid. A 1996 study from the University of Florida found that children aged 6–11 years were more successful at finding the right sites when they marked injection sites on a pair of 'injection teddy bears'.

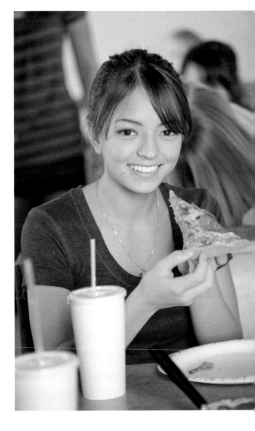

Teenagers with diabetes can learn to manage their condition with confidence

Testing a baby's blood glucose

Babies cannot tell you if they feel hungry or thirsty so you may have to check blood glucose levels more often than you would with an older child. It may be easier to draw blood from a baby's heel or toes. The diabetes nurse can show you how to do this. Keep a record of test results to help you detect patterns of blood glucose levels. This can help you to reduce the number of tests.

GOING IT ALONE

As your child gets older and more independent, he or she may decide to self-inject. Never force this – give your child time to decide when he or she is ready. The diabetes health-care team will help with the transition but you must supervise. Here are some tips:

Help your child to work out how much insulin is needed.

Encourage your child to choose the injection site.

Teach him or her how to draw insulin into the delivery device and inject insulin – it can help to practise on an orange.

USING A PUMP

Insulin pump therapy (continuous subcutaneous insulin infusion) can make diabetes easier to control and enable your child to have a more flexible lifestyle. It's suitable for babies, young children and teenagers but not everyone is eligible for a government-funded pump; the best person to discuss it with is your child's endocrinologist. You can pay for a pump yourself, but it is expensive.

MONITORING BLOOD GLUCOSE

Regular blood glucose monitoring is an important part of blood glucose control (see page 105). Your child's diabetes health-care team can show you how to test blood glucose (see also the panel, left) and advise on devices to take blood from parts of the body other than the finger.

WHEN A CHILD WITH DIABETES BECOMES ILL

If your child becomes ill, his or her blood glucose levels may either rise or fall, so testing is especially important. Be certain always to have the right testing equipment to hand. Here are some suggestions to help maintain your child's diabetic control during bouts of illness:

- Check your child's blood glucose levels frequently.
- If eating or keeping food down is a problem, you can replace

 NURSING KNOW-HOW

Glucose testing made easy

Try to test your child's blood glucose at times when he or she is relaxed and in a good mood. It is important that the test doesn't become a battleground. Here are some tips:

- Make sure your child's hands are warm – it is difficult to draw blood from cold hands and it hurts more.
- Wash your own and your child's hands in water before you begin. Don't use baby wipes as they contain glycerine and could affect the result.
- To minimise pain, prick the side of the finger rather than the middle.
- Avoid pricking the index finger or thumb and use a different finger and part of the finger each time.
- If it is hard to draw blood, ask your child to hold the hand downwards to encourage blood to flow into the fingers.
- Encourage your child to help you put the blood on a testing strip.

meals with drinks that contain carbohydrates, or soft foods such as yoghurt. If your child is being violently or regularly sick, contact your GP or diabetes health-care team.

● If your child has type 1 diabetes, you'll need to test the urine or blood for ketones to find out if the diabetes is uncontrolled. You can obtain the test strips on prescription.

● Continue to give insulin or tablets as normal, but the dose can be adjusted in response to blood glucose test results.

YOUR CHILD'S DIABETES-FRIENDLY DIET

You don't need to feed your child special foods if he or she has diabetes – just provide a healthy, balanced diet as you would for any other child. A registered paediatric dietitian can help you plan your child's meals. Diabetic children should also have a regular review with the dietitian to adjust their diet to meet their needs as they grow. See *Eating your way better,* page 108, for more on eating with diabetes. The following tips may also help:

Keep meals regular Make sure your child eats regularly.

Go low GI Base meals around low-GI (glycaemic index) starchy foods (see *The GI factor*, page 110) and offer plenty of vegetables and fruit.

Reduce fats Cut down on saturated (animal) and trans fats (in processed foods).

Watch sugar intake Keep sugary foods for special treats – and look for low-sugar, low-fat versions of cakes and biscuits, or bake your own. Choose sugar-free or low-sugar drinks as sugar in liquid is absorbed quickly and can push up blood glucose levels.

ACTIVITY MATTERS

Regular physical activity is important for any child and diabetic children are no exception. Aim for your child to have a minimum of an hour of brisk exercise every day. But be aware that physical activity causes a fall in blood glucose and it can take trial and error to balance food intake, insulin and exercise.

If your child is more active than planned, he or she risks having a hypo (see *Managing hypos*, page 107, to find out more about recognising and dealing with hypos). To avoid a hypo:

Check your child's blood glucose before and after activity.

Increase the amount your child eats before exercise.

Reduce your child's insulin dose before exercise.

Teach your child to avoid strenuous activity when insulin action is at its peak – usually up to 2 hours after an insulin injection.

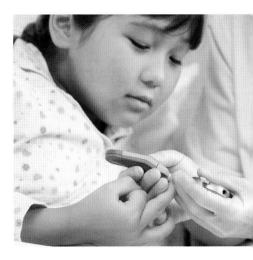

Teach your child to take an interest in the results of his or her blood glucose tests

Encouraging psychological health

Australian research shows that 14 per cent of Australian children and adolescents aged 4 to 17 experience mental health problems. The best chance of a full recovery is when the whole family is involved in the treatment strategy.

It's relatively easy to tell if your child is physically unwell. However, it can be more difficult to detect a psychological problem. Left untreated, psychological difficulties can lead to school failure, alcohol or drug abuse, family discord, violence or even suicide. Bleak though this sounds, the chances of recovery are greatly increased if a supportive parent is actively involved.

A child with ADHD can make progress with the help of specialist teachers

ATTENTION DEFICIT HYPERACTIVITY DISORDER (ADHD)

Attention deficit hyperactivity disorder (ADHD), attention deficit disorder (ADD) or hyperkinetic disorder are the terms used to describe children who are much more active and/or impulsive than you would expect for their age, and whose behaviour affects their relationships as well as their learning.

If you suspect your child has ADHD (see ADHD indicators, facing page), consult your GP, who may refer your child to a child psychologist for assessment. There is no specific test. The psychologist will observe your child; you can help by describing his or her behaviour. The doctor will also request a report from your child's school. The Australian government has a useful information page (www.health.nsw.gov.au/PublicHealth/Pharmaceutical/ adhd/faqs.asp), as do many children's health organisations, such as the Royal Children's Hospital (www.rch.org.au/kidsinfo/fact_sheets/ADHD_an_overview).

HELPING A HYPERACTIVE CHILD

There is much that you as a parent can do to help make life easier for you and your child. Medication (methylphenidate or dexamphetamine) is prescribed for some children with this condition but drug treatment is by no means the only approach. Here are some suggestions for measures you can put in place at home and in partnership with your child's school and GP:

Watch additives Some children with ADHD may be sensitive to sugar and caffeine. Certain food additives may also exacerbate symptoms. Keep a food diary and discuss patterns with a dietitian.

Get fishy According to research, omega-3 supplements can help some children with ADHD, although more studies are needed. Always check with a dietitian before making changes to your child's diet.

Structure it A structured environment and clear understanding of what behaviour is acceptable and what behaviour is not can help your child feel secure.

Work with your child's school Talk to the school about whether they can provide extra help in certain subjects or skills. Obtaining a statement of special educational needs is often a way to access extra help for your child. An educational psychologist may be assigned to monitor your child and suggest ways forward.

Talking it through Your GP or your child's psychiatrist may suggest talking therapy to help your child deal with symptoms such as impulsiveness. Family therapy can also help.

AUTISTIC SPECTRUM DISORDERS

A child with an autistic spectrum disorder (ASD) does not have the same social and communication skills as other children and has difficulty relating to others. As the name suggests, ASDs cover a wide spectrum of difficulties with communication, social development and behaviour. Full-blown autism causes difficulty communicating and interacting with other people and possibly learning difficulties. At the other end of the spectrum, Asperger's syndrome is less severe. Children with Asperger's, while having problems with social interaction and communication, tend to have better language skills, average or above average intelligence and do not have learning disabilities.

RECOGNISING ASD

Although ASD can only be diagnosed by a clinician, parents obviously know their children best and may be the first to realise there's a problem. Clues that a child may have an ASD include:
● Failure to develop speech or non-verbal communication skills (e.g. pointing, clapping, waving) at the usual age. In older children, difficulty understanding meaning and failing to understand jokes or 'read' body language.

ADHD indicators
The following are types of behaviour to look out for that might indicate ADHD, particularly if they are persistent and exaggerated:

● restlessness, fidgeting and overactivity
● talking and interrupting people
● difficulty concentrating (being easily distracted and not finishing tasks)
● impulsiveness ('acting without thinking')
● problems taking turns – in games, conversations or queues
● aggression and disruptive behaviour
● clumsiness
● recklessness
● irritability
● emotional immaturity.

- Problems interacting with others and making friends, which may be linked to difficulties understanding how other people feel (empathy) and adjusting to new situations.
- Finding it hard to understand 'rules', causing problems at school.
- Inability to manage their own emotions, including sudden outbursts of anger or aggression. Resistance to affection.
- Children with an ASD may show little or no interest in social play, such as 'let's pretend' games. Instead they may become interested in repetitive activities and develop obsessive interests such as collecting stamps, plane spotting or storing trivia.
- Other clues include failure to reach developmental milestones such as sitting up, crawling or walking; over or undersensitivity to sensations such as sound, touch, smell or taste; strange behaviour such as rocking backwards and forwards, head banging or walking on tiptoes; clumsiness; and attachment to routine.

HELPING A CHILD WITH ASD

Having a child with ASD can be particularly demanding for a parent. Get all the information you can. Practical advice and information is available from www.autismawareness.com.au and www.autism spectrum.org.au.

Stay on your child's side Recognise his or her difficulties and find ways to structure the environment to minimise challenging behaviour. Praise good behaviour, stay positive and take small steps.

Get help with behaviour Applied behaviour analysis (ABA) begun before the age of five teaches basic social, educational and daily life skills, which can reduce problem behaviour. Ask your doctor to refer you to a child psychologist.

Be a partner in play Learn as much as you can about the best ways to communicate with your child. Be their partner in play and give your child extra time when playing or doing everyday tasks to enable him or her to think about what to say. Speech therapy may also help.

Get support There are many ways of dealing with ASD and lots of help available for parents, so there's no need to feel alone. You may be entitled to benefits such as a carer's pension to help cover the extra expenses involved in caring for your child. Your health professional can advise.

HELPING A CHILD WITH DEPRESSION

All children have ups and downs but if your child or teenager is experiencing more persistent low moods, withdrawal, over or under-eating, sleeping all the time or other changes in behaviour or

Teach your child

A child with ASD should have an educational assessment (statement) and be entitled to educational support whether he or she goes to a mainstream or special school. Many schools now use TEACCH (Treatment and Education of Autistic and Communication-Handicapped Children), which provides the structured environment in which autistic children thrive best. Parents act as 'co-therapists' to ensure consistency between home and school.

personality lasting two weeks or more, he or she could be depressed. Your GP can help and may refer your child to a paediatrician or child psychologist. Here are some tips to enable you to help your child:

Be honest If your child's depression has been sparked off by a family trauma such as a divorce, be honest and keep him or her in touch with what is happening. Hiding what is going on will only make things worse.

Provide the words Young children may not have the vocabulary to express feelings such as sadness, anger or confusion. Help your child to find the words he or she needs to describe feelings.

Provide a shoulder to cry on Let your child know that you are there to talk to. If your child does not want to talk to you, another parent, teacher or family friend may be willing to listen.

Get them moving Exercise can help children get rid of pent-up feelings as it encourages the release of feel-good hormones.

Be alert for changes in eating habits Eating disorders such as anorexia often first occur in the teenage years (see page 254).

Read all about it Many children find it helpful to read about other children who have experienced similar problems – ask your local librarian or children's bookseller for age-appropriate books.

Take a break

Caring for a child with long-term emotional or psychological problems is difficult, so take regular breaks to look after yourself. And you may need a longer respite from your child from time to time. Get in touch with your local social services department to find out what's available in your area.

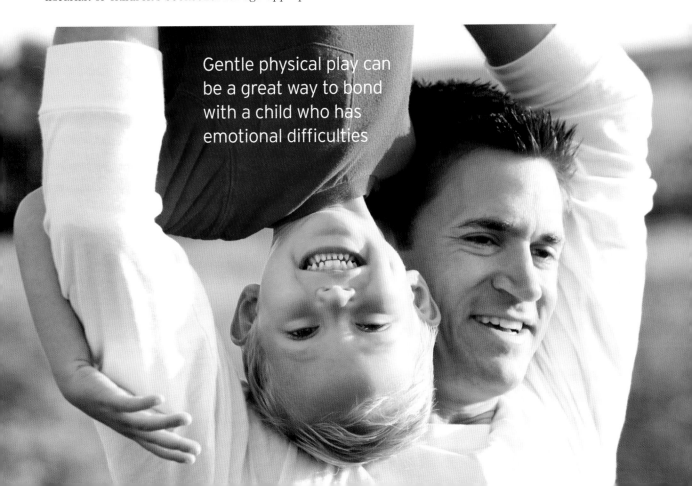

Gentle physical play can be a great way to bond with a child who has emotional difficulties

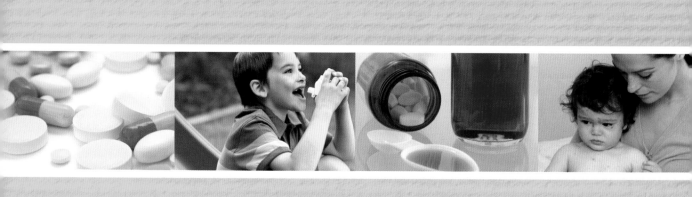

part 3
get the most from your medicine

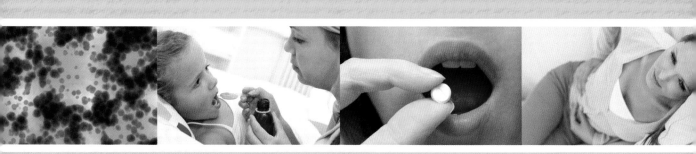

Understanding your medications

Whether you've been given a prescription by your doctor or have bought an over-the-counter medicine for a minor complaint, you need the right information to help you use your medications safely and effectively and give yourself the best chance of a swift recovery.

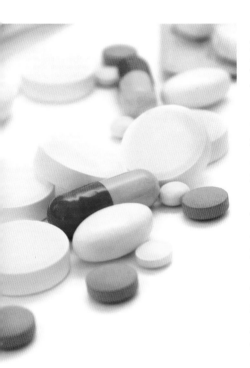

WHAT'S IN A NAME?

Medications can be divided into those that only a doctor (or other health professional) can give you – prescription-only medicines (POM) – and those that you can buy for yourself from a pharmacy, supermarket or corner shop – over-the-counter (OTC) medications. Generally POMs are more powerful than OTC drugs and their use has to be carefully monitored. OTC products can also be prescribed, which may happen if you're entitled to free prescriptions. Or sometimes, your pharmacist may offer you an OTC variant of a prescribed medication if it is cheaper.

In the listings on the following pages, medication names that start with a lower case letter are generic – the official medical name for the active ingredient. The capitalised names in the tables are brand-name products, and there may be more than one of these containing the same generic ingredient. Each drug company that markets a medication will use a different brand name. The tables on the following pages include selected brand names of each generic medication. A separate listing includes medicines that can be bought over the counter. If you want to know whether the medicine you have been prescribed is a generic or brand-name product, ask your pharmacist.

SAME MEDICATION, DIFFERENT APPEARANCE

Most medications for home use are taken by mouth as tablets, capsules or liquids. A notable exception is insulin, which is injected. Medications for skin problems are usually applied topically in the form of a cream, gel or lotion. Other forms of everyday medication include skin patches, nasal drops and sprays, mouth sprays, eye drops, suppositories and pessaries (for vaginal problems). Less commonly, medications for some more serious conditions are administered via a fine tube directly into the blood supply. Some medications are available in more than one form so if you have difficulty swallowing, for example, you might be able to receive your medication by injection or suppository. It is always worth asking your doctor if there is a different form available if you have difficulty taking the medication.

GETTING THE RIGHT DOSAGE

If the medicine has been prescribed, details of the dosage will be clearly printed on the package or container of your medicine. There may also be information about whether to take the medication before, with or after food. Following the guidelines for timing is important as it can help the absorption of the active ingredient and reduce side effects, particularly those affecting the digestive system.

If you accidentally miss a dose, refer to the accompanying leaflet or speak to your doctor or pharmacist. If you mistakenly take too much of a medication, speak to a health professional, but if you develop severe symptoms, go to your nearest emergency department without delay. A prescribed medication should never be stopped without the advice of your doctor. You risk a recurrence of the condition or, in some cases, a reaction to withdrawal from the medication.

WHAT ELSE ARE YOU TAKING?

The vast majority of medications are unaffected by what you eat. There are, however, some groups of medications that can interact with substances in certain foods or drinks. Always check the leaflet that comes with your medicine to find out if there are any food interactions.

You should also be aware that alcohol can interact with some medications. Make sure that you know it is safe to drink before you do so, and bear in mind that the medication can remain in your system for a day or two after you stop taking it.

Interactions with other medications are an important consideration. Always let your doctor or pharmacist know if you are taking any other medicines. This can be particularly important in the elderly who are often taking a variety of medications. It is best to avoid taking any herbal products while you are taking medication prescribed by your doctor, as there is a risk that these could affect the efficacy of the medication. Ask your pharmacist for advice.

SPECIAL CONCERNS FOR WOMEN

If you are pregnant or breastfeeding, there are many medications that can potentially affect your foetus or baby either through your bloodstream or breast milk. It is vital to discuss an existing or new medication

Top Tips

Top tips for taking medicines

Follow these simple rules to avoid problems and give the medicine the best chance of working:

- Always read the leaflet that comes in the pack.

- Never guess or estimate doses for liquid medicines – use the spoon, syringe or pot supplied.

- Take the medicine at the intervals prescribed, even if it means setting your alarm for the middle of the night.

- 'Before food' or 'on an empty stomach' means at least an hour before eating; 'with food' means halfway through or after a meal or snack.

- Do not crush pills that are supposed to be 'swallowed whole'.

- If your medication can be taken at any time, try to have it at the same time of day so you don't forget.

- Never share medicines with other people.

- Always throw away or return to the pharmacy any leftover medicines and drugs that are past their 'use by' date.

regime with your doctor. Women who are on long-term drug treatment for a chronic health condition should also tell their doctor if they plan to stop using contraception in order to start a family. Their medication regime may need to be changed to avoid any unwanted effects on the pregnancy or newly conceived foetus.

If you are taking oral contraceptives, you should mention this to the doctor or pharmacist when any new medication is prescribed, as there may be an interaction that reduces the effectiveness of the contraception. You may be advised to use an alternative method for the duration of the medication treatment.

LONG-TERM HEALTH PROBLEMS

Certain long-term (chronic) health problems – in particular, liver and kidney disease – can affect how the body processes or reacts to certain medications, possibly reducing their effectiveness or leading to an increased risk of adverse effects. And, if you have such a condition, this could be the reason why your doctor may be unwilling to prescribe a particular medication. Always be sure to tell a doctor who may be unfamiliar with your case (for example, any doctor you consult while on holiday) if you have any long-term condition.

HAZARDOUS ACTIVITIES

A large number of medications, especially painkillers, sleeping medications and certain antihistamines, can affect your ability to drive and operate machinery. Check the information leaflet or speak to your doctor or pharmacist if you are unsure about its possible effects.

UNWANTED EFFECTS

Medications are strong chemicals that can affect other parts of your body in addition to the targeted organ or system. The majority of side effects will reduce over time, so unwanted effects from medications taken long term for chronic conditions usually become less noticeable. The aim is always to find the medication that best deals with your symptoms and has the least troublesome side effects. It can sometimes take trial and error to reach a good balance.

Severe and sudden reactions are likely to be allergic reactions and must be dealt with immediately in hospital. A small number of people have life-threatening reactions to certain medications – for example, to penicillins and related antibiotics. If you go into hospital, always make sure you tell the medical staff of any known medication allergies.

Directory of drug groups

On the following pages you will find a listing of the principal groups of drugs, and a selection of common prescription and over-the-counter medicines, used at home for treating the wide variety of conditions covered by this book. They appear under eight headings which reflect the type of disorder, or the part of the body or body system they treat. Cancer drugs have not been included because they are given under the supervision of the hospital oncology team; advice on dealing with the side effects of chemotherapy is given in Chapter 7, *Confronting cancer*, pages 168–195. Contraceptive hormones are also omitted because they are not generally used to promote recovery from an illness.

Antibacterials

Antibacterials (including antibiotics) work by killing the bacteria that cause infection, or preventing them from multiplying, so that the body's natural defences can take over and kill the bacteria. These drugs kill only bacteria and so cannot be used to combat colds and flu, which are caused by a virus (see *Antivirals*, facing page). Antibiotics – a term often used synonymously with antibacterials – were originally extracted from moulds and fungi. Today nearly all antibiotics are synthesised.

TYPES

There are many different types of antibacterial, each of which targets a different range of bacteria. Amoxicillin, for example, belongs to the group of antibacterials called penicillins. It is used to fight a wide range of infections in the ear, nose and throat, the respiratory tract, on the skin, in the kidneys, urinary and genital tracts, and in the bones and joints. Nitrofurantoin, by contrast, has a more limited range of applications and is used mainly to combat urinary tract infections.

In practice, doctors often prescribe initially according to the site of the infection and the nature and severity of the symptoms. The choice of antibacterial is also influenced by the patient's underlying health – for example, if they have poor kidney or liver function, or if pregnant. It is common for the drug to be changed during the course of treatment once the precise cause is known, or if the first choice of antibacterial doesn't have the anticipated effect.

HOW TAKEN

For treatment at home, antibacterials are usually given in tablet or capsule form, but injections are sometimes used for high doses. Some antibacterials can only be administered by intravenous drip in hospital. For children, many of these drugs can be given in liquid form (suspension). Antibacterials are also an ingredient in topical treatments, such as creams or drops, for localised infections of the skin, eyes and ears.

POSSIBLE SIDE EFFECTS

Some people are allergic to specific antibacterials – drugs in the penicillin group are those that most commonly produce an allergic response. Be sure to tell any new doctor if you've previously had a reaction to any antibacterial. Possible side effects for specific groups are:

Aminoglycosides Possible hearing damage, particularly in the elderly.

Anti-tuberculosis drugs Headache, rash, nausea and diarrhoea.

Cephalosporins Allergic reaction (especially in those who are allergic to penicillins), diarrhoea, nausea and headache.

Macrolides Nausea and vomiting, abdominal discomfort and diarrhoea.

Penicillins There is a risk of a severe allergic response, including rash, difficulty breathing and, in extreme cases, collapse. Diarrhoea can also occur.

Quinolones Nausea, indigestion, diarrhoea, joint and muscle pain.

Tetracyclines Dizziness and vertigo, nausea, diarrhoea and discomfort on swallowing. Photosensitivity. Should not be taken by young children.

As I feel much better now, can I stop taking my antibiotics?

Always complete the course of antibiotics you have been prescribed to ensure that the infection has been completely eradicated. If you stop taking them early, there is a risk that the infection will return in a more virulent form.

Antivirals

Antiviral drugs may help to reduce the severity and duration of flu symptoms, and are most effective when taken within a few hours of the first signs of infection. Other viral conditions for which GPs prescribe antiviral drugs include herpes simplex infections of the mouth, lips, eyes and genital region and herpes zoster virus infections (shingles or chickenpox). Antivirals to treat HIV infection are outside the scope of this book.

TYPES

The antiviral drug you are prescribed will depend on the type of infection. Oseltamivir and zanamivir are used to treat flu, aciclovir may be prescribed for herpes simplex infections, and famciclovir is used for herpes zoster infections or genital herpes.

HOW TAKEN

Antiviral drugs are commonly given as tablets, creams or eye ointments. Zanamivir is administered via an inhaler.

POSSIBLE SIDE EFFECTS

Taken by mouth, aciclovir, famciclovir and oseltamivir can cause nausea, vomiting, abdominal pain, diarrhoea and headache. Zanamivir can cause breathing difficulties and rash.

Bronchodilators

These drugs relieve breathlessness by relaxing the muscles surrounding the airways. Bronchodilators are used to treat conditions in which the airways are narrowed or inflamed, including asthma and chronic obstructive pulmonary disease (COPD).

TYPES

Bronchodilators are either short-acting (for the short-term relief of breathlessness) or long-acting (used regularly to help control and prevent symptoms long term). The three main groups are:

Beta-2 agonists These are mainly used to treat asthma attacks. If short-acting, they provide 4–6 hours relief of symptoms; if long-acting, they relieve airway constriction for up to 12 hours.

Anticholinergics or **antimuscarinics** (also called muscarinic antagonists) These drugs are often prescribed to treat COPD.

Xanthines Used in the treatment of COPD and asthma, xanthines are normally prescribed only if other bronchodilators are not effective. This is because of the risk of serious associated side effects (see above right).

HOW TAKEN

Bronchodilators are usually administered via an inhaler or nebuliser, but some are also given as tablets, syrup and injection.

What are the signs that my asthma medication might need to be altered?

If you find that you are needing to use your asthma reliever inhaler more than three times a week, your underlying condition may not be adequately controlled. Ask your GP for a treatment review.

Asthma prevention

Bronchodilators are the mainstay of treatment for asthma attacks but other drugs may be prescribed to prevent attacks. The most common 'preventer' drugs for asthma are corticosteroids (see page 325), administered via an inhaler. These drugs reduce inflammation in the airways and make attacks less likely.

POSSIBLE SIDE EFFECTS

Beta-2 agonists Nervousness, restlessness and trembling, and a dry, irritated throat.

Anticholinergics Dry mouth, constipation, abnormal heart rhythms and headache.

Xanthines Rapid heartbeat, increased blood pressure, restlessness, sleep problems and seizures.

ON PRESCRIPTION

Short-acting beta-2 agonists
salbutamol (Ventolin)
terbutaline (Bricanyl)

Long-acting beta-2 agonists
eformoterol (Foradile, Oxis)
salmeterol (Serevent)

Anticholinergics
ipratropium bromide (Atrovent)
tiotropium (Spiriva)

Xanthines
aminophylline
theophylline (Nuelin SA)

Cough medicines

There is no good evidence that cough suppressants work and they carry a risk of side effects: you're better off with a honey and lemon drink. Expectorants, which are designed to help bring up thick mucus, should only be used if your doctor advises it.

The Therapeutic Goods Administration (TGA) recommends not using cough and cold medicines in children under six years old, while children aged six to 11 should only be given these medicines on the advice of a doctor, pharmacist or nurse practitioner.

HOW TAKEN
Usually as syrup.

POSSIBLE SIDE EFFECTS
Cough suppressants can cause drowsiness.

OVER-THE-COUNTER

Cough suppressants
dextromethorphan (Bisolvon Dry Oral Liquid)
diphenhydramine (Gold Cross Cough Medicine)
pholcodine (Gold Cross Pholcodine Linctus)

Expectorants
guaiphenesin (Robitussin Chest Cough)
ipecacuanha (Gold Cross Ipecacuanha and
   Tolu Mixture)

Is the sugar content of these products a problem for people with diabetes?

Diabetics should choose one of the several sugar-free cough medicines available. Be sure to choose one appropriate for your cough.

Decongestants

A build-up of mucus in the nose, throat, ears and chest is a symptom of disorders such as the common cold, hay fever and other allergies. There are a huge number of proprietary medicines for the relief of colds that contain decongestant drugs to clear mucus from the airways.

TYPES
Over-the-counter decongestants, which work by reducing inflammation in the affected area, can be used to relieve these symptoms.

HOW TAKEN
These preparations are administered for topical application in the form of nasal drops or sprays, or are taken by mouth, usually in multi-ingredient proprietary cold medicines.

POSSIBLE SIDE EFFECTS
Many of these medicines have a stimulant effect, so they should be avoided in the evening. Those who have high blood pressure, a heart condition or thyroid problems should ask the pharmacist for advice before taking a medicine containing decongestants, as they can worsen these conditions. Prolonged (for longer than a week) or over-frequent use can cause further congestion (rebound congestion). Possible side effects of decongestant nasal sprays include irritation to the lining of the nose, headache and nausea.

OVER-THE-COUNTER

Decongestants
phenylephrine (Dimetapp PE Nasal Decongestant,
   Lemsip Cold and Flu)
pseudoephedrine (Sudafed)
xylometazoline (Otrivin)

Antihistamines

Antihistamines are the drugs most commonly used to treat allergic conditions. Examples of the conditions they may be used for include: hay fever; skin allergies; allergic conjunctivitis; insect bites; food allergies. They may also be used to treat nausea (see right) and insomnia (see page 337).

TYPES

All antihistamines work by blocking the effects of a protein called histamine. When histamine is produced, it helps the body to fight infections, but may also lead to other problems, such as swelling or red, swollen and itchy skin. These drugs can be divided into two groups: first and second generation.

HOW TAKEN

They are available in tablet or liquid form and as creams, nasal sprays and eye drops.

POSSIBLE SIDE EFFECTS

Many of the first-generation antihistamines cause drowsiness but second-generation drugs do not have this problem. Other common side effects of first-generation drugs include dry mouth and dizziness. Second-generation antihistamines can have similar effects but these are uncommon.

OVER-THE-COUNTER

First-generation antihistamines
cyclizine (Valoid)
promethazine (Phenergan)

Second-generation antihistamines
cetirizine (Zirtek)
loratadine (Clarityne)

Anti-emetics

Nausea and vomiting are commonly the result of gastrointestinal upsets, but may also be caused by disturbance to the balance mechanism of the inner ear (motion sickness and vertigo) and may accompany migraines.

TYPES

Antihistamines (left) are commonly used to treat nausea and vomiting caused by motion sickness. For nausea caused by other drugs, notably for cancer, you may be prescribed a drug that alters the transmission of nerve signals within the brain.

HOW TAKEN

Most anti-emetics are taken as tablets, but some are given by suppository or injection if vomiting makes administration by mouth ineffective.

POSSIBLE SIDE EFFECTS

Some anti-emetics that act on the brain may cause uncontrolled mouth and tongue movements if taken for a prolonged period.

ON PRESCRIPTION

Drugs that act on neurotransmission
domperidone (Motilium)
granisetron (Kytril)
metoclopramide (Maxolon)
ondansetron (Zofran)
prochlorperazine (Stemetil)

OVER-THE-COUNTER

Antihistamines
promethazine teoclate (Avomine)

Indigestion remedies

Heartburn, nausea and belching are all signs that acid has escaped from the stomach and is causing irritation to other sensitive areas. Healthcare professionals call this indigestion or acid reflux. Indigestion remedies work by reducing or neutralising stomach acid, or by protecting the delicate lining of the digestive tract. Medications within this group are also used in the treatment of peptic ulcers.

Many of these medicines are available over the counter, although some of the stronger preparations may be available only on prescription. Be sure to consult your doctor for a firm diagnosis if you suffer from recurrent indigestion. Even if discomfort is

ON PRESCRIPTION

H2 blockers
cimetidine (Tagamet)
famotidine (Pepcid)

Proton pump inhibitors
esomeprazole (Nexium)
lansoprazole (Zoton)
omeprazole (Losec)
pantoprazole (Somac)
rabeprazole (Pariet)

Ulcer-healing medication
misoprostol (Cytotec)

OVER-THE-COUNTER

Antacids
aluminium hydroxide (Alu-Cap)

H2 blockers
ranitidine (Zantac)

Compound rafting agents
sodium alginate (Gaviscon)

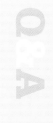

Could other medicines be causing my indigestion?

Several medicines can cause or exacerbate indigestion. Common culprits include aspirin and NSAIDs (see page 335). If you experience symptoms that suggest indigestion in the days or weeks after starting a new medication, be sure to tell your doctor, who may decide to alter your drug treatment.

alleviated by over-the counter remedies, there is a possibility that you have an underlying condition that requires investigation.

TYPES
The most commonly recommended medicines for these conditions fall into two main groups:
Acid reducers These include antacids (which neutralise excess acid), the drug group known as H2 blockers, and proton pump inhibitors (PPIs), which stop acid being produced.
Rafting agents Also known as alginates, these create a thick foam ('raft') that lines the stomach and oesophagus, protecting it from escaping acid. These preparations are usually combined with an antacid.

HOW TAKEN
By mouth. Many of these preparations are taken in liquid form or as chewable tablets.

POSSIBLE SIDE EFFECTS
Serious side effects from indigestion remedies are rare. You may experience the following symptoms: abdominal pain, diarrhoea, constipation, headache, dizziness, rash and tiredness.

Antidiarrhoeals

In treating diarrhoea the priority is to replace lost fluids by drinking plenty of clear fluids. This is particularly important in the very young and the elderly. Antidiarrhoeals are not recommended for the treatment of young children.

TYPES

Treatment is usually with antimotility drugs, which slow down the passage of food through the intestine, giving more time for fluid to be absorbed. Antispasmodics may be prescribed for chronic diarrhoea, which sometimes accompanies long-term bowel disorders such as irritable bowel syndrome.

HOW TAKEN

These drugs are normally taken by mouth (tablets, capsules or in liquid form).

POSSIBLE SIDE EFFECTS

Side effects can include abdominal cramps, dizziness, drowsiness, skin reactions and abdominal bloating. If used excessively, antidiarrhoeals can cause constipation. It is important not to take drugs containing codeine or morphine for prolonged periods as this may lead to dependence.

ON PRESCRIPTION

Antimotility medications
codeine phosphate

Antispasmodics
mebeverine hydrochloride (Colofac)

OVER-THE-COUNTER

Antimotility medications
kaolin and morphine mixture
loperamide (Imodium)

Laxatives

Constipation is characterised by the passing of hard, dry stools, less frequently than normal.

TYPES

There are four main groups: bulking agents, which add bulk to faeces; stimulant laxatives, which speed up passage of faeces through the bowel; faecal softeners, which make the faeces easier to pass; and osmotic laxatives, which work by increasing the amount of water in the large bowel.

HOW TAKEN

Taken by mouth as tablets or in liquid form. It is important to increase fluid intake at the same time as taking laxatives. Some laxatives can take up to 48 hours to act, and they should be used for a maximum of three days, as the body can begin to rely on them.

POSSIBLE SIDE EFFECTS

Laxatives can cause nausea, vomiting, stomach cramps and abdominal pain.

OVER-THE-COUNTER

Bulking agents
ispaghula husk (Fybogel)
sterculia (Normacol)

Stimulant laxatives
bisacodyl (Dulcolax)
docusate sodium (Coloxyl)
senna (Senokot)

Faecal softeners
liquid paraffin

Osmotic laxatives
lactulose (Duphalac)

Antirheumatics

Rheumatoid arthritis is a disease in which the immune system attacks the lining of the joints, causing them to become inflamed. There is no cure for rheumatoid arthritis and treatment aims to reduce pain and stiffness in affected joints as much as possible, prevent further joint damage and minimise any disability. The earlier the drug treatment begins, the more effective it will be.

TYPES

Disease-modifying anti-rheumatic drugs (DMARDs) both help to ease symptoms and slow down the progression of rheumatoid arthritis. It can take 4–6 months before the benefits become noticeable, and some people have to try two or three types before finding the one that works best. Other drugs that may be prescribed are: painkillers (see page 334), including non-steroidal anti-inflammatory drugs (NSAIDs) (see page 335), and corticosteroids (right), to reduce pain, stiffness and swelling.

HOW TAKEN

Most of the drugs in this group are taken as tablets. Etanercept is given by injection.

POSSIBLE SIDE EFFECTS

Loss of appetite, stomach pain and indigestion, stomach ulcers and diarrhoea are among the possible side effects of these drugs.

ON PRESCRIPTION

DMARDs
etanercept (Enbrel)
methotrexate
penicillamine
sulfasalazine (Salazopyrin)

Corticosteroids

Corticosteroid drugs are derivatives or synthetic variants of hormones that are produced naturally by the adrenal glands. They are often simply called steroids and are used to reduce inflammation, suppress allergic reactions and reduce immune system activity.

Corticosteroids reduce inflammation by penetrating certain cells to 'switch off' the mechanisms responsible for releasing inflammatory chemicals. They are commonly prescribed for allergic conditions that cause inflammation, such as asthma, allergic rhinitis (hay fever) and urticaria (hives). Inflammatory skin conditions such as eczema are also often treated with corticosteroids.

These drugs are also used to treat autoimmune disorders, in which the immune system malfunctions and attacks and inflames healthy tissue. These conditions include: rheumatoid arthritis; Crohn's disease, which affects the digestive system; and ulcerative colitis, in which the colon becomes inflamed. Oral corticosteroids are also used to replace or supplement the natural hormones produced by the adrenal glands, when the glands' normal function is reduced.

TYPES

Corticosteroids are subdivided according to whether their action is more similar to that of the natural hormone cortisol (glucocorticoids) or that of aldosterone (mineralocorticoids). Drugs with a strong glucocorticoid action have a more potent anti-inflammatory effect, and are more widely used in the treatment of inflammatory disorders than those with a high mineralocorticoid action.

HOW TAKEN

Corticosteroids are available in a number of different forms including tablets, sprays and inhalers, creams, lotions and injections.

POSSIBLE SIDE EFFECTS

Corticosteroids can have a wide range of side effects, the number and severity depending on the type of corticosteroid and the duration of treatment. Short-term, they can cause an increase in appetite, weight gain, fluid retention, insomnia, and mood changes, such as feeling irritable or anxious.

If used for longer than about two months, oral corticosteroids may cause other changes including acne, the development of a 'moon-shaped' face, osteoporosis, high blood pressure, diabetes, vulnerability to infection, eye disorders, thinning of the skin, bruising and muscle weakness.

If inhaled and used short term, as they generally are to relieve inflammation in the lungs or airways, side effects are rare and mild. In the long term, they can increase susceptibility to oral thrush.

Side effects of topical corticosteroids include thinning of the skin, sometimes resulting in stretch marks, appearance of red spots or lines on the skin (caused by expanded blood vessels), red or purple discoloration of the skin, bruising and vulnerability to skin infections. With the exception of stretch marks, these side effects usually disappear once the treatment has finished. To help reduce side effects, the doctor will prescribe the lowest effective strength. If the corticosteroid has been used for a while, the dose should be reduced slowly to allow the body to adapt and to avoid possibly serious effects.

Injected into a joint or muscle, corticosteroids may cause temporary pain and swelling at the injection site. Other side effects may include a raised heartbeat, stomach irritation, nausea and sleeping problems.

! WARNING

Long-term treatment

If you have been taking steroids by mouth for more than three weeks, you should carry a warning card stating that you are on long-term steroid treatment in case you need emergency medical attention. Always mention that you are on steroids to any health-care professional who is treating you.

Because these drugs suppress the immune system, you should avoid contact with anyone who has an infectious disease. If you have never had chickenpox, see your doctor urgently if you come into contact with someone who has chickenpox or shingles.

ON PRESCRIPTION

Steroid nasal sprays
budesonide (Budamax, Rhinocort)
fluticasone furoate (Avamys)
mometasone furoate (Nasonex)

Steroid inhalers
beclomethasone dipropionate (Qvar)
budesonide (Pulmicort)
ciclesonide (Alvesco)
fluticasone propionate (Flixotide)

Steroid creams
betamethasone dipropionate (Diprosone)
betamethasone valerate (Betnovate)
methylprednisolone aceponate (Advantan)
mometasone furoate (Elocon)
triamcinolone acetonide (Kenacort)

Oral steroids
prednisolone
prednisone

OVER-THE-COUNTER

Steroid cream
hydrocortisone

Steroid nasal sprays
beclomethasone dipropionate (Beconase)
triamcinolone acetonide (Telnase)

Q&A

I've been taking oral corticosteroids for more than three weeks and would like to come off them. Is it safe to stop?

After long-term use, withdrawal from the treatment should then be done gradually under medical supervision to allow the body time to adjust. Withdrawing abruptly can lead to potentially life-threatening collapse.

Medications used in diabetes

Diabetes (diabetes mellitus) is a chronic condition in which there is too much glucose in the blood (see pages 100–119) and is caused by lack of the hormone insulin or resistance to its effects. There are two types of diabetes: type 1 and type 2.

TYPES

Type 1 People with type 1 diabetes must take insulin for life. Insulins fall into three basic groups: short, intermediate and long duration.

Short-duration insulins are generally injected 15–30 minutes before a meal and act for 6–8 hours to cover the rise in blood glucose levels that occurs as the food is digested. Intermediate and long-acting insulins work more slowly and last between 16 and 35 hours; they function as 'background' insulins that maintain glucose levels throughout the day and night. A combination of short- and intermediate- or long-duration insulins is often used.
Type 2 Several types of drug are prescribed for type 2, often in combination. The main ones are metformin, gliptins (DPP-4 inhibitors), glitazones (or thiazolidinediones, TZDs) and sulphonylureas.

Metformin works by reducing the amount of glucose released into the bloodstream by the liver. It also causes an increase in the amount of glucose taken from the blood by the body's cells and makes the cells more responsive to insulin. Sulphonylureas and gliptins increase the amount of insulin produced by the pancreas. Glitazones increase sensitivity to the action of insulin.

HOW TAKEN

Insulin is administered (usually by the patient) by injection. Most treatments for type 2 diabetes are taken as tablets. Exenatide (Byetta), a new drug for type 2, is given by injection.

POSSIBLE SIDE EFFECTS

Side effects of insulin use include hypoglycaemia, which occurs when glucose levels drop too low (see page 107), and lipohypertrophy – a build-up of a lumpy area beneath the skin where an injection site has been used too frequently.

Metformin can sometimes cause mild side effects, such as nausea and diarrhoea. Sulphonylureas may cause side effects that include weight gain, nausea and diarrhoea. These drugs can also increase your risk of hypoglycaemia (low blood glucose).

ON PRESCRIPTION

Short-duration insulins
insulin aspart (NovoRapid)
insulin glulisine (Apidra)
insulin lispro (Humalog)
neutral bovine insulin (Hypurin Neutral)

Intermediate-duration insulins
isophane insulin (Hypurin Isophane)

Long-duration insulins
insulin detemir (Levemir)
insulin glargine (Lantus)
protamine zinc insulin
   (Hypurin Bovine Protamine Zinc)

Gliptins
sitagliptin (Januvia)
vildagliptin (Galvus)

Glitazones (TZDs)
pioglitazone (Actos)
rosiglitazone (Avandia)

Sulphonylureas
glibenclamide (Daonil)
gliclazide (Diamicron)
glimepiride (Amaryl)
glipizide (Melizide)

Other drugs for type 2
acarbose (Glucobay)
exenatide (Byetta)
metformin (Diabex)

Antihypertensives

Hypertension (high blood pressure) is a condition in which the force of the blood flow through the blood vessels is raised beyond healthy limits. Although usually symptomless, this carries a variety of serious risks to health including an increased likelihood of heart attacks, stroke and damage to the kidneys.

TYPES

One or more of a number of different drug groups are the mainstay of treatment for this condition. These drugs lower blood pressure by reducing blood volume or the force of the heartbeat, or by dilating the blood vessels. Drugs used for their anti-hypertensive action include diuretics and beta-blockers (facing page), ACE (angiotensin-converting enzyme) inhibitors, angiotensin-II receptor blockers (ARBs) and calcium-channel blockers. ACE inhibitors and ARBs counter substances in the bloodstream that govern the contraction of the blood vessels, and calcium-channel blockers relax the muscles of the blood vessels.

The choice of treatment depends on the degree of hypertension and what other symptoms or problems you may be experiencing.

HOW TAKEN

By mouth as tablets or capsules.

POSSIBLE SIDE EFFECTS

When starting treatment with any antihypertensive drug, you may experience symptoms of a drop in blood pressure such as dizziness or even fainting. Specific side effects of diuretics and beta-blockers are discussed on the facing page. Other drugs used to treat high blood pressure can cause a build-up of fluid, leading to ankle swelling, as a result of relaxation of the blood vessels. ACE inhibitors can cause a dry cough in some patients. Some people may experience nausea, indigestion, diarrhoea or constipation. Side

Q&A

I have heard that medications used to treat high blood pressure can cause impotence. Is this true?

It is true that some men experience erectile dysfunction when taking antihypertensive medication. However, it is also the case that untreated high blood pressure is a leading cause of impotence as well as being a major health risk. If you are having erectile problems, do not stop your medication treatment. Talk to your doctor, who may be able to suggest a change of medication.

effects of ARBs are usually mild, but include digestive disturbances, headache, and muscle and joint pain. Calcium-channel blockers sometimes cause palpitations or abnormal heart rhythms, digestive disturbances, headache and sleep disturbance.

ON PRESCRIPTION

ACE inhibitors
captopril (Capoten)
enalapril (Renitec)
fosinopril (Monopril)
lisinopril (Prinivil)
perindopril (Coversyl)
quinapril (Accupril)
ramipril (Tritace)
trandolapril (Dolapril)

ARBs
candesartan (Atacand)
eprosartan (Teveten)
irbesartan (Karvea)
losartan (Cozaar)
olmesartan (Olmetec)
telmisartan (Micardis)
valsartan (Diovan)

Calcium-channel blockers
amlodipine (Norvasc)
diltiazem hydrochloride
    (Cardizem)
felodipine (Plendil)
lercanidipine (Zanidip)
nifedipine (Adalat)
verapamil (Isoptin)

Other antihypertensives
hydralazine (Alphapress)
indapamide (Natrilix)
methyldopa (Aldomet)
minoxidil (Loniten)
moxonidine (Physiotens)
prazosin (Minipress)

Diuretics

Diuretics, commonly termed 'water tablets', are often prescribed if you have high blood pressure (see *Antihypertensives*, facing page) or too much fluid in the tissues of the body (known as oedema) as a result of heart failure (see page 331). Diuretics reduce the volume of blood, which lowers blood pressure and eases the workload of the heart.

TYPES

These drugs fall into three main types: thiazides, loop diuretics and potassium-sparing diuretics, so called because they conserve potassium in the body, often lost with other types of diuretic.

HOW TAKEN

By mouth as tablets or capsules.

POSSIBLE SIDE EFFECTS

The immediate effect of diuretics is an increase in the volume of urine produced and the frequency of urination, which can disturb sleep. Other side effects, particularly noticeable with higher doses of diuretics, include dizziness, stomach pain, constipation, diarrhoea, headaches, muscle cramps and weakness, rash and erectile problems.

ON PRESCRIPTION

Thiazides
chlorthalidone (Hygroton)
hydrochlorothiazide (Dithiazide)

Loop diuretics
bumetanide (Burinex)
ethacrynic acid (Edecrin)
furosemide (Lasix)

Potassium-sparing diuretics
amiloride (Kaluril)
eplerenone (Inspra)
spironolactone (Aldactone)

Beta-blockers

These work by blocking the action of a natural substance called noradrenaline at special sites in the arteries, on the heart muscle and on some other muscles and organs. Noradrenaline causes arteries to narrow and the heart to beat faster. By blocking its action, beta-blockers can cause arteries to widen, slow down the heart and decrease the force of its contraction. This results in a drop in blood pressure and less work for the heart.

Beta-blockers are prescribed primarily for disorders of the heart and circulation, specifically high blood pressure, angina, abnormal heart rhythms and heart failure. Less commonly, beta-blockers are used to prevent migraine and to treat the symptoms of overactive thyroid, anxiety, tremor and glaucoma.

TYPES

There are many different beta-blockers. They differ in their duration of action; some need to be taken three times a day, others once a day.

HOW TAKEN

By mouth as tablets or capsules.

POSSIBLE SIDE EFFECTS

Side effects may include tiredness, cold hands and feet, insomnia, dizziness and erectile problems. Be sure to consult a doctor if side effects are a problem. Withdrawal from beta-blockers should be done gradually under medical supervision.

ON PRESCRIPTION

Beta-blockers	
atenolol (Tenormin)	metoprolol (Lopresor)
betaxolol (Betoptic)	nebivolol (Nebilet)
bisoprolol (Bicor)	oxprenolol (Corbeton)
carvedilol (Dilatrend)	pindolol (Visken)
labetalol (Trandate)	propranolol (Inderal)
	sotalol (Sotacor)

Anti-angina drugs

Angina is a symptom of coronary heart disease and occurs when the arteries in the heart narrow. It is characterised by pain or tightening across the chest. The drugs for angina aim to treat both the immediate symptoms and the long-term condition.

TYPES

Drugs for angina fall into four main groups: beta-blockers, nitrates, calcium-channel blockers and potassium-channel activators. Beta-blockers (see page 329) reduce the force and speed of the heartbeat. The other three drug types dilate the coronary arteries and other blood vessels, making it easier for the heart to pump blood.

Immediate treatment Glyceryl trinitrate is used to treat an angina attack in progress. This drug has an immediate relaxing effect on the coronary arteries, allowing more blood to reach the heart muscle.

Angina prevention To prevent angina attacks in the long term, you may also be prescribed one or more of the following: beta-blockers; long-acting nitrates; calcium-channel blockers; and potassium-channel activators. Several of these drugs also lower blood pressure, but additional antihypertensives (see page 328) may also be needed in some cases. Other drugs often prescribed for angina sufferers include aspirin (see *Anticoagulant and antiplatelet drugs*, page 333)

and statins (see page 332) to reduce the likelihood of blood clots and accumulation of fatty deposits in the arteries, and so lower the risk of heart attack.

HOW TAKEN

Glyceryl trinitrate is administered in the form of a spray (used in the mouth) or tablets (placed under the tongue). Long-acting nitrates are available in the form of tablets, spray or patches. Other drugs are taken as tablets or capsules.

POSSIBLE SIDE EFFECTS

The side effects of glyceryl trinitrate include a drop in blood pressure, increased heart rate, throbbing headache and dizziness. Other drugs in this category are known to have a variety of possible side effects, including digestive disturbances, low blood pressure, fluid retention (oedema), erratic heart rhythm, headache, dizziness and lethargy.

Q&A

Since starting medication treatment for angina, I feel tired all the time. Could this be a side effect?

Several of the drugs used in the treatment of angina, including beta-blockers, can cause lethargy and tiredness. Discuss this symptom with your doctor. There may be an alternative drug that has the same benefits, but without the unwanted effects on your energy levels.

ON PRESCRIPTION

Short-acting nitrate
glyceryl trinitrate (Anginine)

Long-acting nitrates
isosorbide dinitrate (Isordil)
isosorbide mononitrate (Imdur)

Calcium-channel blockers
diltiazem hydrochloride (Cardizem)
nifedipine (Adalat)
perhexiline (Pexsig)
verapamil (Cordilox)

Potassium-channel activators
ivabradine (Coralan)
nicorandil (Ikorel)

Medications for heart failure

Heart failure, which is caused by damage to the heart muscle, results in the heart becoming less efficient at pumping blood and therefore less able to meet the body's demands.

TYPES
Heart failure will be treated either with an angiotensin-converting enzyme (ACE) inhibitor or an angiotensin-II receptor blocker (ARB). Along with beta-blockers (page 329), these are the first-line drugs. Diuretics and cardiac glycosides (drugs derived from the foxglove plant – digitalis) may also be prescribed additionally.

HOW TAKEN
Usually by mouth as tablets or capsules.

POSSIBLE SIDE EFFECTS
Side effects of these drugs can include dizziness (caused by low blood pressure) and a dry cough (ACE inhibitors). The most common side effect of digoxin is nausea.

ON PRESCRIPTION

Cardiac glycosides
digoxin (Lanoxin)

ACE inhibitors
captopril (Capoten)
enalapril (Renitec)
fosinopril (Monopril)
lisinopril (Prinivil)
perindopril (Coversyl)
quinapril (Accupril)
ramipril (Tritace)
trandolapril (Dolapril)

ARBs
candesartan (Atacand)
eprosartan (Teveten)
irbesartan (Karvea)
losartan (Cozaar)
olmesartan (Olmetec)
telmisartan (Micardis)
valsartan (Diovan)

Anti-arrhythmics

Treatment for arrhythmia (problems with the rhythm of the heart) depends on the type of arrhythmia (see *Recovering your rhythm*, pages 124–125).

TYPES
Drugs used to regulate the heartbeat can be classified into those that act on supraventricular arrhythmias, including cardiac glycosides (see *Drugs for heart failure*, left) and verapamil (a calcium-channel blocker, see *Antihypertensives*, page 328) and those that act on both supraventricular and ventricular arrhythmias. Beta-blockers (page 329) may be used for both types of arrhythmia.

HOW TAKEN
Usually by mouth as tablets or capsules.

POSSIBLE SIDE EFFECTS
All anti-arrhythmic drugs have potentially serious side effects. They may worsen or provoke the arrhythmia in certain circumstances, and all require close monitoring by a health-care professional. Special care also needs to be taken if anti-arrhythmic drugs are combined.

ON PRESCRIPTION

Supraventricular arrhythmias
adenosine (Adenocor)
digoxin (Lanoxin)
verapamil (Cordilox)

Supraventricular and ventricular arrhythmias
amiodarone (Cordarone X)
disopyramide (Rythmodan)
flecainide (Tambocor)

Lipid regulators

Raised levels of fats (lipids) in the blood including certain forms of cholesterol and triglycerides are a major risk factor for both heart disease and stroke, because fat in the bloodstream can accumulate on the sides of the blood vessels causing often dangerous blockages. In some cases raised blood lipids can be reduced by altering the diet, but drug treatment is usually recommended as well.

TYPES

Statins are the most widely prescribed of the lipid-regulating drugs. They may be used to:

- reduce high levels of cholesterol in the blood due to lifestyle factors such as a high-fat diet or not doing enough exercise (primary hypercholesterolaemia)
- lower cholesterol levels in people genetically predisposed to high cholesterol levels (familial hypercholesterolaemia)
- reduce the risk of heart attack or stroke if you have angina or if you have previously had a heart attack or have other risk factors.

Statins reduce the production of cholesterol by the liver – in particular, that of 'bad' cholesterol called low-density lipoprotein (LDL), which causes furring and narrowing of the arteries.

Before starting statins and during statin treatment, your doctor will give you a blood test to ensure your liver function is normal. Your doctor may also want to check for muscle function.

Other lipid-lowering drugs include the bile acid sequestrants, which promote the conversion of cholesterol in the blood into bile acids in the liver. Ezetimibe inhibits the absorption of cholesterol from food in the bowel.

HOW TAKEN

By mouth as tablets or capsules.

POSSIBLE SIDE EFFECTS

All drugs in this category can cause digestive disturbances, such as nausea, constipation, diarrhoea, indigestion and flatulence. Specific side effects of statins include headache and sleeping problems. Muscle pain and weakness are among the more serious problems associated with statin use in susceptible people. If you notice such symptoms, stop taking the drug and tell your doctor at once; alternative treatment may be advised.

Q&A

I would rather not take medication for my raised cholesterol. Is diet modification an effective alternative?

While it is important for anyone with raised blood cholesterol to adopt a low-fat diet, in most cases dietary measures alone do not reduce blood fats sufficiently. This is because the relationship between fat in food and cholesterol in the bloodstream is not direct. If your doctor has prescribed drug treatment, the best course of action is to take it.

ON PRESCRIPTION

Statins
atorvastatin (Lipitor)
fluvastatin (Lescol)
pravastatin (Lipostat)
rosuvastatin (Crestor)
simvastatin (Zocor)

Bile acid sequestrants
cholestyramine (Questran)
colestipol (Colestid)

Fibrates
fenofibrate (Lipidil)
gemfibrozil (Lopid)

Other medications
ezetimibe (Ezetrol)
nicotinic acid

Anticoagulant and antiplatelet drugs

Drugs in this group are used to treat and prevent the formation of blood clots in the circulation (thrombosis), leading to a risk of blockage of the blood supply to a vital organ such as the heart (causing a heart attack), brain (causing a stroke) or lungs (causing a pulmonary embolism).

TYPES

Antiplatelet drugs reduce the ability of platelets (a type of blood cell) to stick together and form clots. Aspirin is the most commonly used drug of this type. However, because there is some risk of internal bleeding, doctors now prescribe regular doses of aspirin only to people with existing heart problems. Low-dose aspirin is available over the counter, but medical experts now discourage healthy people from taking aspirin regularly.

Anticoagulant drugs block the action of blood clotting factors that bind platelets together. Heparin is the body's natural anticoagulant, and heparin-like drugs are given by injection to dissolve clots that have formed. Oral anticoagulants are given for the prevention of clots following some types of surgery.

HOW TAKEN

Antiplatelet and anticoagulants for home treatment are taken by mouth as tablets or capsules.

POSSIBLE SIDE EFFECTS

Excessive bleeding is a risk of all drugs in this category. Cuts and bruises may take longer to heal. Those taking antiplatelet drugs may experience abdominal pain, diarrhoea, dizziness and headache. Long-term aspirin treatment is associated with an increased risk of stomach ulcers and indigestion. Possible side effects of warfarin include diarrhoea, nausea, jaundice and, with prolonged use, osteoporosis and alopecia.

Testing clotting times

If you are taking warfarin you will need regular testing to monitor how your medication is working. These tests compare the blood-clotting times of people taking and those not taking an anti-coagulant. The test produces a measurement called an international normalisation ratio (INR). If your INR is too high, the blood will not clot quickly enough and you may experience bruising or be at an increased risk of bleeding. In this case, your dose may need to be reduced. If your INR is too low, your medication is not working well enough, in which case the dose may need to be increased.

! WARNING

Excessive bleeding

If you are taking medication that inhibits blood clotting and you need to have surgery, or any kind of invasive procedure (for example, tooth extraction), tell the health-care professional, as you may experience excessive bleeding during surgery and poorer healing afterwards.

ON PRESCRIPTION

Antiplatelet medications
aspirin
clopidogrel (Plavix)
dipyridamole (Persantin)

Oral anticoagulants
dabigatran (Pradaxa)
rivaroxaban (Xarelto)
warfarin

Painkillers

Drugs to alleviate pain, also called analgesics, are found in most home medicine cabinets. Numerous over-the-counter medicines are available for the relief of minor problems such as headaches. Stronger, prescription-only drugs are available for the relief of more severe pain. See also *Banishing pain*, pages 214–239.

TYPES

Painkillers fall into two main categories: opioid and non-opioid. Some opiods can be delivered by patch.
Opioids work by blocking pain receptors in the brain, so that it fails to register the pain 'signals' that the body is sending out.
Non-opioid painkillers work by stopping the production of prostaglandins – messenger molecules that are involved in producing pain, inflammation and fever. Many of these drugs are available in limited quantities or in low-strength formulations without prescription, and are often included in combined formulations and in proprietary cold remedies.

- **Aspirin** is a non-opioid that is useful for treating headaches, toothache, sore throat and fever.
- **Non-steroidal anti-inflammatory drugs (NSAIDs)** are particularly useful for painful inflammatory conditions such as arthritis or dental problems (see facing page).
- **Paracetamol** works in a different way to other non-opioid drugs, acting on the brain only to reduce the sensation of pain. It does not reduce inflammation.
- **Tricyclic antidepressants (TCAs)** (see facing page) and **anti-epileptics** (drugs usually used in the treatment of epilepsy) are sometimes prescribed for neuropathic (nerve) pain.
- **Triptans** are a group of drugs that act specifically to relieve the pain of migraine.

HOW TAKEN

Opioid drugs can be administered by mouth, by injection or via a pump into the bloodstream. Non-opioids are usually taken by mouth.

POSSIBLE SIDE EFFECTS

Side effects of opioid painkillers include nausea and vomiting, constipation and dry mouth. Some people also experience drowsiness, muscle stiffness, low blood pressure and breathing problems. Long-term use of opioids may lead to dependence.

Aspirin and NSAIDs may inflame the stomach lining, which makes these drugs unsuitable for people with stomach ulcers. Buffered aspirin preparations can offer protection to the stomach. A paracetamol overdose can cause potentially fatal liver damage.

Tricyclic antidepressants, anti-epileptics and triptans may cause drowsiness and dizziness.

ON PRESCRIPTION

Opioids	Anti-epileptics
codeine phosphate	carbamazepine
fentanyl (Durogesic)	(Tegretol)
morphine (Oramorph,	gabapentin (Neurontin)
Sevredol)	
oxycodone (Oxycontin)	**Triptans**
tramadol (Tramal)	eletriptan (Relpax)
	naratriptan (Naramig)
Antidepressants	rizatriptan (Maxalt)
amitriptyline (Endep)	sumatriptan (Imigran)
	zolmitriptan (Zomig)

OVER-THE-COUNTER

Non-opioids
aspirin
ibuprofen (Nurofen)
mefenamic acid (Ponstan)
naproxen sodium (Naprogesic)
paracetamol (Panadol)

Non-steroidal anti-inflammatory drugs

This large group of drugs, generally referred to as NSAIDs, are widely used as painkillers, but they also have a role in reducing inflammation in a range of disorders affecting the joints, such as rheumatoid arthritis, or damage resulting from an injury.

TYPES

NSAIDs inhibit the effect of an enzyme that promotes the production of the inflammation-producing hormone prostaglandin. They are categorised according to the degree of selectivity for this enzyme.

HOW TAKEN

NSAIDS are available as tablets or capsules, injections, topical gels, and suppositories.

POSSIBLE SIDE EFFECTS

The main side effect of NSAIDs taken by mouth is inflammation of the stomach lining. Other possible side effects include worsening of asthma and an increased risk of blood clots (selective NSAIDs).

ON PRESCRIPTION

Selective NSAIDs
celecoxib (Celebrex)
diclofenac (Voltaren)
etoricoxib (Arcoxia)
indomethacin (Indocid)
ketoprofen (Orudis)
ketorolac (Toradol)
meloxicam (Mobic)
naproxen (Naprosyn)
parecoxib (Dynastat)
piroxicam (Feldene)
sulindac (Acin)

OVER-THE-COUNTER

Non-selective NSAIDS
aspirin
diclofenac (Voltarol)
ibuprofen (Nurofen)
ketoprofen (Oruvail, Oruvail Gel)
mefenamic acid (Ponstan)
naproxen sodium (Naprogesic)
piroxicam (Feldene, Feldene P Gel)

Antidepressants

Drug treatment for depression is usually given only after self-help measures and 'talking therapies' such as counselling have been unsuccessful. Medication is usually reserved for mild depression that has not improved for at least two years, or for moderate or severe depression. See also *Coping with depression*, pages 244–247.

TYPES

The different types of antidepressants all work by altering levels of chemicals in the brain that are responsible for mood, known as excitatory neurotransmitters. These include serotonin and noradrenaline, both of which are linked to feelings of wellbeing.

Selective serotonin reuptake inhibitors (SSRIs) are usually the first choice of drug treatment, being effective and producing fewer side effects than other antidepressants. They work by reducing the natural breakdown of serotonin, thereby raising its levels in the brain. Selective serotonin and noradrenaline reuptake inhibitors (SNRIs) and noradrenaline reuptake inhibitors are newer agents with roughly similar effects.

Q&A

I want to stop taking my antidepressants – what should I do?

If you want to stop taking these medications, be sure to discuss this with your doctor first to make sure that the timing is right. Antidepressants are not addictive, but if you stop taking them suddenly, you may experience unpleasant symptoms, including intense anxiety. Your doctor will probably want you to decrease the dosage gradually, over several weeks or even months.

Diet and MAOIs

With these medications it is essential to avoid food containing the chemical tyramine, which when ingested while taking an MAOI causes a sudden and dangerous rise in blood pressure. Tyramine is normally found in foods that have been fermented or cured, such as cheese, pickled meat or fish, yeast extract products (Vegemite) and alcohol. Your GP or other health-care professional will advise on food and other substances to avoid.

Tricyclic antidepressants (TCAs) work by raising the levels of both serotonin and noradrenaline in the brain. Many drugs within this group have a marked sedative effect and may be most appropriate for those whose depression is accompanied by feelings of anxiety.

Monoamine oxidase inhibitors (MAOIs) work by reducing the activity of an enzyme that breaks down excitatory neurotransmitters. These drugs are prescribed infrequently because they can cause a severe adverse reaction when taken with certain foods (see above). They are used only when treatment with other types of antidepressant has been unsuccessful.

St John's wort It is not known exactly how this herb works but it appears to be as effective as prescription medications for mild-to-moderate depression and is very safe.

HOW TAKEN

These drugs are usually taken as tablets or capsules. Some are also available in liquid form.

POSSIBLE SIDE EFFECTS

The positive effects of antidepressants may take some time to become apparent, whereas unpleasant side effects may be noticed earlier. Some people find that during the first couple of weeks of taking the medication, their depressive symptoms worsen.

Each group of antidepressant drugs has its own side effects, and the extent to which they are experienced varies greatly between individuals.

The side effects of SSRIs initially may include nausea, headache, sleep problems, anxiety and sexual difficulties. Such symptoms usually improve over time.

Common side effects of TCAs usually subside within a few weeks. These include dry mouth, constipation, sweating, problems passing urine, slight blurring of vision and drowsiness. You should not smoke cannabis if you are taking TCAs because the combination can cause your heart to beat alarmingly rapidly.

Possible side effects of MAOIs include blurred vision, dizziness, drowsiness, increased appetite, nausea, restlessness, shaking or trembling, and difficulty sleeping. Some side effects of MAOIs are serious and require immediate emergency medical attention. Symptoms of this type of reaction include stiff neck, severe headache, chest pains, vomiting or nausea, and a fast heartbeat.

ON PRESCRIPTION

SSRIs
citalopram (Celapram)
escitalopram (Lexapro)
fluoxetine (Prozac)
fluvoxamine (Luvox)
paroxetine (Aropax)
sertraline (Zoloft)

SNRIs
desvenlafaxine (Pristiq)
duloxetine (Cymbalta)
venlafaxine (Efexor)

Noradrenaline reuptake inhibitor
reboxetine (Edronax)

TCAs
amitriptyline (Endep)
clomipramine (Anafranil)
dothiepin (Prothiaden)
doxepin (Deptran)
imipramine (Tofranil)
nortriptyline (Allegron)
trimipramine (Surmontil)

MAOIs
moclobemide (Aurorix)
phenelzine (Nardil)
tranylcypromine (Parnate)

Other
mianserin (Lumin)
mirtazapine (Avanza)
St John's wort

Drugs for anxiety and insomnia

Anxiety and sleeping problems are often closely related and are often treated with similar drugs.

TYPES

The two main types of drug prescribed for these conditions are benzodiazepines or the newer non-benzodiazepines, both of which work by slowing down brain activity. They do this by increasing the action of a 'go-slow' chemical, called gamma-aminobutyric acid (GABA), the presence of which promotes sleep and reduces anxiety.

Benzodiazepines can have both a sedative and anxiolytic (anti-anxiety) effect and, due to their potential for making people dependent on them, they are prescribed only for very short courses, to avoid any danger of such dependence.

Non-benzodiazepines used for treating insomnia are also prescribed only for short courses.

Melatonin is a naturally occurring hormone involved in the sleep cycle (also known as the circadian rhythm). It is sometimes prescribed for short-term insomnia in older people.

HOW TAKEN

These drugs are usually taken as tablets or capsules. Some are available in liquid form.

POSSIBLE SIDE EFFECTS

Benzodiazepines can cause a range of side effects, including confusion, stumbling, memory loss, lightheadedness and aggression, and they may cause you to feel 'hung over' and drowsy during the day. Do not drive or operate dangerous machinery until you know how these drugs affect you.

Drugs of this type can cause physical and psychological dependence if taken for more than a few weeks, or sometimes even days, which is why they are prescribed for only limited periods. The effects of withdrawal can be unpleasant and include confusion, insomnia, anxiety, loss of appetite and weight, shaking, sweating and ringing in the ears. Another reason to avoid long-term use is that over a prolonged period, people can develop a tolerance for the drug and then need to take more for it to have the same effect.

Non-benzodiazepines have fewer side effects than benzodiazepines, but can cause drowsiness, nausea and memory loss. Less commonly, these drugs can cause confusion, difficulty concentrating, dizziness and changes to your senses of smell, hearing, speech and vision.

Both benzodiazepines and non-benzodiazepines can temporarily affect your coordination and reasoning skills.

Melatonin supplements may also make you feel irritable and dizzy and may cause migraine, constipation, stomach pain and weight gain.

ON PRESCRIPTION

Benzodiazepines used for insomnia	Benzodiazepines used for anxiety
flunitrazepam (Hypnoderm)	alprazolam (Xanax)
lormetazepam	bromazepam (Lexoton)
nitrazepam (Mogadon)	clobazam (Frisium)
temazepam (Normison)	diazepam (Valium)
triazolam (Halcion)	lorazepam (Ativan)
	oxazepam (Serepax)

Non-benzodiazepines	Hormones
zaleplon (Sonata)	melatonin (Circadin)
zolpidem (Stilnox)	
zopiclone (Zimovane)	

OVER-THE-COUNTER

diphenhydramine (Snuzaid)
doxylamine (Restavit)

Antipsychotics

Antipsychotic drugs (formerly referred to as major tranquillisers) are used to treat psychosis – mental disorders that affect the sufferer's ability to think clearly, behave rationally or perceive reality. These disorders include schizophrenia and paranoia. The drugs work by increasing or reducing the effects of natural chemicals in your brain. These chemicals are involved in regulating behaviour, setting your mood and emotions, control of sleeping and wakefulness and appetite. The brain chemicals affected by these medicines are dopamine, serotonin, noradrenaline and acetylcholine.

TYPES

Antipsychotic drugs are generally classified into two broad types: typical, first-generation, or conventional antipsychotics; and the newer atypical, or second-generation antipsychotics.

Antimanic, or mood-stabilising, drugs are used to treat the symptoms of bipolar disorder, a condition characterised by excessive mood highs and lows. Treatment may include antidepressants (see page 335). All mood-stabilising drugs, including lithium, require careful monitoring to ensure the patient receives an appropriate dose.

HOW TAKEN

Most of these drugs are taken by mouth in tablet or capsule form. Some are also available as a liquid medicine. Long-acting injections, known as depot injections, may be offered to those who have difficulty remembering to take their medication. In some cases antipsychotics may be injected for a rapid effect to calm someone whose behaviour has become violent.

POSSIBLE SIDE EFFECTS

A range of side effects is commonly associated with the use of antipsychotic drugs including involuntary movements of the muscles (less so with atypical antipsychotics), restlessness, dry mouth, blurred vision, constipation, dizziness or lightheadedness, and weight gain. Taking antipsychotics increases the risk of a stroke in elderly people with dementia and in patients with other risk factors for stroke.

Side effects of lithium are closely related to dosage. Too high a dose may lead to nausea, slurred speech and staggering. Other possible side effects include weight gain, tremors and feeling thirsty. Prolonged use may eventually lead to impaired kidney function.

ON PRESCRIPTION

Typical antipsychotics
chlorpromazine (Largactil)
flupenthixol (Fluanxol)
haloperidol (Haldol)

Atypical antipsychotics
amisulpride (Solian)
aripiprazole (Abilify)
asenapine (Saphris)
clozapine (Clozaril)
olanzapine (Zyprexa)
paliperidone (Invega)
quetiapine (Seroquel)
risperidone (Risperdal)
ziprasidone (Zeldox)

Mood stabilisers
carbamazepine (Tegretol)
lamotrigine (Lamictal)
lithium (Lithicarb)
sodium valproate (Epilim)

Q&A

My relative needs to take antipsychotics to stay well, but I am worried that he often forgets to take them.

If possible, talk to his doctor about the problem. Long-acting 'depot' injections of the medication may be the answer.

Medications for thyroid disorders

The thyroid gland at the front of the neck produces the hormones thyroxine and triiodothyronine, which are released into the bloodstream to control the body's growth and metabolism. Sometimes the thyroid gland malfunctions, becoming either overactive (hyperthyroidism) or underactive (hypothyroidism).

TYPES

The treatment for hyperthyroidism aims to stop the thyroid gland producing excessive amounts of hormones and return the level of thyroid hormones in your blood to normal.

Anti-thyroid drugs may be used to lower the level of thyroid hormones produced. They take 4–8 weeks before hormone production returns to normal levels.

Beta-blockers (see page 329) may also be used to relieve the symptoms of an overactive thyroid, which can include tremor (shaking and trembling), rapid heartbeat and restlessness.

Radio-iodine treatment may also be used. It works by building up in the thyroid gland and shrinking it by destroying tissue, reducing the amount of thyroid hormone that it can make. The dose of radioactivity contained in the radio-iodine is very low and is not harmful.

An underactive thyroid (hypothyroidism) is treated with levothyroxine, a synthetic form of the hormone thyroxine, which is taken for life.

HOW TAKEN

Most of these drugs are given by mouth as tablets or liquid medicine. Radio-iodine is usually given in liquid form. Some people, such as those who are very ill and newborns, may be given levothyroxine by injection.

POSSIBLE SIDE EFFECTS

Side effects of anti-thyroid hormones are rare and usually mild and include mild skin rash, pain in the joints, nausea and itchy skin. However, in rare cases there may be a problem affecting the white blood cells (see *Immune system damage*, below).

If the dose of levothyroxine is too high, side effects, including diarrhoea, vomiting, palpitations, restlessness, insomnia, headache, flushing, sweating and fever, may occur until the dose is adjusted. Annual blood tests are advised to check that the prescribed dose is at the right level.

! WARNING

Immune system damage

Occasionally there may be a sudden drop in white blood cells in those taking anti-thyroid medications. Consult your doctor as a matter of urgency if you develop any of the following symptoms while taking these medications:

- fever
- sore throat
- mouth ulcers
- other signs of infection.

ON PRESCRIPTION

Anti-thyroid dugs
carbimazole (Neo-Mercazole)
propylthiouracil

Beta-blockers
propranolol (Inderal)

Drugs for hypothyroidism
levothyroxine

Helpful organisations

Here you will find a selection of charities and other organisations that can provide further information and advice.

ALCOHOL
Al-Anon Provides support for people with a family member affected by alcohol. www.al-anon.alateen.org

Alcoholics Anonymous (AA) AA provides support for anyone wanting to stop drinking.
www.aa.org.au
www.aa.org.nz

CANCER
Cancer Council Australia The experts on cancer prevention and treatment.
Tel: 13 11 20 www.cancer.org.au

Cancer Society of New Zealand Dedicated to reducing the incidence of cancer and ensuring the best in cancer care.
Tel: 0800 226 237 www.cancernz.org.nz

CARERS
Carers Australia The national peak body representing Australia's carers.
Tel: 1800 242 636
www.carersaustralia.com.au

Carers New Zealand National charity providing information, advice, learning and support for families with health and disability needs.
Tel: 0800 777 797
www.carers.net.nz

DIABETES
Diabetes Australia The national peak body for diabetes in Australia, helping people living with diabetes, their families and carers.
Tel: 1300 136 588 www.diabetesaustralia.com.au

Diabetes New Zealand Provides support, advocacy and information to people living with diabetes.
Tel: 0800 342 238 www.diabetes.org.nz

FIRST AID TRAINING AND ADVICE
Australian Red Cross First aid training.
www.redcross.org.au
www.redcross.org.nz

St John Ambulance First aid training.
www.stjohn.org.au
www.stjohn.org.nz

GENERAL INFORMATION
Better Health Channel Top-quality Australian health information.
www.betterhealth.vic.gov.au

National Health and Medical Research Council Australia's leading expert body promoting the development and maintenance of public and individual health standards.
www.nhmrc.gov.au

HEART DISEASE
Heart Foundation (Australia) These national experts advise doctors and patients about preventing and treating heart disease.
Tel: 1300 362 787
www.heartfoundation.org.au

Heart Foundation New Zealand Funds research and promotes heart health.
Tel: 0800 863 375
www.heartfoundation.org.nz

JOINT PROBLEMS
Arthritis Australia Learn simple measures that can help anyone manage their symptoms.
Tel: 1800 011 041
www.arthritisaustralia.com.au

Arthritis Foundation Valuable information about all types of arthritis and how to get support.
www.arthritis.org

Arthritis New Zealand Learn simple measures that can help anyone manage their symptoms.
Tel: 0800 663 463 www.arthritis.org.nz

MENTAL HEALTH
beyondblue Empowering people with depression and anxiety to seek help, and supporting recovery, management and resilience.
Tel: 1300 224 636 www.beyondblue.org.au

Black Dog Institute World leader in the diagnosis, treatment and prevention of mood disorders such as depression and bipolar disorder.
www.blackdoginstitute.org.au

Lifeline (Australia) Provides around-the-clock crisis support and suicide prevention services.
Tel: 13 11 14 www.lifeline.org.au

Lifeline (New Zealand) Provides around-the-clock crisis support and suicide prevention services. Tel: 0800 543 354; www.lifeline.co.nz

Pathways (New Zealand) National provider of community-based mental health and wellness services. www.pathways.co.nz

SANE Australia Helping all Australians affected by mental illness lead a better life.
www.sane.org

PAIN MANAGEMENT
Australian Pain Management Association Provides pain-management options and information for people living with pain and their carers. www.painmanagement.org.au

RESPIRATORY CONDITIONS
Asthma Foundation (Australia) Information on treatment and prevention, how to use puffers and inhalers properly, and how to develop an action plan. Tel: 1800 645 130; www.asthmafoundation.org.au

Asthma Foundation (New Zealand) Information and resources for people with asthma and respiratory diseases.
www.asthmafoundation.org.nz

Lung Foundation Information and support for people with a range of lung conditions, including COPD.
Tel: 1800 654 301 www.lungfoundation.com.au

SMOKING
Quitline (New Zealand) All the help you need to quit smoking.
Tel: 0800 778 778 www.quit.org.nz

QuitNow (Australia) All the help you need to quit smoking. Tel: 13 78 48; www.quitnow.gov.au

STROKE
Stroke Foundation (Australia) These national experts advise doctors and patients about preventing and treating stroke.
Tel: 1800 787 653
www.strokefoundation.com.au

Stroke Foundation of New Zealand Dedicated to reducing the incidence of stroke, improving treatment outcomes, and supporting those affected by stroke
Tel: 0800 78 76 53 www.stroke.org.nz

Index

Page numbers in **bold print** refer to main entries

Acknowledgements

Cover (front and back) all Shutterstock **2** Getty Images (top right), all others Shutterstock **3** Getty Images (bottom left), all others Shutterstock **4** Shutterstock **5** Shutterstock **6-7** Shutterstock **8** Shutterstock, Shutterstock, Shutterstock, Thinkstock **9** Getty Images, Thinkstock, Shutterstock, Shutterstock **11** Shutterstock **13** Thinkstock **14** iStockphoto **15** Shutterstock **16** Shutterstock **21** iStockphoto **22** Shutterstock **24** Shutterstock, Shutterstock, Shutterstock **25** Shutterstock, Shutterstock, Shutterstock **27** iStockphoto **28** Getty Images **29** Getty Images **30** iStockphoto **31** Getty Images **32** Thinkstock **34** Shutterstock, Shutterstock, Shutterstock, iStockphoto **35** Shutterstock, Getty Images, iStockphoto, Shutterstock **36** Shutterstock **39** Getty Images **40** Shutterstock **41** Getty Images **42** Shutterstock **43** Shutterstock **47** Getty Images **48** Shutterstock **49** Shutterstock **51** Shutterstock **52** Shutterstock **53** Shutterstock **54** Getty Images **55** Shutterstock **56** Shutterstock **57** Getty Images **58** Shutterstock **59** Getty Images **60** Shutterstock **61** Shutterstock **61** Shutterstock **63** Shutterstock **64** Shutterstock **66** Shutterstock **69** Getty Images **70** Science Photo Library **71** Science Photo Library **72** iStockphoto **73** Shutterstock **73** Shutterstock **75** Shutterstock **76** Shutterstock **79** Getty Images **81** Shutterstock **82** Shutterstock **83** Science Photo Library **84** Getty Images **85** Shutterstock **87** Shutterstock **88** Getty Images **91** Shutterstock **92** Science Photo Library **92** both Science Photo Library **93** Shutterstock **94** Getty Images **95** Shutterstock **97** Getty Images **100** Getty Images **101** Shutterstock **102** Shutterstock **106** Shutterstock **108** Shutterstock **109** Shutterstock **109** Shutterstock **109** Shutterstock **110** Shutterstock **111** Shutterstock **113** Shutterstock **115** Shutterstock, Packshotfactory.co.uk/Paul Snell **117** Getty Images **118** Shutterstock **119** Shutterstock **120** Shutterstock **121** Shutterstock **122** both Science Photo Library **122** Shutterstock **123** Shutterstock **123** Shutterstock **125** Getty Images **125** Shutterstock **125** Shutterstock **126** iStockphoto **127** Shutterstock **128** Shutterstock **128** Shutterstock **129** Getty Images **130** Shutterstock **131** Shutterstock **131** Shutterstock **133** Shutterstock **134** Getty Images **135** Shutterstock **136** Getty Images **137** Shutterstock **138** Shutterstock **139** Getty Images **140** Shutterstock **141** Shutterstock **142** Getty Images **145** Getty Images **146** Science Photo Library **147** both Science Photo Library **148** Shutterstock **149** Shutterstock **150** Getty Images **151** Shutterstock **154** Getty Images/Jupiterimages **155** Shutterstock **157** Getty Images **159** Getty Images **163** Shutterstock **164** Shutterstock **165** iStockphoto **166** Shutterstock **167** Shutterstock **168** Getty Images **169** Science Photo Library **171** Getty Images **173** Shutterstock **174** Shutterstock **175** Shutterstock **176** Shutterstock **177** Getty Images **179** Shutterstock **180** Shutterstock **182** iStockphoto **183** Science Photo Library **186** Shutterstock **187** Shutterstock **187** Shutterstock **189** Shutterstock **190** Shutterstock **192** Shutterstock **193** Shutterstock **195** Shutterstock **196** Getty Images **198** Science Photo Library **201** Shutterstock **202** Shutterstock **204** Shutterstock **204** Shutterstock **205** iStockphoto **207** Science Photo Library **209** Shutterstock **210** Shutterstock **211** Shutterstock **212** Shutterstock **213** Shutterstock **214** Science Photo Library **215** Corbis Images **217** Getty Images **219** Getty Images **220** Shutterstock **221** Shutterstock **222** Getty Images **224** Alamy **225** Shutterstock **228** Shutterstock **229** Shutterstock, Getty Images **230** Getty Images **231** Shutterstock **233** Shutterstock **234** Science Photo Library **235** Getty Images **236** Shutterstock **238** Shutterstock **238** Getty Images **239** Shutterstock **240** Getty Images **241** Shutterstock **243** Shutterstock **245** Shutterstock **247** Science Photo Library **248** Shutterstock **251** Getty Images **252** Getty Images **255** Shutterstock **256** Getty Images **257** Getty Images **258** Shutterstock **259** Shutterstock **262** Shutterstock **266** Getty Images **267** Getty Images **269** Getty Images **270** Getty Images **272** Shutterstock/**273** Shutterstock **277** Shutterstock **278** iStockphoto **281** iStockphoto **283** Getty Images **284** Getty Images **285** Shutterstock **287** Shutterstock **289** Shutterstock **291** Shutterstock **292** Shutterstock **294** Shutterstock **296** Shutterstock, all others Science Photo Library **297** Science Photo Library **298** Shutterstock **301** Science Photo Library **303** iStockphoto **304** Science Photo Library **305** iStockphoto **307** Shutterstock **308** Shutterstock **311** Shutterstock **312** iStockphoto, all others Shutterstock **313** all Shutterstock **314** Thinkstock

1001 Great Ways to Get Better

CONSULTANTS

Dr Sue Davidson MB BS MRCP MRGCP DRCOG
Associate specialist in diabetes
Brian Dolan MSc (Oxon) MSc (Nurs) RMN RGN
Nurse consultant
Michele Harms PhD MSc MCSP
Editor of *Physiotherapy*
Dr Joan Hester MBBS FRCA MSc FFPMRCA
Consultant in pain medicine, King's College Hospital, London
Fiona Hunter BSc Nutrition Dip Dietetics
Nutritionist
Ciarán Hurley RN MA BMedSci PGDipE
Senior lecturer in adult nursing, Sheffield Hallam University
Dr Chris Irons DClinPsy PhD BSc
Clinical psychologist, Mile End Hospital, London
Graham Jackson FRCP FESC FACC
Consultant cardiologist, Guy's & St Thomas' Hospital, London
Dr Kathy Kramer GP BA/MBBS BSc(Med) (Hons) (USyd)
General practitioner
Dr Christian D Mallen BMedSci BMBS MMedSci MPhil MRCGP PhD
Senior lecturer in general practice, Keele University, UK
Pamela Mason BSc (pharmacy) MSc PhD (nutrition)
Pharmaceutical and nutrition consultant
Professor Tony Rudd MA MB BChir FRCP
Professor of stroke medicine, Guy's & St Thomas' Foundation Trust, London
Professor Karol Sikora MB PhD MA FRCP FRCR FFPM
Medical director, CancerPartnersUK and Dean, University of Buckingham Medical School
Dr Frances Williams MB BChir MRCP MRCPCH
General practitioner, London

Writers Ailsa Colquhoun, Jane Feinmann, Jane Garton, Claire Gillman, Barbara Lantin, Sheena Meredith MB BS, Patsy Westcott
Project editor Samantha Kent
Cover designer Joanne Buckley
Indexer Diane Harriman
Senior production controller Martin Milat

READER'S DIGEST GENERAL BOOKS

Editorial Director Lynn Lewis
Managing Editor Rosemary McDonald

1001 Great Ways to Get Better is published by
Reader's Digest (Australia) Pty Limited
80 Bay Street, Ultimo, NSW, 2007
www.readersdigest.com.au; www.readersdigest.co.nz; www.rdasia.com;

First published in 2011 in the United Kingdom by Vivat Direct Limited (t/a Reader's Digest), 157 Edgware Road, London W2 2HR.
1001 Great Ways to Get Better is owned and under licence from The Reader's Digest Association, Inc.

This edition first published 2014

National Library of Australia Cataloguing-in-Publication entry
Title: 1001 great ways to get better.
ISBN: 978-1-922085-32-0 (hardback)
Notes: Includes index.
Subjects: Health–Popular works. Medicine, Popular. Self-care, Health.
Other Authors/Contributors: Reader's Digest (Australia)
Dewey Number: 613.0424

Prepress by Colourpedia, Sydney
Printed and bound by Leo Paper Products, China

We are interested in receiving your comments on the content of this book. Write to: The Editor, General Books Editorial, Reader's Digest (Australia) Pty Limited, GPO Box 4353, Sydney, NSW 2001, or email us at: bookeditors.au@readersdigest.com

To order additional copies of *1001 Great Ways to Get Better*, please contact us at:
www.readersdigest.com.au or phone 1300 300 030 (Australia)
www.readersdigest.co.nz or phone 0800 400 060 (New Zealand)
or email us at customerservice@readersdigest.com.au

While the creators of this work have made every effort to be as accurate and up to date as possible, medical and pharmacological knowledge is constantly changing. Readers are recommended to consult a qualified medical specialist for individual advice. The writers, researchers, editors and publishers of this work cannot be held liable for any errors and omissions, or actions that may be taken as a consequence of information contained within this work.

Emergency contact telephone numbers:
Australia: 000
Malaysia: 999
New Zealand: 111
Singapore: 999 (police);
  995 (ambulance, fire)

Concept code: UK2084/1C
Product code: 041 5365